"I believe that Alzheimer's disease can be delayed and prevented. I believe that age-associated memory impairment can be eradicated. I believe that people in their forties, fifties, sixties—and beyond—can retain not only an almost perfect memory, but can have 'youthful minds,' characterized by the dynamic brain power, learning ability, creativity, and emotional zest usually found only in young people. Ten years ago, almost no one in medicine sub-scribed to these ideas; I certainly didn't. But now I'm positive they're true."
—from *Brain Longevity*

PRAISE FOR DR. DHARMA SINGH KHALSA'S
BRAIN LONGEVITY

"A wonderfully sensible regimen. . . . A charming bookside manner. . . . An accessible, smart guide to living a healthier life."
—*Publishers Weekly*

"BRAIN LONGEVITY reveals the brain's vulnerability to physical abuse and stress, as well as its incredible ability to revitalize and regenerate."
—*Light Connection*

"Finally, a practical solution to the problem of brain aging in the baby boomer age wave. This is one of the few books that can actually change your life."
—Ken Dychtwald, Ph.D., author of *Age Wave*

"Khalsa presents his case in calm, medically persuasive prose."
—*Fort Lauderdale Sun-Sentinel*

"[BRAIN LONGEVITY] uses medicine, science, and spirituality to educate, inspire, and point the way to a more hopeful future."
—*Tacoma News Tribune* (WA)

"BRAIN LONGEVITY covers all the technical bases, yet is easy to read and readily accessible to members of the lay public. . . . Reveals that brain-specific nutrients, pharmaceutical medications and exercise, combined with yogic mind-body exercises and other protocols, have a synergistically powerful effect on improving brain function."
—*Life Extension Review*

"BRAIN LONGEVITY is well written, easy to understand, and inspiring. Its simple presentation of technical material makes it a great book for cognitive enhancement novices. Its presentation of a balanced program provides some food for thought for the smart-drug aficionado. Its passionate call for a wise old age of continued productivity . . . is a missive I think none of us baby boomers should miss."
—*Smart Drug News*

DHARMA SINGH KHALSA, M.D., graduated from Creighton University School of Medicine and trained at the University of California at San Francisco School of Medicine, Harvard Medical School, and UCLA School of Medicine. He is Board Certified by the American Academy of Anti-Aging Medicine, of which he is also a founding member.

CAMERON STAUTH is the author of nine critically acclaimed books, a former editor in chief of the *Journal of Health Science*, and a journalist who has written more than a hundred articles for the *New York Times Magazine, Prevention, Natural Health* and other publications.

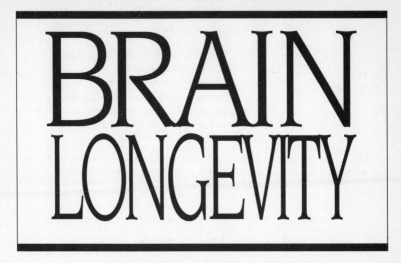

BRAIN
LONGEVITY

The Breakthrough Medical
Program that Improves Your
Mind and Memory

DHARMA SINGH KHALSA, M.D.
with Cameron Stauth

WARNER BOOKS

A Time Warner Company

For the One Divine Creator who is the doer of all things.
—Dharma Singh Khalsa, M.D.

For Shari and Gabriel . . .
and for the family of Dr. Benjamin Shawver,
in honor of all families of Alzheimer's disease victims.
—Cameron Stauth

The program described in this book is not intended to be a substitute for medical care and advice. You are advised to consult with your health care professional with regard to matters relating to your health, including matters which may require diagnosis or medical attention. In particular, if you have been diagnosed with senile dementia of the Alzheimer's type, other cognitive impairment, or have any other special conditions requiring medical attention, or if you are taking or have been advised to take any medication, you should consult regularly with your physician regarding possible modification of the program contained in this book.

The identity of the patients referred to in this book, and certain details about them, have been modified. Conversations included in this book are not necessarily verbatim accounts, but rather are set forth to Dr. Khalsa's best recollection.

The information provided in this book is based upon sources that the authors believe to be reliable. All such information regarding specific products and companies is current as of December 1996.

If you are interested in the scientific articles that support the research mentioned in this book, please write or call the Alzheimer's Prevention Foundation (see page 446) and Dr. Khalsa will be happy to send you a scientific bibliography.

Copyright © 1997 by Dharma Singh Khalsa, M.D., with Cameron Stauth
Introduction copyright © 1999 by Dharma Singh Khalsa, M.D.
All rights reserved.

Warner Books, Inc., 1271 Avenue of the Americas, New York, NY 10020
Visit our web site at www.warnerbooks.com

W A Time Warner Company

Printed in the United States of America
First Trade Printing: May 1999
10 9 8 7 6 5 4

The Library of Congress has cataloged the hardcover edition as follows:
Library of Congress Cataloging-in-Publication Data

Khalsa, Dharma Singh.
   Brain longevity : the breakthrough medical program that improves your mind and memory / Dharma Singh Khalsa, with Cameron Stauth.
       p.   cm.
   Includes bibliographical references.
   ISBN 0-446-52067-5
   1. Brain—Aging.   2. Hydrocortisone—Physiological effect.
3. Longevity.   4. Memory.   5. Alzheimer's disease—Prevention.
I. Stauth, Cameron.   II. Title.
QP376.S634   1997
612.8'2—dc21   96-45376
                                                                                    CIP

ISBN: 0-446-67373-0 (pbk.)
Book design by H. Roberts

Contents

Acknowledgments

This book is the product of the hard work and the vision of many people. Beyond that, it is the result of blessings and grace.

I would like to first thank my teacher, Yogi Bhajan, for his strength, his guidance, and his infinite love.

When it comes to hard work, I must salute my co-author, Cameron Stauth. He never wavered in his work ethic or intensity. His obsession with creativity and quality is impeccable.

Cam and I also wish to thank Maureen Egen, editor of this book, for her enthusiasm, her ideas, and her dedication to this long and arduous project. Maureen's insight, as well as that of Laurence Kirshbaum, CEO of Warner Books, was clear right from the start. To them and all their great staff—including Jackie Joiner, Harvey-Jane Kowal, David Smith, Karen Torres, Bruce Paonessa, Debbie Stier, and Martha Otis— we say thank you.

The vision of our agent, Richard Pine, of Arthur Pine Associates, exceeded even our own. He was instrumental in the creation of this book, and we will always be grateful for his important contributions. I'd like to thank Sabine and Andrew Weil, M.D., for directing me to him. Arthur Pine was also very encouraging and his advice, as always, was astute.

My personal thanks go out to Hal Zina Bennett, Ph.D., who helped me tremendously in the preparation of the initial proposal. I'd like also to thank and acknowledge Jerry M. Calkins, Ph.D., M.D., for his ongoing support, and Somers and Susan White, for their friendship and wise counsel.

Many other people were also of great help, including Jeanne Withrow, Meaghen Porte, Sandra Stahl, Nicole Hunscher, Joanne Yearout, Goldie Vickers, and Diane Paulson.

My heartfelt love and thanks to my wife, Kirti, who worked with me around the clock to bring our vision to fruition, and to the rest of my family: Hari, Sat, and Ethel.

The authors would also like to gratefully acknowledge the many physicians and scientists who generously cooperated with our research efforts. We especially want to express our appreciation to the patients who agreed to tell their stories in this book. After all, it is for them that we have worked so tirelessly.

—**Dharma Singh Khalsa, M.D.**
Tucson, Arizona

Introduction

Since the publication of the hardcover edition of *Brain Longevity* in May 1997, I have received many letters, faxes, and e-mails from people all over the world about how much they appreciate the book. In fact, this has led me to develop a series of three-day seminar consultations in Tucson, Arizona, in which we continue to prove that it is possible to not only combat brain aging but also enhance all levels of cognitive function and impact Alzheimer's disease. For that I am eternally grateful.

As discussed in *Brain Longevity*, the key to understanding the program is to realize that your brain is flesh and blood like the rest of your body. And it will respond to lifestyle measures you take to strengthen it. If you can recognize the power that the integrated medical approach has on the whole brain, not just on one isolated chemical or gene, it becomes clear why the program is so successful.

The program presented in *Brain Longevity* was well ahead of its time. Since then, however, additional scientific research and clinical studies have added to our knowledge. I would like to share some of this new work in this introduction, as well as preview a few key principles in the book.

The Brain Longevity Diet

The fifteen- to twenty-percent fat, nutrient-dense diet recommended in the book has recently been confirmed by two new exciting research projects. The first is an extension of the work by Roy Walford, M.D., and his colleagues in Biosphere II, which is discussed in chapter 11. The diet's anti-aging benefits are very powerful because they help lower your blood cholesterol and lipids. This is very beneficial for long-term brain function.

The most dynamic research in this field was done by William B. Grant, Ph.D. He is a NASA scientist who has the interesting job of traveling to exotic locations around the world to study such environmental conditions as global warming. When Dr. Grant's mother developed Alzheimer's he became inspired to try and spare others the pain of watching a family member suffer. He therefore began investigating the link between Alzheimer's and nutrition. While reviewing the literature of the World Health Organization, he discovered that the countries of the world with the highest intake of total calories and fat also have the greatest incidence of cognitive decline. He also learned that the addition of fish, such as salmon and tuna, as well as grains to your diet will help limit the destructive effects of fat.

This research is also important because of the recently discovered intimate relationship between cardiovascular disease and cognitive decline. As I say in *Brain Longevity,* "What works for the heart, works for the head." Now more than ever, this key fact must be addressed if you want to prevent Alzheimer's disease. Moreover, this is another scientifically proven reason to follow the total brain longevity program.

Although I present a complete array of supplements to maximize your nutritional program, several of these supplements are especially helpful.

B Vitamins: The complete family of B vitamins help your brain cells create energy. Additionally, the B vitamins, especially B_{12} and folic acid, work to lower and control levels of the heart-harmful amino acid homocysteine. You can find the optimal dosages in chapter 13.

Vitamin E: A daily dose of 2000 IU of vitamin E has been found to slow the progression of Alzheimer's disease. According to Professor Marguerite Kay of the University of Arizona Health Sciences Center, however, the dose of vitamin E needed for neuroprotection is only 800 IU, especially when incorporated into a full-spectrum brain longevity program.

Coenzyme Q-10: Further studies have shown this to be a major neuroprotective compound. The ideal dose is discussed in the text of *Brain Longevity.*

Ginkgo biloba: Recent dynamic research was published in the prestigious *Journal of the American Medical Association.* In a year-long multicentered placebo-controlled study of more than three hundred patients with either Alzheimer's or multi-infarct dementia, ginkgo helped. In fact, it helped as much as the drugs used by many neurologists, without the risk and at a lower cost.

Conquering Stress

We are living in incredibly stressful times. Since the publication of *Brain Longevity* the research of Dr. Sonia Lupien at McGill University in Canada has been extended. We now know that the early forms of stress-related memory loss described in the book can contribute to the development of Alzheimer's. Stress produces a toxic chemical that acts like battery acid on your brain's memory center. The stress-relieving techniques presented in chapter 15 and mind-body exercises in chapter 18 are therefore of paramount importance. I agree with the thousands of people who have told me that these techniques are the key to the success of their program. In the words of one of my patients, starting each day in a positive way is "like putting on a suit of armor against stress."

Exercise and Physical Activity

Most neurologists would agree that keeping the mind active goes a long way toward the prevention and reversal of memory loss. Ways to do so are highlighted in chapter 17. Moreover, a new study supports the information on physical exercise in chapter 16. In this retrospective analysis of subjects between the ages of forty and sixty, it was shown that a regular exercise program may slow the aging of your brain and prevent Alzheimer's disease.

Medication

The drug deprenyl has proven to be even more effective than described in the hardcover edition. It is a true anti-aging and cognitive-enhancing drug. Patients with Alzheimer's who are taking the drug Aricept have benefited, in some cases achieving moderate, short-term improvements in memory. Unfortunately, Aricept does not affect the progression of the disease. A new drug called Exalon will soon be available in America. It may have greater benefits without as many side effects. Another new drug, propentofylline, may be more beneficial in fighting Alzheimer's disease. In a multinational study it was effective in helping memory as well as activities of daily living. Propentofylline has a good safety profile and is a drug soon to be prescribed by those doctors working with patients suffering from dementia.

Benefits of Brain Longevity

Patients who practice the complete brain longevity program enjoy a benefit substantiated by work done at Harvard Medical School. My patients have not only improved their physical and brain health but have also developed a newfound relationship with their spirit. This realization leads to greater happiness, more wisdom, and better medical outcomes. It is my most profound prayer that by helping you to develop wisdom and achieve the perfect combination of age, experience, and intelligence, we can call give back to society and make this world of ours a much better place to live.

Wishing you blessings for a lifetime of peak mental performance.

—Dharma Singh Khalsa, M.D.
Tucson, Arizona

PART ONE

The Discovery of Brain Longevity Therapy

1

The Cortisol Connection

The Cry of the Wounded Boomer

My first patient of the day tried to settle into his chair, but he was so tense that he just teetered on the edge of it, his arms clamped to his sides. He was a block of rigid muscles and right angles.

He was afraid that he had early symptoms of Alzheimer's disease, and feared that I would soon doom him with that diagnosis. He knew that if he did have Alzheimer's, conventional medicine could do little to help him. He would simply have to wait for the terrible progression of symptoms to begin.

This man hated the idea of waiting passively while his brain disintegrated. He was a fit, fiery man of considerable success, who was accustomed to *grappling* with his problems until he *solved* them. He wanted to *fight* for his mental acuity, and that's why he'd come to me. He'd read in a medical update newsletter that I had developed a treatment program for memory loss and optimal mental function.

Before he had arrived, I'd done an extensive review of his medical records. Based upon what I'd seen, I was not at all convinced that this fifty-one-year-old man was indeed in the early stages of Alzheimer's. It appeared much more likely that he had a type of memory loss that is common among people his age. In most people, this type of memory loss does not lead to Alzheimer's.

When I explained this to the man, he seemed very relieved, and he let out a sigh. I could hear the air hiss out of him.

"Then what's going *on* with me?" he asked. "How come I've started to get so absentminded?"

I told him that, in all likelihood, he had some degree of what neurologists call "age-associated memory impairment," a condition that is virtually pandemic among people of approximately age fifty. Theoretically, according to most neurologists, losing some brain capacity at fifty is a "normal" sign of aging, just like diminished eyesight at age forty.

I told him I was pleased that he'd come to see me before his symptoms had become more pronounced, because *preventing* mental decline is much easier than *reversing* it.

If his memory problems were indeed relatively mild, I told him, he could probably regain full use of his ability to remember. He could also greatly increase his ability to concentrate. With improvements in memory and concentration, his learning ability would almost certainly improve. In all likelihood, he would experience a rebirth of brain power, as had many of my other patients.

Then I asked him how his memory problems were affecting his life.

He launched into a passionate litany of complaints. He said that over the past couple of years he'd begun to forget people's names, and to forget important items when he packed for business trips. Lately he'd had to stop being a referee at his daughter's soccer games, because he often forgot which team had last touched the ball when it went out of bounds. The girls on his daughter's team had been getting angry at him, and his daughter was becoming increasingly embarrassed.

His life at home was also suffering, he said, because he was often irritable. He didn't have much patience with his daughters, and he was tense so often that it was creating distance between him and his wife.

Almost every day now, he said, he had problems with what he called his "fuzzy brain."

In the morning he'd be unable to find his car keys, and at lunch he'd forget his wallet. He often forgot where he'd parked his car, and when he dialed a number, he'd have to recheck his Rolodex in mid-dial.

Years before, he said—when he'd had a steel-trap mind—these things had rarely happened.

At work, his memory was stunting his career. For twenty years he had sacrificed to reach his current lofty level, but now his job was in jeopardy. Before important meetings, he said, he would be given long legal briefs and be expected to read them, learn them, retain them, and then discuss them intelligently. He couldn't do this as well as he once had. He said he couldn't "shut out the world" anymore. Even without deadline pressure, it was harder for him to learn new information, such as his firm's new software system. He was relying increasingly on his secretary and his assistant. His secretary would remind him who he was having lunch with, and his assistant would preview his briefs and highlight the key points. They both covered for him when he tired out in midafternoon, and his assistant would return calls that he should have been handling himself.

Net result: His superiors were getting impatient with him.

The competitive atmosphere "inside the Beltway," as he put it, was intense. Some of the ambitious young lawyers in his firm, he said, were trying to grab his job. They seized an advantage every time he forgot a detail or made a slip of the tongue. He felt as if they were circling him in a pack.

I knew full well what he was talking about. I often heard similar versions of the same complaint. I even had a name for it: The Cry of the Wounded Boomer.

Baby boomers, who were just now hitting the "memory barrier" of their late forties and early fifties, were consulting me with increasing frequency. They were *shocked* by the sudden onset of age-associated memory impairment, and by the corresponding declines in their hormonal systems. They were suddenly losing the mental sharpness that had propelled their careers, and had allowed them to juggle families and jobs. They were also losing their endocrinological spark as their "youth hormones" dried up. Their sexual urges were flattening out, they were gaining weight, losing muscle and hair, and needing more and stronger coffee just to slog through the day. The boomers' loss was Starbuck's gain.

Most of them had the "dual curse": memory impairment, combined with decreased ability to concentrate. Each of these problems exacerbated the other, and both impaired learning ability. My midlife patients often told me that they just couldn't "soak up" facts as they had during their peak learning years. And they *missed* this wonderfully vital state of mind, just as much as they missed other aspects of their younger years.

But the worst thing of all, according to many of them, was that they were losing the inner fire that had once made them jump out of bed in the morning ready for action and full of fun. Now they pushed the "snooze" button, and got up grudgingly. Their lives had become dull. Fun was too much trouble. So was sex. Action was a chore. Life was . . . work.

Many of them had tried to rationalize their recent declines with talk about "acceptance" and "maturity" and "lowered expectations." Others had tried to deny their deterioration by pumping weights, dyeing their hair, and getting their tummies tucked. Many were self-medicating with caffeine, nicotine, alcohol, and megadoses of vitamins.

Nonetheless, what I saw was a frightened generation.

And they had good reason to be scared. For years they'd struggled to build a foundation of security and prosperity for the last half of their lives, but now they were smacking headlong into an unexpected roadblock: the decline of their brain power and energy at the very peak of their career curves and family demands. Early burnout was *not* something they'd planned for.

In addition, I had discovered, almost all baby boomers with age-associated memory impairment were haunted by a dark fear: the specter of Alzheimer's disease. They knew that Alzheimer's—

which usually takes about twenty years to develop fully—reduces people to virtual infancy. It renders them unable to speak, use the toilet, remember family members, or even smile. They also often become paranoid and hostile. And in that pathetic condition, patients often survive for up to ten years.

When these baby boomers had gone to their local doctors for help, however, they'd been told that no medical protocol existed for arresting or preventing Alzheimer's disease, or for treating age-associated memory impairment.

In general, the medical profession takes a lamentably passive approach to cognitive decline. According to long-standing conventional wisdom, *nothing* can stop Alzheimer's, or relieve age-associated memory impairment.

Supposedly, some memory loss is inevitable for virtually *everyone,* starting at about age forty-five to fifty. Age-associated memory impairment is one of the most common medical problems of people in midlife.

Alzheimer's disease is also commonly considered inevitable for a great many people. Today, Alzheimer's strikes *up to 50 percent of all people who live to age eighty-five.* Because of this high incidence, Alzheimer's is the third-highest cause of death by disease in America, after cardiovascular disease and cancer.

But I don't accept the inescapability of Alzheimer's, or of age-associated memory impairment.

I believe that Alzheimer's disease can be delayed and prevented.

I believe that age-associated memory impairment can be eradicated.

I believe that people in their forties, fifties, sixties—and beyond—can retain not only an almost perfect memory, but can also have "youthful minds," characterized by the dynamic brain power, learning ability, creativity, and emotional zest usually found only in young people.

These beliefs of mine—now shared by other cutting-edge researchers and clinicians—are absolutely revolutionary. Ten years ago, almost no one in medicine subscribed to these ideas; I certainly didn't. But now I'm positive they're true, for one central reason: the clinical results I have achieved. For a number of years I have been applying to the brain a unique medical regeneration program that is at the white-hot forefront of anti-aging medicine. This program employs *complementary medicine,* a relatively new clinical approach that combines Western technological medicine with the most powerful proven techniques from Eastern medicine.

I have become, to some extent, a medical pioneer, implementing a program that creates "mental fitness" and "brain longevity."

The results have been astounding. My patients have, quite literally, achieved the impossible.

I have helped people regain the minds they once had. Rejecting the assumption that all minds must deteriorate with age, I have helped many patients regain "youthful minds."

I have been able to achieve this, in part, because I have begun addressing an element of memory loss that has only recently emerged from the laboratories of brain research: the "cortisol connection."

The Cortisol Connection

Cortisol is one of the hormones secreted by the adrenal glands. It's secreted in response to stress. In moderate amounts, cortisol is not harmful. But when produced in excess, day after day—as a result of chronic, unrelenting stress—*this hormone is so toxic to the brain that it kills and injures brain cells by the billions.*

I am now certain that chronic exposure of the brain to toxic levels of cortisol is a primary cause of brain degeneration during the aging process. Over decades, excessive cortisol destroys the biochemical integrity of the brain.

I believe, further, that cortisol toxicity is one of the primary causes of Alzheimer's disease.

Defined very simply, Alzheimer's is a mental condition characterized by extensive death of brain cells. I am convinced, based upon my research and clinical work, that excessive cortisol production is one of the primary causes of death of those cells. The other causes appear to be genetic factors, environmental factors, metabolic factors, and decreased blood flow to the brain.

The genetic causes of brain cell death cannot be readily influenced yet, but the other causative factors *can* be.

I therefore believe that many of the primary causes of Alzheimer's disease and age-associated memory impairment can be avoided, and compensated for.

Not all brain researchers agree on the causes of brain cell death. Alzheimer's causation is still being debated. But all brain researchers do agree on one thing: *The brain is just flesh and blood.* That sounds obvious, but the general public tends to overlook this simple fact. People often confuse the *brain* with the *mind,* even though the brain and the mind are two distinctly different entities. The mind is "software," the mystical and mysterious product of all that we are. The brain is "hardware," a bodily organ that requires nutrition, rest, use, and proper medical care.

Because people tend to forget that their brains are flesh and blood, they often overlook the physical care and maintenance of their brains. Millions of us expend enormous energy in physical fitness programs for our hearts and muscles—but we totally ignore the most important organ in the body: the brain.

What's the result of this neglect? Slow brain death. In almost all people, 20 percent of all brain cells die over the course of a lifetime. The size of the brain shrivels significantly. Brain power diminishes.

Furthermore, during the same years that your brain cells are dying, excess cortisol is causing a decline in the day-to-day function of your brain. Cortisol robs your brain of its only source of fuel: glucose. It also wreaks havoc on your brain's chemical messengers—your neurotransmitters—which carry your thoughts from one brain cell to the next. When your neurotransmitter function is disrupted, and when your brain's fuel supply plummets, it's difficult for you to concentrate and to remember.

Over the years, as your brain physically degenerates, it also loses its ability to properly orchestrate your hormone-secreting endocrine glands, which are a primary link between your body and your mind. When this happens, you suffer declines in energy, mood, sex drive, and immune function.

Unfortunately, many aging people passively accept such factors as diminished brain power, reduced sex drive, lowered immunity to disease, and loss of youthful exuberance. After all, they reason, aren't these problems a natural part of growing old?

No. They do not *have* to be.

Rebuilding the Brain

Modern medicine is entering a thrilling new era. New techniques are yielding incredible results. We no longer have to accept the same kind of decline that our grandparents did.

Especially encouraging are the results achieved by modern complementary medicine, with its panoply of treatment resources, ranging from ancient herbal remedies to the latest high-tech wizardry. Using this type of medicine, I have achieved clinical successes that are literally astonishing.

I explained all this to the Beltway attorney, telling him why I believed he was suffering from mental decline. In summary, I told him that the special problem with life in the fast lane—with all its excessive stress and cortisol overproduction—is that many hard-driving people experience neurological burnout before they are able to achieve their goals in life.

As I talked, the attorney grew increasingly gloomy.

But then I gave him the good news. I told him about "brain plasticity."

Until not long ago, researchers thought the brain was essentially static, that once damage was done, it couldn't be undone. But all the new technology of the past few decades, such as CAT, PET, and MRI, has shown that, because of the brain's unique regenerative power, blighted areas of the brain can be brought back to life.

The attorney became encouraged. His competitive fires began to burn.

The human brain, I told him, is the most complex, powerful

organism in the universe. It has an unparalleled capacity for restoring its own function. Why? Because the brain doesn't store each of its memories in single, separate brain cells, or *neurons*. Instead, memories exist in *networks* of connected neurons—just as phone calls exist in networks of wires and stations. If one neuron is killed, the brain can switch its memory connection through another neuron, and retain the memory. Neurologists call this *redundant circuitry*.

The Beltway attorney, though, feared that perhaps too many of his brain cells had died, and that not enough redundant circuits were left.

So I gave him an illustration, as I often do, of just how many healthy, interconnected neurons he still had. I told him that if he started counting connections in just his higher-thought area alone, at the rate of one connection per second, he wouldn't finish counting for 32 million years.

In addition, I told him, each brain cell has "branches" that reach out to other brain cells, to make memory connections. As we age, our brain cells grow more and more branches, just as a growing tree keeps sprouting branches. Therefore, by middle age, we have *far* more branches than we did in our younger years. Those extra branches powerfully compensate for brain cell death.

Besides, I told the attorney, he already had far more knowledge in his brain than did any of his young competitors. Most of the millions of facts he had once learned were still in his brain. He just needed to have better access to those facts—and he could achieve that access by improving the biochemical function of his brain.

Also, not only did he *know* more than his young associates, but he probably had far better judgment than most of them did, simply because he had far more experience from which to draw wisdom. But he needed to be able to recall his experiences efficiently, so that he could skillfully apply the lessons that life had taught him.

I assured the attorney that he still had a lot left to work with and that if he worked hard at his brain longevity program, as had other patients before him, he would probably soon begin to feel better than he had in years. His memory would, in all likelihood, return to practically full capacity within about one month. His concentration would become much sharper. As his memory and concentration improved, his learning ability would increase. As the left and right hemispheres of his brain began to function with improved coordination, his problem-solving creativity would expand. Also, his endocrine function would probably stabilize, and he'd stop tiring out in the middle of the afternoon, and also start to feel more cheerful and buoyant.

Eventually, I said, he would probably begin to feel like he had as a youngster. This would happen when his brain, nervous system, endocrine system, and metabolism became physically recharged.

When that happened, I said, he'd be able to stop worrying about the younger attorneys in his office—and they'd start worrying about *him*. He would regain the powerful memory and crystal-clear focus that had once vaulted him to the top of his profession. And he would regain the emotional zest that had made his family love him.

If he successfully completed his brain longevity program, I said, he might even achieve a mental condition that I refer to as a "twenty-first-century mind"—a mind that knows how to continually *regenerate itself*. He might no longer be locked into the old linear pattern of aging ➔ degeneration ➔ death.

If he could achieve that, he would, in a critically important way, be freed from the awful tyranny of time.

When I finished telling him about what my brain regeneration program would entail—and what it could reasonably hope to offer—he sounded tremendously relieved. His voice no longer seemed as if it were trapped in his chest. I had returned to him a very precious thing: hope.

Good Science and Good Sense

Before my next patient consultation, I stepped outside into the crackling dry air of Tucson, Arizona, where my clinic was located.

I sat by the fountain outside my office and soaked up the sun's golden radiation.

As I sat there, I reflexively began to do a powerful Eastern-medicine technique—an ancient yogic mind/body exercise that increases blood flow and energy flow to the brain.

Within minutes I could feel an almost magical surge of energy and calm. If I'd taken a blood test at that moment, it would have indicated a marked reduction in my serum cortisol. If I'd taken a cognitive function test, it would have shown that my ability to concentrate had become elevated.

I took advantage of my mental boost by focusing on a problem I needed to solve. I could feel my mind zeroing in on the problem, to the exclusion of everything else, and I began to formulate some creative solutions. For a few minutes time fell away, and it felt fantastic. When you can focus completely, you're able to experience your life fully in the here and now, free of worry, regret, and boredom. You march to the beat of your own heart, instead of the ticking of the clock. You're able to discover alternatives that your harried mind has overlooked.

I gradually pulled out of my problem-solving reverie, and enjoyed a few minutes of gazing at the beautiful setting around me.

My clinic was part of a lovely, sunny campus of physicians and other health practitioners who collaborated on cases. Even by the standards of advanced complementary medicine, our medical complex was extraordinary. Our campus housed the offices of a medical doctor, a chiropractor, a clinical nutritionist, a message therapist, and an herbalist. The doctors here gave each patient access to each practitioner, to ensure an all-encompassing treatment program.

The Western medical paradigm has one major fault: It's too fragmented. Specialists tend to focus too narrowly, often addressing only single, isolated elements of complex health problems. Western medicine constantly strives to reduce each illness to a specific, isolated cause with a single "magic bullet" cure.

For example, in conventional Alzheimer's research, there is a strong tendency to search for a single cause, such as aluminum toxicity or a genetic predisposition. This reductionist approach, while very effective in many scientific endeavors, overlooks a fundamental fact of biology: that most degenerative diseases, including Alzheimer's, have a number of different causes, and may have different causes in different people.

Even though I believe that excessive cortisol production is probably an important cause of Alzheimer's in many people, I think that other factors also play significant roles.

By the same token, I am convinced that no *single* drug will ever cure Alzheimer's, stop age-associated memory impairment, or create optimal mental function. The only effective way that I have found to combat Alzheimer's and age-associated memory impairment, and to optimize brain power, is to apply a *multifactorial* treatment program. My program includes nutritional therapy; supplementation with specific vitamins, minerals, and trace elements; administration of natural medicinal tonics; cardiovascular exercise; mental exercise; yogic mind/body exercises; stress management; and administration of certain pharmaceutical medications.

Each element of the program works synergistically with the other elements; no single aspect of the program would be completely effective if used alone.

As you might imagine, this concerted program has a therapeutic effect on more than just memory and concentration. It helps virtually every aspect of cognitive ability, especially creativity and learning.

Furthermore, people with very mild cognitive impairment, or *no* cognitive impairment, have used my mental fitness program to develop "super minds"—that is, minds that can focus and learn with incredible efficiency. To put it simply, I have helped smart people become smarter.

My brain longevity program has also worked miracles for accident victims with brain damage, who were supposedly beyond the help of medicine. I have, for example, helped patients recover from cerebral damage caused by car wrecks and by high-altitude pulmonary edema.

In addition, my program has a remarkably positive effect

upon energy and mood, because of its benefit to the endocrine system. Some patients say it's like having a "second childhood."

Also, because the program is a broad-based, health-inducing regimen, it generally boosts immune power and can help the body to overcome various illnesses and degenerative conditions.

Finally, it's an excellent general program to slow signs of aging and promote longevity. Many things that help the brain to regenerate also help the rest of the body to restore itself.

My program may sound almost magical, but it's not. It's just good science and good sense. The magic lies within my patients. The healing ability of their bodies and brains is nothing short of miraculous.

By the time I got back to my office after my short break, my next patient was waiting. One look told me she would be a tough case.

She was a beautifully mature woman, with porcelain skin and lustrous silver hair, but she looked absolutely exhausted. She was droopy. She looked as if someone had molded her out of modeling clay, and then left her out in the sun. As I introduced myself, she cradled her chin in her palm, as if she didn't have the energy to hold up her head.

She was too young to look so exhausted. At sixty-four, she should still have had a hard kernel of vitality in her. But her zest for life was gone.

Shortly after we began talking, she told me that she'd been diagnosed with clinical depression. According to her doctor, her memory loss was one of the symptoms of her depression.

It's true that clinical depression often causes memory loss. But this woman, according to her records, had not responded positively to any of a number of antidepressant medications. This was an indication that depression might have been a misdiagnosis. Doctors frequently label patients as depressive when they can't pinpoint any specific, organic problem. It's a convenient, catch-all diagnosis.

I told her that I had some doubts about the viability of her diagnosis. I clearly recall what she said to me in response: "Whatever." What she meant was, "Fix me, Doc, and don't bother me with the details."

I was concerned that she might have early-stage Alzheimer's, symptoms that sometimes mimic those of clinical depression. So I gave her a fundamental intake screening test, the Mini-Mental State Exam, to measure her cognitive function. First I tested her orientation: Who are you, where are you, and what day is it? She had no problem with those questions. Thus she did not have frank, advanced Alzheimer's.

Then I gave her the "immediate recall" test. I named three objects—book, apple, and shoe—and she was able to repeat them.

I then asked her to count backward from one hundred, by sevens. When I asked her to do that, she looked at me as if I'd sentenced her to hard labor.

When she finished counting, I asked her to name the three objects. She could only remember two. That response is common among patients with age-associated memory impairment, and with early-stage Alzheimer's. I repeated the words to her, and she mouthed them to herself. Instinctively, she was using a memory trick, establishing an aural memory. Patients with memory loss generally use dozens of mnemonic devices; often they're not even aware that they're using them, or that people with intact memories don't use them.

Then I asked her to fill out a questionnaire. Here's what was on it:

ARE YOU EXPERIENCING COGNITIVE DECLINE?

T   F

☐ ☐ From time to time, I forget what day of the week it is.

☐ ☐ Sometimes when I'm looking for something, I forget what it is that I'm looking for.

☐ ☐ My friends and family seem to think I'm more forgetful now than I used to be.

☐ ☐ Sometimes I forget the names of my friends.

☐ ☐ It's hard for me to add two-digit numbers without writing them down.

T   F

☐   ☐   I frequently miss appointments because I forget them.

☐   ☐   I rarely feel energetic.

☐   ☐   Small problems upset me more than they once did.

☐   ☐   It's hard for me to concentrate for even an hour.

☐   ☐   I often misplace my keys, and when I find them, I often can't remember putting them there.

☐   ☐   I frequently repeat myself.

☐   ☐   Sometimes I get lost, even when I'm driving somewhere I've been before.

☐   ☐   I often forget the point I'm trying to make.

☐   ☐   To feel mentally sharp, I depend upon caffeine.

☐   ☐   It takes longer for me to learn things than it used to.

She scored ten "trues." Anybody with nine or more may have age-associated memory impairment. If people score twelve or more, they're probably in trouble. They may have early-stage Alzheimer's disease, and will require more extensive testing.

I then asked her to try to recall the three objects I'd named. She was able to name only the last one—shoe.

She realized she was not performing well on the intake tests, and became upset. On the verge of tears, she said that she was afraid she was becoming senile. She said her memory was "shot," and that she couldn't concentrate hard for more than a few minutes at a time.

I told her that senility was an essentially outdated term, and that the correct technical word for what she was experiencing was *benign senescent forgetfulness.* Basically, that's the same thing as age-associated memory impairment. Hearing that she wasn't "senile" made her feel better. Older people hate that label.

No matter what you called this woman's problem, though, it was becoming clear to me that she had a significant impairment of cognitive function. She probably did not have early-stage Alzheimer's at this point; her symptoms were not yet that severe.

It was possible, though, that she might soon develop Alzheimer's if she did nothing to stop the physical degeneration of her brain.

A growing number of medical practitioners now believe that age-associated memory impairment and early-stage Alzheimer's disease are often linked. Until as late as the mid-1990s, most researchers thought that age-associated memory impairment and Alzheimer's were distinct, separate maladies. Very recently, though, researchers at the federal Alzheimer's Disease Research Centers discovered that many people with age-associated memory impairment soon develop Alzheimer's. Each year, about 15 percent of patients with progressive memory impairment convert to frank Alzheimer's. In comparison, only about 0.3 percent of cognitively healthy people aged sixty-five to seventy annually develop Alzheimer's.

Thus, not everyone who has age-associated memory impairment will develop Alzheimer's. But many will.

Therefore, in my clinical practice, I generally treat Alzheimer's and age-associated memory impairment with similar medical protocols. The more severe the symptoms, however, the more aggressive the treatment.

My primary clinical goal is to intervene in the earliest possible stages of cognitive decline. This, I believe, helps to *prevent* frank, late-stage Alzheimer's. It is much easier to prevent cognitive decline than to reverse it.

I cannot "cure" Alzheimer's. No one can. Based upon my clinical work, however, I believe I can slow the *progression* of Alzheimer's. In so doing, I may be able to spare many Alzheimer's patients from suffering the worst, most painful symptoms of advanced, late-stage Alzheimer's, which may take twenty years or longer to develop. If there is anything "good" about Alzheimer's, it is that it generally strikes only elderly people. Therefore, if I can delay the disease's progression, patients may be able to live their full lives without suffering from the worst symptoms of advanced Alzheimer's, which are far more heartbreaking and destructive than the early symptoms.

The reason I believe I can slow Alzheimer's progression is

that many of my patients seem to be "holding their own" against the disease.

I explained these ideas, as well as my theories about cortisol, to my patient. But she had a hard time processing the information. Processing problems are common among people with age-associated memory impairment. They just can't hold thoughts long enough to make sense of them. Nor can they retain a clear picture of their "menu" of options, which hampers their ability to solve problems creatively.

To provide a graphic context for the information, I told the woman a story, one that I first heard from a great neurological researcher, Dr. Robert Sapolsky, whom I'll tell you about later. The story, which I often tell new patients, clearly describes the neurotoxic assault of cortisol. I call it the "fish story." It goes like this:

No journey is more dramatic in the animal kingdom than that of salmon fighting their way upstream to spawn. They battle the current, and leap past dams and up waterfalls. Where do they get all this energy? Mostly, they get it from cortisol, secreted by their adrenals. At the time when salmon make this epic journey, their normal control over cortisol production stops working, and they oversecrete massive quantities of it. This overproduction exhausts their adrenal glands and disrupts their metabolisms. Just after they spawn, they have enormous, swollen adrenal glands, and their hormonal balance is completely destroyed. They have peptic ulcers, their immune systems are degraded, they appear disoriented, they have lesions on their kidneys, and they're easily overcome by parasites and infections. They quickly die.

But when researchers remove their adrenal glands right after they spawn, and stop cortisol production, the salmon return to health, behave normally, and live for another full year.

The moral of the "fish story" is that cortisol overproduction—*which also happens to stressed-out people*—wreaks havoc upon the body, the brain, and the nervous system. It ruins hormonal balance, and throws the brain and nervous system into a tailspin.

When I finished the story, my patient nodded vigorously. She said she often felt like the salmon in their fight against the current. She told me about the stress she'd endured over the past thirty years, and it sounded as if it had been intense.

I told her that there was a good possibility that I could help her to remember better and to concentrate better—but that she would have to work hard.

She said she was willing to apply herself, but she said it with no real conviction. It was obvious that her willpower had been sapped long ago. And that was a problem, because some aspects of my program, such as dietary change and the mind/body exercises, require determination.

I began to outline the general program for her, and she seemed to shrink before my eyes. She just didn't seem to have enough willpower left to help herself.

As I described the program, I showed her one of the mind/body exercises. It was not a difficult exercise, so I asked her to try it with me.

Her effort was halfhearted. I was beginning to wonder if I could help this patient.

In the midst of the exercise, my receptionist buzzed me, and told me that some of the results of this woman's lab work had arrived.

When I saw the lab report, I was stunned. She had astonishingly low levels of a hormone called DHEA, which generally exists in the body in inverse proportion with cortisol. DHEA is called the "mother steroid hormone," and it's absolutely vital for energy, immunity, and proper neurological function.

This woman desperately needed hormonal replacement therapy; it would be the logical first step to take to stop the degeneration of her brain and endocrine system. If the hormonal therapy worked the way I thought it would, it would revive her dormant willpower. Then she would have the strength to participate in the more difficult parts of the program. She would, in all probability, regain her memory and her ability to concentrate and to solve problems creatively.

People often don't think of such an intangible thing as willpower as being partly biochemical, but it is. So is creativity. We think of creativity as something we're born with, but that's not entirely true. By stimulating the brain's *corpus callosum,* which links the left and right hemispheres, creativity can be significantly increased. To me, it's amazing that so many intangible mental aspects can be influenced biochemically. To paraphrase Mies van der Rohe, God is in the molecules.

I felt very encouraged. I was almost certain that hormonal replacement therapy would prove to be the linchpin in this patient's recovery. It would enable her to take the first step on the long journey toward health.

I began to explain to her how, by working together, she and I could dramatically improve the way she felt.

For the first time since entering my office, her eyes began to glow with hope.

A Case in Point

There's No Such Thing As a Hopeless Case

S.L. was told by her neurologist that nothing could be done for her. Her doctor told her she would have to learn to accept the fact that she had brain damage, and that she would never again attain a high level of mental function. But S.L. did not accept this pronouncement of doom and gloom. She simply was not a quitter.

All her life, S.L. had been extremely aggressive about making her dreams become reality. She came from an accomplished family of high achievers. Her father was a prominent doctor in West Virginia, and her mother held a Ph.D. in biochemistry. S.L., who was bright and also very attractive, had become a CPA and had also been accepted into Harvard's MBA program. However, she had a great interest in the environment, and had begun studying forestry instead of business administration. She'd received a master's degree in forestry, and had become a regional manager of the U.S. Forest Service.

Then disaster struck.

A car she was driving was hit on the driver's side by another automobile, and she suffered a crushed pelvis, broken ribs, and a collapsed lung.

She also suffered a severe head injury (as do 2 million other Americans every year).

S.L. was in a complete coma for six days. When she finally emerged from the coma, she suffered from retrograde amnesia, and was unable to remember the events immediately before her accident. The cluster of symptoms associated with her amnesia included a gross inability to concentrate, and difficulty in maintaining a logical train of thought.

Only rarely do people with amnesia suffer *only* from memory loss, and not from intellectual impairment. This type of "classic" amnesia occurs mostly in soap operas.

Besides her intellectual problems, she'd also developed a seizure disorder, which was revealed as epileptic activity on her EEG tests.

She also had an extreme case of vertigo, apparently caused by injuries to her inner ear, and to her cerebellum (the part of the brain that governs movement).

Because of this debilitating constellation of symptoms, she had become unemployable, and was not even able to manage her own living situation. The state welfare system had placed her with a case manager who helped coordinate her daily activities. Her caseworker helped her to remain living at home, arranged for her to receive Social Security disability payments, and scheduled her medical appointments. She was receiving speech therapy, occupational therapy, and physical therapy.

After she had reached a minimal level of recovery, her physician recommended no further treatment. He knew of nothing else that might benefit S.L.

The caseworker, who is a colleague of mine, asked me to come visit her.

One of my most vivid recollections of that first meeting was seeing that, in early spring, she still had not taken down her Christmas lights, inside or outside. She just didn't have the focus she needed to carry out even that simple task. When she spoke, her words gushed out "a mile a minute," moving in a thousand directions at once. Her eyes darted around the room, and she had absolutely no ability to focus her conversation.

She soon began a full-spectrum brain longevity program, engaging enthusiastically in the four primary aspects of the program: (1) nutritional therapy (including dietary change, nutritional supplementation, and administration of natural medicinal tonics); (2) exercise (including cardiovascular exercise, mental exercise, and mind/body exercises); (3) stress management; and (4) pharmacology. Like all of my patients, she received a program that was tailored to her own needs, biochemical makeup, and lifestyle.

She stopped eating her regular high-fat diet, and began ingesting a nutrient-dense "cleansing" diet, which contained a relatively high amount of chlorophyl-rich foodstuffs, and fresh juices. She took the herb *Ginkgo biloba,* as well as a broad spectrum of vitamins and minerals. She also took a homeopathic remedy for vertigo, in pills and injections.

In addition, she underwent a regimen of advanced medical acupuncture, and each day she performed a series of mind/body exercises designed to increase her ability to focus, and to improve her vertigo.

The acupuncture treatment, focused primarily on points in her scalp, was somewhat similar to another treatment that has elicited remarkable results among thousands of amnesia patients: transcranial electrical brain stimulation. This therapy is employed by physicians in the treatment of severe brain damage.

Within a few weeks her eyes stopped darting distractedly when she talked, and she began to be more focused in her conversation. There was clinical evidence that her brain biochemistry had begun to shift back into balance.

By the end of six months she had made an almost miraculous recovery. Her ability to concentrate had returned, and she no longer required any assistance in managing her life. She soon began studying at a nearby university, in a master's degree program of music therapy.

Less than a year after beginning her brain longevity program, she had lost virtually all recognizable symptoms of brain damage. Her life was once again whole and happy.

In her words, she had "returned to her center."

She had, in fact, been transformed—into her "old" self.

2

The Development
of Brain Longevity
Therapy

My long day of consulting with patients continued. But it did not get easier.

When I first saw my last patient of the day, my heart went out to him.

This sad-eyed man sitting before me—once he'd been one of John F. Kennedy's "best and brightest." In the 1960s, he'd been an important member of the legendary American Camelot—a man of vigor, power, and brilliance.

What a life he'd built! Year after year, he'd piled up the kind of achievements that he'd thought would make him proud until the day he died.

But now his past—his *life*—was being ripped away. Now, with sickening speed, his past was receding into a dull tangle of vague recollections, shadows, and black holes. Now his only link to the life he'd so loved—his memory—was turning to dust. Day by day he could feel his vital spark, his very selfhood, leaving him. Much of the time now, he felt empty. It was almost as if he'd never achieved anything. As if he'd never been married, never had children. Never worked in the White House.

It was as if he had never lived.

And there was even more to his pain than that. He was also losing his ability to function on a day-to-day basis. Many simple tasks were now becoming hard. He held a Ph.D., and had recently run a large bank, but now, most of the time, he felt stupid. His mind was dull and confused, as if it were tied in knots. He couldn't concentrate on a complex problem for more than a minute or two. Virtually every day he had to rely on other people to help him perform routine jobs. Sometimes these people were patient with him; sometimes they were condescending. He was beginning to feel like a dim-witted child, and it made him hate being alive.

But this unhappy man in the wrinkled suit was fighting like a warrior to hang on to his mental faculties and cling to his life. Each day he tried to concentrate on specific events from his past, attempting to reignite the vivid memories that had once filled him so full.

And that's what he was doing at this moment, as he sat in the main office of my clinic. Outside, the crystalline fountain burbled in the yellow Arizona sun, as he and I gradually became acquainted.

As we chatted, he began telling me about the initial meeting of JFK's campaign team, when they had kicked off their run for the White House. He seemed to be talking as much to himself as to me—as if to remind himself of his past. Often, patients with memory impairment try to "memorize" the events of their lives, to lay down a memory of a memory. This enables them to "play tapes" of past events, and helps them avoid the pain and humiliation of forgetfulness.

When he forgot a detail, his eyes would dart uncomfortably around my office, as if he were looking for his life in the corners of the room. This happened frequently, because his memory was pocked with areas that I call "Swiss cheese": formerly vivid memories that were now riddled with holes, due to neuronal loss.

He also had a pronounced tendency toward aphasia, the inability to recall specific words. Like many people with aphasia, which is one of the first signs of memory decline, he'd learned to quickly substitute synonyms for missing words.

At one point, when he was telling me about the first campaign meeting, which had been at Joseph Kennedy's mansion in Palm Beach, Florida, he told an anecdote about the Kennedy patriarch. All the other advisers at the meeting, he said, had been very concerned about the fact that JFK was a Catholic. "But not old Joe," he said. "Joe just kept yelling, 'Run against the other *candidates,* Jack, not *God*!' "

He told the story perfectly, without hesitation or aphasic episodes. Apparently that incident had made a powerful impression on him at the time, allowing him to biochemically create an almost indelible memory of it. When emotion accompanies an event, we produce more of the neurological chemicals that create memories. That's why we can easily remember traumatic events.

As we talked, he mentioned that his neurologist in Chicago had told him that, although experimental drugs were being developed, nothing could be done to halt the ebb of his memory. His doctor had told him that, in all probability, his situation was hopeless. Within seven or eight years, the doctor had said, he might not even be able to remember his own wife.

But this man, whom I will call D.S., simply refused to accept this prognosis. He told me that he "didn't believe" in the concept of hopelessness—and that's why he'd come to me.

"Well," I told him, "I don't believe in hopelessness either. No one entity on earth is without hope. Not even," I intoned gravely, "the Chicago Cubs."

That got a little laugh out of him, partly because most people don't expect me to be aware of down-to-earth things like sports. They see my turban, which I wear because I'm a member of the Sikh religion, and assume I have my head in the clouds.

It was no coincidence that D.S. was at my clinic. He was simply not the type to accept passively a doctor's pronouncement of doom. During his prime, he and his associates had ushered in an era of activism that had changed the world; they'd believed that *nothing was inevitable.* Like many other baby boomers, I'd been inspired by that attitude, and was now applying it to my own work.

I pulled a copy of the "Global Deterioration Scale" out of my desk, and began going over it with D.S. This scale, developed by Barry Reisberg, M.D., of the New York University School of Medicine, is what neurologists often use to assess the severity of the brain's decline.

It looks like this:

GLOBAL DETERIORATION SCALE

Stage	Characteristics	Diagnosis	Duration
1	No memory decline.	Normal	—
2	Forgetting names of associates; forgetting placement of familiar objects.	Age-associated memory impairment	—
3	Decreased retention of written material; forgetting placement of valuable objects; concentration decline; anxiety accompanying forgetfulness; deficits noted in demanding employment situations.	Mild neurocognitive disorder	7 years
4	Decreased knowledge of current events; decreased ability to travel, handle finances, perform complex tasks; lack of emotion.	Mild Alzheimer's disease	2 years
5	Inability to recall major event in current life; moderate time disorientation; forgetting names of family members.	Moderate Alzheimer's disease	18 months
6	Forgetting name of spouse; forgetting most recent life events; requiring assistance with daily living; delusional and paranoid behavior; anxiety and agitation; urinary and fecal incontinence.	Moderately severe Alzheimer's disease	2 years
7	In chronological order: loss of speech; loss of ability to walk; loss of ability to sit up; loss of ability to smile.	Severe Alzheimer's disease	7–10 years

The Current Era of Super-Stress

Judging from D.S.'s medical records, he was at an indeterminate point in stage three of this scale. I hoped he was still in an *early* phase of stage three. I told him that if his mental fitness program was successful, he could reasonably hope to remain in the stage-three condition indefinitely, with no further deterioration.

I also told him that he might even be able to improve to an early stage-two status. If this happened, his memory would improve, and he would again be able to focus the considerable powers of his learned mind.

That information pleased him very much. He had a close friend with Alzheimer's, he said, and had been appalled at this friend's precipitous decline.

He told me that a number of his peers had contracted Alzheimer's, even though some were only in their late sixties. He wanted to know if the incidence of the disease was rising, or if there was simply an increase in reportage of the disease.

I told him that public health records indicated that incidence was, indeed, rising rapidly—even when increased reportage was factored in. Our current generations are being ravaged by the disease.

One major reason for the increase is that people are living longer. The older you get, the greater your chances are of developing Alzheimer's.

I also believe, however, that the incidence of Alzheimer's is rising because of factors related to the cortisol connection. More than previous generations, it appears, our present population is being decimated by stress and its biochemical ramifications. Why? Because there are simply more neurological stressors these days than there were in the past.

To some extent, our current generations are "guinea pigs." No one is certain about the eventual biological impact of life in the postindustrial age. There are now many stressors on the nervous system that never before existed.

One is the "mega-information syndrome," the daily bombardment of information upon our brains. For example, guess how many advertisements alone the average American sees each day, including logos and labels? Guess high.

The answer is sixteen thousand. Each ad, of course, does not send us into a screaming panic—but it *does* register upon our brain's nervous system, taxing our brain cells and neurotransmitters, and sometimes causing release of stress hormones. And these are just *ads*—not news messages, radio programs, Muzak, job-related information, movies, books, magazines, and so on. If you doubt that the effects of the mega-information syndrome are profound, go spend five days in a cabin in the woods, and take note of the monumental changes in your nervous system and thinking patterns. You'll feel reborn.

Similarly, technology-induced exhaustion is also now at a historic high. The around-the-clock assault of phones, faxes, computers, TVs, voice mail, portable stereos, car radios, and just plain old *noise* creates a formidable burden on the nervous system, sending out jolts of cortisol every few minutes. In modern life, it's uncommon for a person to sit in peaceful silence for even ten minutes each day. Furthermore, much of the information that's blasted at us originates from distant corners of the world, destroying any sense of geographic security that we might have.

Also, in this era of two-salary families, most people end up playing at least two roles each day, and survive only through "multitasking"—doing two or more things at once. We've all become adept at this, but it takes a heavy neurological toll.

Please don't misunderstand me, though: I don't believe that life today is more difficult than ever before. In many ways it's much easier. Many of us live in luxury. But life is currently more stressful in terms of its effect upon the brain and nervous system. I'll give you an example. In the early 1900s, if someone had to walk outside his or her home to draw a bucket of water from the well, it was physically difficult, but was generally a peaceful experience. These days, a person walking down the block to buy a bottle of uncontaminated water might be subjected to honking horns, flashing lights, irritable clerks, hundreds of ads, and loud rap music. Buying the bottled water is physically easier than fetching a bucket of water, but more neurologically taxing.

Unfortunately for us these days, our complex environments are almost constantly stressful, and it's the constancy of this attack that creates chronically high cortisol levels. In a way, this assault is like the "death of a thousand cuts."

Sad to say, life will almost certainly get even more stressful in the future, particularly for the baby-boom generation. The demographic cards are stacked against the boomers.

Current economic trends are already making life more worrisome. Corporate downsizing is killing so many full-time, family-wage jobs that now 75 percent of the workforce, according to a recent poll, fears job loss. This restructuring means more competition for jobs, and less consideration for older workers who fall slightly off the pace. It also means many people are having to learn new careers in midlife.

Further, in the years to come, as aging boomers' earning abilities begin to decline, they will find fewer "safety nets" to cushion their falls. The Social Security system is in jeopardy. Medicare is on the verge of bankruptcy. Clearly the trend in government is to provide fewer social services to the elderly and ill.

Nor can people these days depend upon their own families for long-term elder care. Though families once took full responsibility for their aging members, that social custom is much less prevalent now, after fifty years of the government assuming this responsibility.

Consequently, many millions of the 78 million baby boomers are simply going to have to take care of themselves as they age.

But within about fifteen years, up to 10 million people, according to one prediction from the National Institute of Aging, may not be able to take care of themselves, because they may have Alzheimer's disease. This is more than twice our current Alzheimer's population of 4 million—and, already, Alzheimer's accounts for almost 50 percent of all admissions to nursing homes. Alzheimer's strikes up to half of all people over age eighty-five, and increased life expectancy is quickly ballooning that seg-

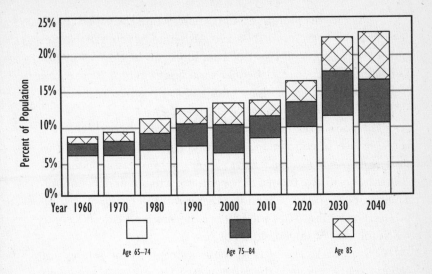

Figure I
Over the next few decades, an unprecedented number of people will join the ranks of the elderly. Unless current trends in cognitive decline are reversed, this "graying of America" will create a public health crisis.

ment of the population. Within twenty-five years, the number of eighty-five-year-olds in America will double.

If all the worst-case scenarios come true, and if there is no society-wide Alzheimer's prevention program put into place, it is quite possible that in the year 2030—when most of us will still be alive—*up to 20 percent of the population over age sixty-five will have Alzheimer's.*

To me, that notion is absolutely horrifying. If it happens, it will be a social holocaust. It conjures images of vast storehouses of pathetic people, millions of them little more than zombies.

Who will they be? The first, smaller, wave of them will be the World War II generation. That generation is already hitting prime Alzheimer's age. The second wave—inordinately larger, a virtual tidal wave—will be the baby boomers, the flower children—the former "younger generation."

As bad as this sounds, though, there is one clear mechanism for clinical intervention. Because Alzheimer's generally strikes only elderly people, if onset of symptoms can be delayed by just five years, incidence of Alzheimer's will be cut in half. If onset can be delayed by ten years, which I think is very possible, Alzheimer's will once again become a relatively rare disease.

The people rescued from Alzheimer's will also experience a very positive phenomenon. They won't grow less intelligent as they age; *they'll just grow wiser.* Their ever-increasing neuronal "branches" will give them a rich, complex sense of understanding. Their vast experience will endow them with a deep, abiding comprehension of life. They will achieve the status all elderly people yearn for, that of valued elder adviser.

D.S. and I kicked around these concepts as the setting sun began to glow orange in the purpling sky. He was well schooled in public policy, and the societal implications of all this were obvious to him.

I described to him the clinical successes I was having with my brain longevity program. As I spoke, he began to grow more optimistic.

When I finished, he told me that he felt lucky.

I asked him why.

"Because now I have something I can *do,*" he said.

I knew exactly what he meant. He *was* lucky.

Ten years ago, no medical treatment program for memory disorder existed. Nor was there any medical program to help people achieve optimal mental function.

Ten years ago, all people could do was *wait*—for "the inevitable."

Discovering the Good News:
A Detective Story

Ten years ago, I had yet to unravel the mystery of the "cortisol connection," and I had yet to devise a medical program for memory loss. But, even at that time, I strongly suspected that there was a link between adrenal hormones and neurological degeneration.

But what *kind* of link? How did it work? And what could be done to break the link?

This mystery is one that has preoccupied me for over twenty-five years. Ever since medical school, I've been studying the link between stress hormones and brain dysfunction.

My interest in this mystery is rooted in my own childhood. During my birth, I suffered from oxygen deprivation, and it caused a minor physical insult to my brain. Because of this, as a child, I had mild learning disabilities. I was prone to slight hyper-activity, and sometimes had difficulty concentrating. At an early age I noticed that when I was under stress, I had a much harder time focusing. But I eventually found that, with proper medica-tion, I could concentrate effectively, and I became able to excel in school.

When I began medical school at Creighton University, I started doing hatha yoga—just basic stretching. I began doing yoga because I was curious about it, and I soon found that I enjoyed it. I noticed that when I did the yoga exercises regularly, my sense of stress declined, and I was able to focus with greater clarity. I began doing yoga very conscientiously, and was able to discontinue the medication that helped me concentrate.

When I became an intern at Alameda County Hospital in Oakland, California, I took my yogic studies one step further: I started doing transcendental meditation. I thought that if TM was good enough for the Beatles, it was good enough for me. I thought it might help me get away with working all day and so-cializing all night. It did. It gave me a lot of energy, and it had a powerful effect on my ability to learn. Soon I was named chief resident and "most improved resident" at UC San Francisco.

At that time my primary intellectual interest was physiology, and my primary professional satisfaction came from helping relieve distress. Therefore I became fascinated by anesthesiology and pain management.

As I studied anesthesiology, I gained a true reverence for the amazing sensitivity of the body, and for its incredible powers of restoration and adaptability. Just one example: When you make an incision on an anesthetized patient, his or her blood pressure and pulse will spike up, as the body automatically defends itself against physical stressors. To me, that's amazing. It's as if the body has a mind of its own.

As I became adept at anesthesiology, I was struck by how severely my patients' mental faculties were hurt by stress, such as that caused by chronic pain, or by an operation. Very intelligent people would become markedly less cogent as their stress mounted. Some of this mental decline seemed to come from worry, but some of it seemed to be biochemical. I wondered if this decline in cognitive function was similar to the stress-related concentration problems I'd suffered as a child.

I became increasingly interested in the biochemistry of stress, and read the book that was then the "bible" on the subject, *The Relaxation Response*, by Harvard's Herbert Benson, M.D. The book had a profound effect upon me. Benson, a cardiologist specializing in hypertension, offered an exact description of the physiology of stress, and explained how it helped cause degenerative disease (particularly cardiovascular disease).

Extremely intrigued, I took postgraduate training at Harvard Medical School, where I studied behavioral medicine under the famous Dr. Benson. Those studies changed my professional life, as I began to appreciate fully the effect of lifestyle on health. Thus I took a giant step toward becoming a physician who treated his patients holistically rather than symptomatically. I began to realize that such elements as stress and nutrition were of vital importance in preventing diseases of degeneration, which may take decades to develop.

While studying with Dr. Benson, I read *Peak Performance*, by Charles Garfield, Ph.D., and Hal Zina Bennett, Ph.D., and that book also contributed to my clinical approach. Dr. Garfield demonstrated clearly that various mental training techniques, such as voluntary relaxation and mental rehearsal, could greatly improve physical performance, and alter brain waves, heartbeat, and respiration.

Armed with my new knowledge of the detrimental effect of

stress—and how to overcome it—I took my anesthesia board exams. Using yoga, meditation, and Benson's and Garfield's stress-reduction techniques, I psyched myself into a state of unparalleled mental energy, and did better on the test, according to the panel of examiners, than anyone else in the country that year. I'd like to think I did so well because I was one of America's smartest doctors—but I doubt it. My success, I am certain, resulted from my use of stress-reduction techniques and mental training.

Excited by these methods, I began teaching an exam-preparation course to doctors who were taking their board exams. The average pass rate for these exams is about 50 percent, even though almost all doctors take prep courses for the exams. Our pass rate was 90 percent. Obviously, our program had helped people achieve states of elevated focus, mental clarity, and advanced problem-solving creativity. I knew I was on the trail of something important, but I wasn't sure exactly what it was, or how best to use it. All I knew for certain was that stress had a negative impact on mental performance.

Spurred on by Dr. Benson's approach to degenerative disease, I began an earnest and systematic study of complementary medicine. I took advanced training in clinical nutrition, and enrolled in UCLA's Medical Acupuncture for Physicians program. I found that many Eastern methods, though lacking the scientific rationale of Western modalities, were extremely effective. Those techniques often achieved success where Western medicine failed. As a pragmatist, I embraced these methods; my sole interest was in serving my patients, and I was willing to do whatever I could to help them.

For example, a stroke victim came to me suffering from ophthalmoplegia—paralysis of an eye muscle. One of his eyes was virtually useless. No doctor had been able to help him. But with one acupuncture treatment—just one needle, using "Yamamoto new scalp acupuncture"—I completely and immediately cured the problem. It was a remarkable clinical success, which I could never have achieved with any Western method.

After a number of years of working as an anesthesiologist, I was recruited by the University of Arizona's teaching hospital in Phoenix to become the founding director of their Acupuncture, Stress Medicine, and Chronic Pain program. My pain control program was one of the first complementary medicine pain programs in America, and we achieved some extremely dramatic results, using such techniques as acupuncture and nutrition, in conjunction with conventional Western modalities. I loved this stage of my life. Helping people in pain was extremely rewarding to me.

As I directed the pain program, I became ever more aware of the terrible toll that the stress of chronic pain takes on mental function. I'd expected chronic pain to affect the emotions, of course, but I was continually surprised at how much it also hurt mental clarity and intellectual capacity. It made me even more interested in my long-standing preoccupation: the relationship between mental decline and chronic stress. But I still didn't understand the physiology of that mysterious connection.

For years I constantly reviewed the medical literature, seeking clues to the mystery. Gradually the clues began to mount. It became obvious to me that one or more of the physical by-products of stress negatively impacted cognition. The most likely factor was either a hormone, an endocrine secretion, or a brain chemical called a *neuropeptide*. Whatever this factor was, it appeared to cause both temporary damage to memory (presumably because it interfered with neurotransmitter function) and permanent damage (presumably because of death of brain cells).

But what was this mysterious, brain-damaging compound? And through what mechanism did it exert its destructive power?

My search for the answers was often frustrating. But I didn't give up. I'd grown up in an era of activism, and felt in my heart that no problem was ever insoluble. Besides, when you're constantly around people in great pain, you gain a sense of responsibility that won't let you give up.

In the absence of a complete understanding of why stress was biologically toxic to the brain, I began, nevertheless, to devise a treatment program for chronic stress. My patients, particularly my pain patients, were in dire need of a protocol to help with their high levels of stress.

I began to incorporate everything I had learned about the physiology of relaxation into a fledgling anti-stress program. This treatment prototype eventually evolved into the therapeutic regime I use today.

As I had hoped, the program began to improve the cognitive function of a great many of my patients. They showed fewer symptoms of confusion, and were more adept at processing information. The improvement in mental clarity that many of my pain patients achieved was extremely gratifying to them—almost as pleasing as the diminution of their pain.

In my continuing study of yoga, I took a class in kundalini yoga. Kundalini is a strenuous, energy-focusing form of yoga that makes conventional "stretching yoga" seem about as sophisticated as Richard Simmons's "Sweatin' to the Oldies."

Because kundalini yoga and meditation are central practices of the Sikh religion, I was introduced to that religion and found myself drawn to it. Sikhism is a very simple religion, short on dogma, that believes there is one creator, and that no one has a franchise on this creator. The fifth-largest religion in the world, it started in northern India, and focuses on helping people who are suffering and working hard at being happy and healthy. To me, part of the religion's appeal is that it calls for discipline and effort; Sikhs don't believe in passively waiting for paradise, but in struggling to create joy in their own daily lives.

As my work with pain patients grew increasingly complex and successful, I returned to Harvard for advanced training in behavioral medicine. By this time, having treated hundreds of patients suffering from severe stress, I had developed an unshakable belief that the cognitive decline caused by stress could be alleviated, and even prevented. I still wasn't sure, though, exactly *why* my anti-stress program was so effective at regenerating brain function. As a Western physician, this was very irritating to me. I wasn't satisfied with just utilizing a phenomenon. I had to *understand* it.

After several years of running my pain program, I decided to broaden my practice. I began treating patients with a wide array of illnesses—everything from clinical depression to drug addiction to heart disease. I placed a great many of these patients on my anti-stress program, and the program elicited very encouraging results. The stress-control program not only helped ameliorate the physical symptoms of patients' primary illnesses, but also generated the improvements in cognitive function that I had come to expect.

All the while, I continued an ambitious clinical research agenda, seeking to understand the exact biochemical effect of stress upon mental function.

Finally, one day, after years of searching, I found it: the "smoking gun." In a scientific journal I discovered an article by Robert Sapolsky, Ph.D., of Stanford University, about the biochemical effect of stress upon cognitive function.

Within two days I was in Palo Alto, California. I had an appointment with Dr. Sapolsky.

I drove straight to Stanford's biology building, where I began to wend my way through the maze of hallways. The Stanford biology department is probably the finest in the world, and you could practically smell the intelligence in the long, winding halls. You could also smell the aroma of Thai food, because this was the kind of place where obsessive geniuses hibernated for days at a time, cooking meals on their Bunsen burners to keep from having to leave their microscopes.

I found Dr. Sapolsky half-buried in a rat's nest of papers and books. His office looked like a library after an earthquake.

Though a full professor, and a man in much renown in the academic world, Sapolsky was much younger than I'd imagined. The first thing I thought when I saw him was—Banana! He looked just like the piano player named Banana, from the old rock group the Youngbloods. If that cultural reference is a little too arcane for you, suffice it to say he looked like a cross between Simon and Garfunkel: youthful-looking, with a glob of curly hair, and an outfit that could best be described as "Birkenstock chic." However casual he might have looked, though, I'd discovered over the past couple of days that Robert Sapolsky was an absolute god to neuroscientists.

I introduced myself. "Yes!" he said. "You're the doctor who wants to look at my stress and memory stuff! Got just what you need."

Then, in one of the most adroit acts of Zen I've ever seen, he stuck his arm behind his back, reached into a haystack of papers behind him, and, *without looking back,* grabbed precisely the article he needed.

As casually as if he were talking about the weather—"it's eighty-eight degrees today, it's sunny, a little humid"—he said, "There are three basic reasons stress affects memory; the first is by decreasing glucose utilization, the second—"

"Wait! Let me write this down."

I grabbed a pen off his desk and started madly making notes in the margins of the research paper he'd given me. I felt electrified, as if I were suddenly peering over the peak of a mountain I'd been climbing for twenty years.

In a nutshell, what he told me was this: There are three essential ways that stress destroys optimal function of the brain, and blots out memory.

First, when cortisol is released in a stressful situation, it *inhibits the utilization of blood sugar* by the brain's primary memory center, the *hippocampus*. If there isn't enough blood sugar in the hippocampus, it suffers an energy shortage, and the brain has no way to chemically lay down a memory. A person can experience an event, but have almost no recall of it. This accounts for the immediate, short-term memory deficit of people under stress.

Second, cortisol overproduction *interferes with the function of the brain's neurotransmitters*. Thus, even if a memory *has* been properly laid down in the past, it can no longer be easily accessed. In effect, the "lines are down," just like downed telephone lines in a storm. Brain cells just can't communicate with one another, and the mind becomes muddled. This is why I call cortisol the "concentration killer." It's why people often become temporarily befuddled in high-stress situations.

Third, too much cortisol *kills brain cells*. This happens when cortisol disrupts normal brain cell metabolism, and causes excessive amounts of calcium to enter brain cells. That excess of calcium eventually produces molecules called *free radicals,* which kill brain cells from within. Over long periods, excess cortisol can kill billions of brain cells this way.

By the time I finished my note-taking, my hands were trembling with excitement. My many years of study told me that everything he was saying was completely logical. Every word had the ring of truth.

"You understand," said Dr. Sapolsky, "these concepts are based on the results of animal testing. Maybe they won't carry over to humans. Besides, even if the same phenomenon applies to humans, it may not be possible to intervene clinically."

"But you're certain of these findings?" I asked.

"Every experiment we've done supports our thesis. And we've done numerous experiments. The science holds up perfectly."

I probed him for every possible detail. It quickly became apparent to me that he was, indeed, a brilliant scientist.

The clinical implications of what Dr. Sapolsky had outlined were staggering: There might be a way to help prevent, and even arrest, Alzheimer's disease and age-associated memory impairment.

I hurried off. I had patients waiting—patients who were suffering from mental decline—and now I was certain I could help them. By combining this new biochemical information with what I already knew about stress management, I believed I could achieve the most profound breakthrough yet in the treatment of Alzheimer's disease and age-associated memory impairment, and in the attainment of optimal mental function.

As I stepped onto the massive Stanford quadrangle, I felt alive with joy. I said a quick prayer of thanks.

In the months to come, I would focus my research primarily on cortisol, and would soon uncover further academic work that corroborated Dr. Sapolsky's findings. In Montreal, two biologists proved that Sapolsky's animal studies did carry over to humans. And at the University of Arizona, psychology professor Alfred Kazniak showed that stress levels in elderly people correlated directly with their levels of memory loss. Both of these discoveries would prove to be tremendously gratifying to me. They would confirm my theories, and contribute to the clinical approach I was developing. That approach, based on my prototypical stress-management program, would soon achieve unparalleled clinical success.

My emerging brain longevity programs would, for example, enable me literally to work wonders with all three of the patients I've mentioned, as we'll see in chapter 4. With all three—who were supposedly beyond the reach of medical help—I was literally able to achieve "the impossible."

But for pure excitement, nothing ever matched the climactic thrill of my day at Stanford, when I finally found the key piece to the elaborate puzzle of cognitive impairment.

I can't fully describe the mingling of satisfaction and optimism that I felt. All I can say is that for the next few hours the world had a golden glow to it, the way it does during a spectacular sunrise.

A new day was dawning.

A Case in Point

Added Stress Can Destroy the Balance of a Healthy Brain

C.B., fifty-four years old, had lived a life full of hard work and heavy demands. He was an important European industrialist, and many people had long depended upon him.

C.B. had never considered his life very stressful, however. And, by my definition, his life had not been excessively full of stress. My definition of stress—which I learned from Dr. Herbert Benson—is very simple: *Stress is feeling that your ability to perform is exceeded by the demands you must meet.*

A man of considerable ability, C.B. had always been confident that he could successfully handle the demands that were placed upon him. Therefore, he had always perceived these demands as challenges—not stressors—and he had faced them eagerly and happily. He had rarely felt the overwhelming, restless feeling of stress.

As handsome as a movie star, with sparkling blue eyes and a wide smile, he was sophisticated and wealthy. Educated in the finest European schools, he'd done postgraduate work at an Ivy League university and then had begun a meteoric rise through the ranks of industry. At fifty, he had become president of a very prominent company.

But then, two years later, he'd been named director of the largest company in his country. Shortly after that, his problems had begun.

It was at this point that I was brought in to consult with him. I was consulting in Europe, and a member of C.B.'s family was aware of my work. C.B.'s doctor had become unable to offer any substantive help to C.B., so I was asked for my input.

After intake testing, it became clear to me that C.B. had finally encountered a series of problems—all tied to his new job—that he didn't think he could solve. Thus for the first time in his career, he was perceiving his work as a stressor instead of a challenge.

This change in perception had taken a profound toll upon him. He no longer looked forward to going to work each day. He sometimes felt paralyzed by the monumental decisions he had to make. He had begun to avoid decisions that he felt unable to resolve. He often became frustrated and agitated. Frequently he felt nervous, and he often overreacted to minor annoyances.

He was exhibiting many of the classic symptoms of a man who was chronically experiencing the "stress-response" mechanism. The stress he was experiencing was affecting him both mentally and physically.

C.B. told me that he had two primary symptoms of cognitive dysfunction. The one that was most distressing to him was memory loss. He had many of the symptoms of age-associated memory impairment. Often he would grope for certain words, but would be unable to remember them. Also, details would sometimes fade from his mind. He had a classic case of "Swiss cheese" memory, in which his memory systems were mostly still intact, but his recall ability had many "holes" in it.

In addition to memory problems, he also had difficulty maintaining a high level of concentration throughout the day. He would frequently become mentally fatigued in late afternoon. Almost every afternoon his focus would slip, his mood would sour, and he would become irritable with the people around him.

His longtime associates, he said, were very aware of his mental and emotional changes. They said he was no longer acting like "himself."

In addition to his cognitive problems, he was also troubled by recent weight gain. Ever since he'd begun directing his country's largest corporation, he'd steadily packed on extra pounds. He did not feel as if he were eating a great deal more than usual, or exercising less. Nonetheless, his stomach and hips had begun to balloon.

The weight gain and emotional stress were contributing to another physical problem—severe lower-back pain. His back hurt almost constantly.

This pain was causing him further stress. Thus he was locked into a cycle of stress degeneration.

As I began to implement his brain longevity program, I performed a series of acupuncture treatments on him. These treatments were aimed at quelling his back pain. Soon the pain diminished, and he began to feel revitalized.

According to the Western interpretation, the acupuncture had relieved inflammation in his lumbar nerves, and he had been energized by the resulting relief from pain. According to the Eastern interpretation, I had balanced the "yang energy" in his kidney-adrenal area (which is where I had focused my treatments). Eastern practitioners believe that kidney yang energy is the primary source of overall vitality. The restoration of this vital force, according to the Eastern perspective, had not only energized him, but had also relieved his back pain. Both of these interpretations, I believe, are valid—and are not contradictory.

As C.B. began to participate in other aspects of his brain longevity program, he started to lose weight, and to experience improvements in cognitive function.

He received tremendous value from his program's emphasis on stress management. He finally recognized that, for the first time in his life, he often faced stressful situations. When he accepted the fact that stress had become an inescapable part of his life, he began to develop effective strategies for dealing with the stress. When he found himself in an "impossible" situation, he no longer tried to "do the impossible"; instead, he did what *was* possible, and tried hard not to worry about controlling what was beyond his control.

When worry did begin to get the best of him, he was generally able to calm down by doing simple relaxation techniques, and by quietly meditating for a few minutes.

After his back pain completely disappeared, he became more physically active. This activity also helped relieve his stress. In addition, it stimulated the release of energizing catecholamine neurotransmitters. His weight soon normalized.

He recovered from his memory problems relatively quickly. The speed of his recovery prompted me to believe that his memory problems had been primarily caused by neurotransmitter dysfunction—caused by cortisol—and not by the death of brain cells.

After C.B. became fully rejuvenated, he began functioning with the greatest efficiency and zest he'd ever experienced. He was grateful for my therapeutic help.

But I was also grateful to him, just as I am grateful to all of my patients who work hard to get better. As my patients recover, I always learn something new. From C.B. I learned that no matter how well a person deals with stress, there is always a threshold of stress that must not be exceeded, a "straw that breaks the camel's back."

For many years, C.B. had been able to maintain mental and physical equilibrium by balancing his work with his energy. But when he had taken on a job that tipped the balance, he had lost the optimal function of his brain and body.

From C.B., I learned an important lesson. All people must find their *own* balance. And they must *maintain* it.

3

How the
Program Works

As I flew home from Palo Alto—with the amazing information about cortisol still percolating in my brain—I began to develop a full-scale protocol for brain longevity.

I threw myself into this task heart and soul, and found it the most rewarding and exciting work of my life.

For months I focused the entirety of my intellect and spirit on this challenge. I pored through volumes of medical textbooks. I consulted with a number of researchers. I began following the latest trends in memory research and neurogeriatrics. I also intensified my study of complementary medicine, because I was convinced that Eastern medicine, with its emphasis on the integration of mind and body, offered special therapeutic insights into a physical disease that destroyed the mind.

Almost every day, pieces of the puzzle of cognitive dysfunction came together. Each new discovery filled me with joy. Because my pilgrimage into the world of brain aging was motivated by the desire to help others, and because it consumed every fiber of my intellect and emotions, it became, quite literally, a spiritual experience. I emerged from it, I believe, a more whole person.

I also emerged with a comprehensive, consolidated medical program for the treatment of age-associated memory impairment, for the prevention and delay of Alzheimer's disease, and for the creation of optimal mental function.

Even before I began applying this program clinically, I was confident that it would prove efficacious, because I had *already* achieved positive responses with various *individual* elements of the program. Putting all of these elements together, I was virtually certain, would synergistically increase the power of each individual element.

This presumption soon proved to be true. From its inception, my brain longevity program consistently elicited remarkable results—often even in "hopeless" cases.

The Four Basic Elements

I strove to create a program that would be characterized by simplicity and common sense, for a specific reason: This therapy would be a *lifestyle program*—not a "magic bullet" treatment—and would therefore be relatively more patient-managed than physician-managed. The program had to be something the average person could comprehend and coordinate. As a physician I could offer specific, individualized programs, and monitor the progress of each patient, but it was up to the patients themselves to direct the daily management of their programs.

This patient-managed approach was a practical necessity. I simply didn't have time to micromanage each patient's life. But this approach also fit perfectly with my philosophy of healing: Each patient is ultimately responsible for his or her own healing; all a doctor can do is inaugurate and monitor the process.

Thus I consolidated the brain longevity program into just four major areas: (1) *nutritional therapy* (including dietary therapy; supplementation with vitamins, minerals, and trace elements; and use of natural medicinal tonics); (2) *stress management* (including meditation and removal of lifestyle stressors); (3) *exercise therapy* (including aerobic exercise, mental exercise, and mind/body exercises), and (4) *pharmacology* (including administration of various cognitive-enhancement medications, and hormone-replacement therapy).

The underlying medical assumption behind this program was that stress was a primary cause of accelerated brain aging, because of the cortisol connection.

The program was designed, however, to be of therapeutic value *even if stress was not a major causative factor* of a particular patient's problem. Why? Because, first of all, no two patients are exactly alike. In one patient, stress might be a major cause of cognitive impairment, while, in another, it might be only a minor cause. Nonetheless, both patients may well have ended up with the same result: death of neurons, and a poorly functioning brain biochemistry. Therefore, both patients could benefit from an essentially similar course of treatment: one that "rescues" and restores neurons, and that optimizes the biochemistry of the brain.

This "nonspecific" clinical philosophy is also appropriate for many other degenerative diseases. I believe that virtually all degenerative diseases—including cancer, cardiovascular disease, and Alzheimer's—have *multiple* causes, and require a multimodality approach. Consider, for example, heart disease. In a given patient, heart disease may have been caused mostly by stress, mostly by bad diet, mostly by a genetic predisposition, or mostly by lack of exercise. Regardless of the primary cause, though, the patient will almost certainly benefit from a broad therapeutic regime that includes stress reduction, dietary modification, exercise, and pharmacology.

A weakness of the Western medical paradigm is its relentless quest for a one-to-one cause/effect relationship. Using deductivist logic—which is the driving force of modern science—Western practitioners too often try to reduce a patient's pathology to a single, isolated cause. Then they treat this pathology with a single, isolated modality. But this approach is simply not realistic when it's applied to complex biological organisms. It's almost like asking, "What does a human being need to survive—food or water?"

There is also another excellent reason to apply a broad-based therapeutic regime to patients with memory loss and cognitive impairment, regardless of the specific *cause* of the problem: Memory loss and cognitive impairment have a multitude of causes that have *nothing* to do with the effects of aging. I have found that many patients with symptoms similar to those of early-stage Alzheimer's or of age-associated memory-impairment, do not suffer from *either* of these maladies. Approximately 50 percent of all memory disorder patients actually suffer from a range of non-Alzheimer's problems, including depression, repeated minor strokes, toxic reactions to drugs, long-term effects of alcoholism, brain injury, chronic fatigue syndrome, and severe allergies.

Even though this array of problems has a wide variety of origins, most of them respond quite positively to my brain longevity programs. The reason, of course, is that my programs were not designed to have a specific *anti-disease* function, but, instead, to have a general *pro-health* function. The brain longevity programs provide an optimal biological milieu for the brain and the body, and therefore encourage activation of a panorama of self-healing powers.

Because of this overall positive effect, brain longevity programs help not just the brain, but also the body. The programs can help reverse such problems as high blood pressure and immune dysfunction, to name just two.

Within this philosophical framework, then, let's take a quick look at the four major aspects of my brain longevity programs. (I will explain each of these aspects more fully in later chapters.)

Nutritional Therapy and Brain Regeneration

Nutritional therapy, applied properly, can help repair damaged neurons, protect neurons and neurotransmitters from further damage, and improve day-to-day biochemical function in even a damaged brain.

In a healthy patient, dietary therapy and supplementation with specific nutrients and natural medicinal tonics can help create a virtual "super brain."

The single most important dietary rule for brain longevity is: "What's good for the heart is good for the head." It is vitally important for all brain longevity patients to optimize their blood circulation. Age-associated memory problems are often exacerbated by poor circulation. Neurons killed by cortisol and other negative factors almost always impede blood flow to healthy neurons, increasing memory loss and concentration problems. Also, vascular plaque caused by excessive dietary fat contributes to decreased blood flow to brain cells. The brain is critically dependent upon abundant blood flow, *because it requires about 25 percent of all blood pumped by the heart.* Therefore, any disruption of cerebral circulation has a profoundly negative effect upon the brain.

Furthermore, elevated blood pressure—often a direct result of a poor diet—is quite damaging to optimal cognitive function. In the brain, high blood pressure creates a subtle shunt effect, drawing blood away from where it is needed. This "anti–Robin Hood effect" disrupts memory and concentration.

Also, excessive dietary fat greatly increases free radical production, which causes billions of neurons to die.

Therefore, I recommend a commonsense, low-fat diet, high in complex carbohydrates, with adequate protein.

It is critical that this diet be "nutrient dense," delivering high amounts of key nutrients, while causing minimal stress upon the organs of digestion and assimilation.

A healthy diet also stabilizes blood sugar levels, a factor that is of critical importance to the brain. Low blood sugar significantly interferes with proper brain function, because blood sugar is the only source of fuel for the brain. Low blood sugar disrupts concentration and can biochemically prevent the brain from storing new memories.

Many of the people who are most prone to memory loss and concentration difficulty—because of chronic stress—are also prone to dietary deficiencies, for a simple reason: Stress increases nutritional needs. People under high stress require extra nutrients, just as athletes do. Frequently, however, they do not receive these nutrients, and substitute for this loss with caffeine, sugar, nicotine, and alcohol. These substances, in turn, not only damage neurons and neurotransmitters, but also decrease ability to deal successfully with stress, thus a degenerative spiral begins.

The Brain Longevity Diet is not severe or restrictive, but it is certainly different from the standard American diet, which consists of 35 to 40 percent fat, and includes an abundance of processed foods and refined sugars. I recommend a diet that revolves around whole grains, vegetables, non-animal protein, fruits, and an occasional serving of fish. In general, this diet is tailored to fit individual needs and preferences. Some people, for example, find it very difficult to abstain from eating meat. Often the diet is somewhat less flexible in the early days of a brain longevity program (to get brain regeneration off to a strong start).

An absolutely vital adjunct to nutritional therapy from dietary sources is concentrated nutrition in supplement form. Supplements I recommend include the antioxidant battery of vitamins A, C, and E; B-complex vitamins; choline-rich lecithin; and a trace mineral combination that includes magnesium. A newer antioxidant I have begun using is coenzyme Q-10, which has proven effective in protecting the brain.

Antioxidants are crucial, because they can protect neurons from the damaging effects of cortisol and other destructive elements. Antioxidants are known as "free radical scavengers," because they inhibit the free radical molecules (created by cortisol and other factors) that kill neurons from within. Other free radical scavengers include the minerals selenium, zinc, and chromium.

Some supplements also have direct positive influence on cognitive function. Vitamin C, for example, has a calming effect.

Magnesium also produces a calming effect; its deficiency is sometimes implicated in anxiety. Furthermore, people with so-called Type A personalities are prone to accelerated magnesium depletion. In one study, Type A people in a stressful situation excreted almost 100 percent more magnesium than a control group of Type B people.

Magnesium also plays an important role in keeping brain cells alive in that it minimizes the negative effects of reduced blood flow, and increases the ability of neurons to receive nutrients (by increasing cell membrane fluidity). Also, it helps prevent calcium buildup in brain cells—a phenomenon that frequently kills brain cells. Calcium buildup in brain cells is common in Alzheimer's patients. One study of Alzheimer's patients found that they had an abnormally high ratio of calcium to magnesium.

B vitamins are absolutely critical for proper neurological function. I recommend at least 50 mg daily of the entire B-complex series. Depletion of serum B vitamins typically causes memory loss, disorientation, lethargy, mood swings, and depression.

Choline is also of special importance, because it is the nutritional precursor, or "building block," of the neurotransmitter acetylcholine—the primary "carrier" of memory. Choline, found in lecithin, is also important in maintaining "brain plasticity"—the ability of the brain to find new thought "pathways" when old pathways are destroyed. Choline protects and restores the brain cell "branches" that reach out to other brain cells, to create memory pathways. Therefore, choline helps these branches—which are called *dendrites*—to make new connections for memories when old connections are broken. In one study, patients with memory loss experienced up to 50 percent improvement just from choline supplementation.

I have also noted tremendous benefit from several natural medicinal tonics—powerful nutritional substances that improve, or tonify, the function of various organs and systems. These include such nutrients as *Ginkgo biloba* and various other herbs from the Asian pharmacopeia, such as ginseng. Other natural medicinal tonics that are of particular benefit are phosphatidyl serine, phosphatidyl choline, and acetyl-L-carnitine.

Another nutritional tonic I often recommend is a "green juice" that includes such ingredients as blue-green algae, wheat grass, and spirulina. These products are the richest possible sources of partial proteins called peptides, which the brain converts to neuropeptides (such as the well-known beta endorphins).

Many of these natural medicinal tonics have dramatic effects upon cognitive function—almost like the effects of powerful pharmaceutical medicines rather than nutrients. For example, in a recent double-blind study of early-stage Alzheimer's patients, an herbal extract of *Ginkgo biloba* exhibited remarkable therapeutic properties. Patients were tested for cognitive function, memory, and concentration, and those taking *Ginkgo biloba* improved significantly in all categories over a one-month period.

As you can see, relatively simple nutritional changes can have a profound effect upon the function of the brain.

Stress Management and Brain Regeneration

It is critically important for people suffering from memory loss to reduce their stress levels. Continued stress creates further neurological damage.

In one of the crucial ironies of age-associated memory impairment, the more damage to the brain a person has suffered, the harder it is for him or her to "turn off" stress. The part of the brain that "shuts off" cortisol production—thereby reducing the detrimental effects of stress—commonly deteriorates with age. When this happens, the person reacts even more strongly to stress—and therefore suffers even more damage to the shut-off mechanism. Thus a deadly downward spiral occurs.

There are, however, a number of ways to reduce stress, and to reduce the body's *reaction* to stress, even in the presence of this unfortunate biological spiral.

Recently researchers have discovered several fascinating new things about the body's physical reaction to stress. One thing they have found is that the physical effects of stress are greatly magnified when people feel "out of control." Although is it currently in vogue to criticize people who are "control freaks," the fact is, we are *all* control freaks.

Another recent finding is that stress seems much worse when

no attempt has been made to prepare for it. Stress that comes as a surprise evokes a much greater physical stress response than stress that was predicted.

Still another recent discovery is that most of the negative physical impact of stress can be avoided if a person doesn't "hold it in." If one can "let go" of stress, it usually has a minimal physical impact.

It has also been demonstrated recently that the physical effects of stress can be greatly reduced if a person has a social support system—friends or family. In one interesting experiment, monkeys were subjected to a flashing light, followed by an electric shock. Soon they began to react to the flashing light with a copious secretion of cortisol. If a monkey had one companion, however, the cortisol secretion was markedly lower. And if a monkey had *five* companions, no cortisol secretion at all occurred.

Of course, some of these findings about stress merely reflect common sense. But that's good! If something makes sense to patients, they'll do it.

An even more commonsense approach to stress management—but one that can be extremely challenging—is to reduce the actual number of stressors in your life. In brain longevity programs, patients are urged to examine their lives and note the situations that cause them the most stress. In one of the self-tests in this book, you'll get some help in determining what causes you the greatest degree of stress. You'll also be given advice on how to refine your lifestyle to minimize exposure to stressors. Minimizing stressful events is like exercising—it's hard to do at first, but the more you do it, the easier it gets.

Another extremely powerful tool against stress is meditation. There are many forms of meditation, and you probably do some of them already, without even thinking about it. For example, you probably fall into a meditative state much of the time when you watch television. Research indicates that when people watch television, their brain waves tend to shift to what is called the alpha state, which is a meditative condition. This is why TV often has a hypnotic effect, like the effect of watching a fire. It's why people often watch TV "mindlessly," with little regard for the actual content of the program.

There are many ways to meditate, all of which evoke the physical effect called the "relaxation response," which is the exact opposite of the adrenal-driven "stress response." When you achieve the relaxation response, blood pressure decreases; alpha waves are elicited; oxygen consumption declines; cortisol output decreases, as does muscle tension; immunity is heightened; alertness is increased; and memory is potentiated. Also, blood flow to the brain is increased by up to 25 percent.

Further, if the relaxation response is elicited regularly, your body will remain much less *vulnerable* to the stress response, even when you are not meditating.

The most common forms of meditation are transcendental meditation and various forms of voluntary relaxation (including progressive muscle relaxation and "autogenic training"). Prayer is also a powerful form of meditation.

I also teach my brain longevity patients a very unique and special form of meditation called *naad yoga*. This is an ancient and highly effective form of Eastern meditation that I have adapted specifically for healing the brain and nervous system. I consider naad yoga, which employs the chanting of specific mantras, to be the most advanced form of meditation. For over five thousand years, Indian yogis have used naad yoga to achieve states of elevated focus, mental acuity, and well-being.

Using naad yoga as a neurological modality may seem futuristic to you. That's ironic, of course, considering how many millennia it has been employed for that specific purpose. Nonetheless, my clinical experience with it has confirmed my belief that it can be one of the most effective elements in a brain longevity program. I believe it strongly validates my theory that the most dynamic approach to modern healing comes from complementary medicine.

Any technique that can decrease a patient's stress is a valuable tool in a brain longevity program. Stress is a highly subjective experience, and no method of managing it should be dismissed.

Exercise Therapy and Brain Regeneration

In my clinical application of brain longevity programs, I have found that general aerobic exercise can produce great benefits neurologically. Mental exercise, as well as specific mind/body exercises, can also be of value.

Aerobic exercise has *direct* beneficial effects upon the brain and endocrine system. It increases blood flow to the brain, and even spurs growth of new brain cell "branches." It also has powerful *indirect* benefits. It physically protects the body against the stress response, and also "burns off" harmful stress hormones.

One of the most beneficial direct cognitive effects of exercise is to increase blood flow to the brain. Not only can this create an *immediate* improvement in your neurological function, but it can also help your brain to thrive over the course of your lifetime. Because about one-fourth of all the blood in the body is used by the brain, almost any exercise that increases blood flow will help the brain. In fact, the commonly mentioned phenomenon called "runner's high"—which is usually ascribed to the secretion of endorphins—is partially a result of increased blood flow.

Another direct benefit of exercise is that it causes the release of various neurological and endocrinological secretions, including *norepinephrine,* the stimulating brain chemical that acts as a neurotransmitter. Norepinephrine is one of the most important neurotransmitters in the laying down of new memories, and is especially important in moving memories from short-term to long-term storage. Norepinephrine is also extremely important in the maintenance of a good mood.

Exercise can also directly benefit your mood. Because exercise increases norepinephrine and also the production of endorphins, exercise often relieves depression. Depression is not only emotionally painful in itself, but is also extremely destructive to memory. It is one of the most common causes of memory loss (along with age-associated memory impairment, Alzheimer's, and multiple minor strokes). A number of studies have indicated, however, that exercise is unequivocally effective at dispelling depression. Often it is even more effective than traditional therapies, including psychological counseling.

Exercise is also an effective buffer against stress. People who exercise are not as vulnerable to the stress response as are sedentary people. For approximately four hours following exercise, people experience a "tranquilizer effect" that diminishes their physical responses to stress.

To best achieve the tranquilizer effect, a person needs to exercise for the right length of time. Too little exercise (less than half an hour) doesn't effectively evoke the tranquilizer effect; nor does too much exercise (over an hour). In one study of runners, those who best achieved the tranquilizer effect ran about twenty-four miles a week. Runners didn't achieve the effect nearly as effectively if they ran significantly less (fifteen miles a week), or significantly more (fifty-two miles a week).

Some researchers also think that it's a mistake to exercise too strenuously. These researchers say that extremely fast-paced, strenuous exercise keeps people from achieving the high levels of longevity and immunity that are enjoyed by more-moderate exercisers. These researchers theorize that strenuous exercise actually increases formation of free radical cells, through "oxygen toxicity." Too much oxygen, they say, increases the formation of free radicals.

Other researchers disagree with the theory; they say that the more strenuously you exercise, the healthier you get. Because this debate is still raging, I take a middle-of-the-road position. I advise patients generally not to exceed more than about 50 to 75 percent of their maximal aerobic capacity. Further, when patients do exercise very strenuously, I advise them to compensate for possible free radical formation by taking supplements that are free radical scavengers, such as vitamins C and E.

The eminent physician Andrew Weil, M.D., also espouses a moderate approach. In his excellent book *Spontaneous Healing*, he recommends that people make walking their primary form of exercise.

Exercise is especially beneficial for people who have a primarily physical reaction to stress, rather than a primarily psychological reaction. A "physical reactor" is someone who reacts to stress with headaches, stomachaches, pacing, and other physical manifestations of anxiety. For these people, exercise is helpful in relaxing tense muscles, which "lock in" stress.

Exercise is also helpful in dispersing excess adrenal hormones, including cortisol.

All brain longevity patients are advised to make exercise as playful as possible. This not only encourages regular participation, but also provides a psychological oasis of relaxation.

Even more effective than standard aerobic exercise, however, is use of a series of yogic mind/body exercises that I have adapted specifically for my brain longevity programs. The book you are now reading may be the only source of these exercises in Western literature.

My clinical experience strongly indicates that these unique mind/body exercises increase mental fitness. The mind/body exercises restore the brain's biochemical ability to lay down new memories, and to focus intensely for extended periods. They also stimulate access to existing "remote" memories of long-past events.

For most patients, I recommend four to five mind/body exercises, derived from a group of approximately forty ancient yogic exercises that were developed specifically to enhance brain power. I discovered these exercises in the course of my seventeen-year study of the physiology of yoga, during which I examined more than two thousand yogic exercises.

The exercises I recommend most often were chosen because of their power, and because of their relative ease. Each of them is part of a *kriya:* a sequence of specific movements linked to a breathing pattern, a posture, and a mantra. Each kriya also incorporates elements of meditation, which amplify the effectiveness of the exercises.

The primary purpose of the mind/body exercises is to drive nutrient-rich blood to the brain and to particular endocrine glands. This creates an immediate surge of mental energy, increasing concentration, short-term memory, and learning ability. Many patients say these exercises give them an immediate burst of energy. Aftereffects of this burst of energy can last up to twenty-four hours. Because of this prolonged effect, I recommend some of these exercises as part of a daily wake-up routine.

Personally, I love these mind/body exercises, which I've been doing for about fifteen years. I receive a profound sense of rejuvenation from them, and consider them not just an important contributor to my physical well-being, but also to my spiritual well-being.

Another extremely important form of exercise is mental exercise. A number of very recent experiments have proven that just *using* the brain actually increases its size and also increases the number of dendritic branches of brain cells.

One of the world's premiere brain researchers, Dr. Marian Diamond of the University of California, Berkeley, recently discovered in animal experiments that intellectual enrichment can even help rebuild the brain after it has suffered physical damage. She also discovered that if a brain is not regularly engaged in mental exercise, it can atrophy physically, just as an unused muscle can waste away. This atrophy appears to be most pronounced in an area of the brain closely associated with memory; atrophy of up to 25 percent was noted in that area.

I recommend, therefore, that all my brain longevity patients spend at least a couple of hours each day doing some form of mental exercise. This mental exercise can include anything from reading to playing cards to playing along with quiz shows on television.

Mental enrichment is especially valuable for older people, because the brain cells that are most influenced by it are the ones with the most dendritic branches; the mature brain cells of older adults.

Studies have shown that when people do engage in moderate pleasant forms of mental exercise, it increases not just their knowledge, but also the efficiency and power of their brains.

Pharmacology and Brain Regeneration

Because Alzheimer's is considered to be incurable, and because its cause is still being debated, it is common for physicians to take an essentially passive pharmacological approach to its treatment. Patients are sometimes given only sedatives, which make them more manageable for their caregivers. At other times, patients are administered single, isolated drugs, as their doctors search for a "magic bullet" to cure the disease. Currently the FDA has approved only two drugs, tacrine and Aricept, for Alzheimer's disease. Tacrine, which slightly decreases symptoms in some patients, has possible serious side effects. It helps only a limited number of people for a limited period of time. Aricept has fewer side effects.

Frequently, patients are treated by their doctors with drugs that are not specifically approved for Alzheimer's, but that have shown beneficial effects. Often, however, the dosage levels are too low to elicit significant positive responses. Also, it is rare for physicians to prescribe aggressive treatment during the very early stages of the disease, when it may be manifested as age-associated memory impairment. Many neurologists consider age-associated memory impairment to be benign, so they refuse to offer treatment for it.

It is extremely uncommon for physicians to prescribe medications aimed solely at achieving optimal mental function, in the absence of a diagnosable pathology.

I have achieved significant clinical successes, however, with an aggressive pharmacological approach, used as part of my multi-modality program. With this aggressive approach, I have been able to help not only patients who have frank Alzheimer's, but also those who suffer from age-associated memory impairment. I have also helped people who have no negative symptoms to optimize their cognitive function.

In some instances the drugs I prescribe, while FDA-approved, are not commonly used for Alzheimer's, or for age-associated memory impairment. Nonetheless, I have achieved some notable clinical successes with these medications. Also, some of the drugs I recommend are much more widely prescribed in Europe than in the United States. Of course, you should check with your physician before taking any medication.

Very frequently, I prescribe combinations of drugs, each of which has a different mechanism of action. One drug, for example, might improve neurotransmitter function, while another might improve overall brain metabolism.

Based upon my own clinical experience, as well as double-blind studies performed by many researchers, I have come to believe that Alzheimer's progression can be significantly retarded, in some cases, with vigorous pharmacological intervention. It also appears as if symptoms of early-stage age-associated memory impairment can often be completely eradicated with proper medication. Furthermore, certain medications help some patients without frank cognitive pathology to achieve very high levels of concentration, learning ability, and creativity.

Drugs that have contributed to some of my patients' most remarkable recoveries include deprenyl, piracetam, Hydergine, and various hormonal replacement agents (including pregnenolone and DHEA). Frequently these *nootropic* (mental enhancement) drugs are most effective when applied in careful combinations. All have no or very few documented side effects. Currently, nootropics are the fourth-largest class of pharmaceutical drugs on a worldwide basis.

One of the drugs that has proven to be of particular benefit in cognitive enhancement, and in slowing progression of Alzheimer's, is deprenyl. Because it is virtually free of side effects, I often prescribe it to patients with age-associated memory impairment and early Alzheimer's. Thus it may well prove to be an effective preventive agent for Alzheimer's. It is now being used successfully in Europe as a treatment for Alzheimer's and is presently being used for Alzheimer's in the U.S. in a large multi-center study. However, the drug is usually used in the United States as a treatment for Parkinson's disease.

Deprenyl has the ability to "rescue" damaged neurons before those neurons die. In one remarkable experiment, mice were injected with a neurotoxin, then treated with deprenyl, which rescued 69 percent of the toxified neurons. Without deprenyl, virtually all of those brain cells would have died.

Deprenyl is an "MAO-B inhibitor"—a drug that prevents the destruction of the neurotransmitter dopamine. It also increases the levels of other neurotransmitters. That's why it is of special value to early-stage memory-loss patients, whose primary problem is often neurotransmitter dysfunction, rather than dead brain cells. It can facilitate access to established "remote" memory of long-past events, which may be clouded only because of neuro-transmitter dysfunction. Deprenyl is also of significant value for concentration difficulties, which are often caused by neurotrans-mitter dysfunction.

Piracetam is a controversial drug because—alone among the pharmaceuticals that I recommend—it has not yet been approved by the FDA. It is, however, widely prescribed in Europe, where I frequently travel to study and consult, and is easily available in America through various "buyers' clubs." Piracetam, which has no known toxicity, has the unique and fascinating ability to enhance function of the brain's corpus callosum, the band of nerve fibers that coordinates the brain's left and right hemispheres. Piracetam is thus considered valuable in the stimulation of creativity, and is widely used by European writers and artists. In several European double-blind studies of Alzheimer's patients, use of the drug sig-nificantly increased scores on mental function tests.

Lucidril is a powerful free-radical scavenger that enjoys a rep-utation as an intelligence-booster. It has a demonstrated effect of increasing learning ability. Because of its aggressive action against free radicals, Lucidril, like deprenyl, has been shown in labora-tory experiments not only to increase mental function, but also to increase the lifespans of animals by an average of 30 percent.

Another drug I have used with extremely encouraging results is Hydergine. I owe my success with Hydergine in part to the fact that I commonly increase the drug's dosage from the standard American level of 3 mg daily to the common European level of 9 mg. Hydergine is very valuable in stabilizing the brain's glucose metabolism; therefore it helps protect against the glucose disrup-tion caused by excessive cortisol production. Because of this ef-fect on glucose metabolism, it enhances concentration as well as memory.

Another pharmaceutical approach that has achieved no-table clinical success in patients with memory loss is hormone-replacement therapy. Estrogen replacement in females is being studied as a therapeutic agent for memory disorders, apparently because, as shown in recent research at Rockefeller University, estrogen increases the number of neuronal connections in the brain's "memory center," the hippocampus.

Estrogen also increases the production of acetylcholine, the neurotransmitter that is vital for memory, and which is uniformly depressed in Alzheimer's patients.

The nootropic power of estrogen replacement therapy was recently demonstrated at New York's Mount Sinai Medical Center, where women with early-stage Alzheimer's showed marked improvement after just three weeks of estrogen-replacement therapy. Estrogen is also effective at improving mood, and increasing a subjective sense of well-being.

Some researchers, though, believe that estrogen administration may have some negative side effects, and may be related to the onset of some forms of cancer. I take a very cautious approach to estrogen-replacement therapy, as I do to the administration of *all* pharmaceutical drugs. I much prefer to administer a far safer hormonal replacement agent called *pregnenolone,* which can be converted by the body into estrogen, and also into other hormones. I believe it is even more effective than estrogen. Many of my patients have achieved dramatic improvements in cognitive function, and in mood stability, following administration of pregnenolone.

Another hormone that I commonly amplify is DHEA, which generally exists in the body in inverse proportion to cortisol. DHEA, the "mother steroid hormone," is one of the most accurate biomarkers of aging, because production of it decreases regularly during each year of life. In fact, at age eighty, people commonly produce only 10 to 20 percent of the levels of DHEA that they produced during their twenties. Furthermore, serum DHEA levels in Alzheimer's patients are almost always far lower than those of the general population of elderly people. Because the brain and endocrine system need DHEA for optimal function, even slightly lowered levels of DHEA can result in decreased ability to concentrate, and in diminished sex drive.

A common clinical mistake made by many physicians is to assume that if an older patient's DHEA levels are similar to those of most people in his or her age group, the levels are adequate. I believe, instead, that DHEA levels are optimal only if they approximate the levels of a person in his or her late twenties, before the decline of DHEA has begun.

Obviously, I believe that a great deal of good can come from proper use of pharmacology.

To me, though, one of the most impressive things about my brain longevity programs is that they do not rely extensively upon the use of pharmaceutical drugs. Instead, I try to stimulate the patient's body to heal itself.

I frequently recommend pharmaceutical agents more aggressively in the early phases of patients' programs. Then I gradually prescribe fewer drugs, in lower dosages, as my patients' bodies and minds regain their former powers.

Thus far, we have looked at the four major components of my brain longevity program. As you can see, my program is nothing more than, as I've stated, good science and good sense.

There is nothing very difficult about the program. If you're already pursuing a healthy lifestyle, you may not have to make many changes in the way you live.

If you *do* need to make substantial changes, though, don't be discouraged. You'll notice the benefits almost immediately. Your mind will become clearer and more powerful, your general mood will elevate, and you'll begin to glow with energy.

When all this happens, you'll be motivated to continue your program—and to achieve a lifetime of peak mental performance.

A Case in Point

Multi-Modality Brain Longevity Programs Are Synergistic

I met D.G., a forty-nine-year-old physician, at a medical conference that we were both attending. He was a remarkably intelligent man; besides being a family practitioner, he also held a degree in electrical engineering. In addition, he was very active in the business world, and was developing a series of medical care franchises. He was extremely successful. But D.G. was worried. He was certain that his keen intellect was starting to slip.

He sometimes had brief memory lapses, and frequently had episodes of anomia—the inability to remember names. Even so, his memory was still better than most people's.

His general cognitive function was also well above average. He was decisive, quick-witted, and good at creative problem-solving.

But he was not at all satisfied with being "above average" in his cognitive ability. For most of his life, his cognitive function had been virtually brilliant. He wanted to keep it that way.

For many years, D.G. had been able to grasp quickly the most arcane of abstract principles. He had been able to absorb medical knowledge at a lightning-swift pace, and then to transcend this knowledge by creating unique theories of his own. Over the course of a single day he had been able to swoop mentally from one discipline to another—from medicine to engineering to business. His mind had held a vast range of details, and he'd been able to retrieve them at will. He had also been able to concentrate with laser-sharp focus for hours at a time, without becoming mentally exhausted.

But in his mid-forties, when he became very active in business, he noticed that he was gradually losing some of his exceptional cognitive abilities. He didn't really enjoy the business world, and was stressed by his involvement in it. For him, practicing medicine was a challenge, but doing business was a burden. His heavy involvement with business made him feel as if his life were no longer his own. He felt as if he were just "observing" his life.

As he approached fifty, his wondrous mental abilities clearly began to fade. He began to mistrust his memory, and relied increasingly upon various systems of information retrieval. He could still focus sharply, but he told me that he no longer had the ability to "lose himself" in concentration for hours at a time.

In short, he still had a good brain—but it wasn't as good as it had been. And for him that wasn't good enough.

After the convention, he consulted me as a patient. Intake testing revealed that his cognitive function was quite normal; indeed, it was well above average. Even so, I placed him in the stage-two level in the Global Deterioration Scale. Why? Because he had reported a *subjective decline* in mental performance, and that is one of the indices of stage two. It's important to remember that if *you* think you're not as sharp as you once were, you probably aren't.

Part of the reason D.G. was so worried about his declining cognitive function was that he felt that he was already doing everything he could to stay mentally and physically healthy. He worked out religiously, and was obviously in excellent physical condition. His diet was good, his cholesterol level was acceptable, and his circulation was functioning adequately. On a regular basis, he took a number of brain nutrients: vitamins, minerals herbs, *Ginkgo biloba,* lecithin, and the brain-cell nutrient DMAE. Also, he told me that he tried his best to moderate his exposure to stressors, and that he didn't have any overtly negative habits, such as drinking too much alcohol. He was already taking the pharmaceutical hormone replacement substance DHEA.

It was very apparent that he was investing a significant amount of time and energy in being mentally fit. But somehow the various pieces of his "puzzle" of brain regeneration just weren't fitting together.

While we were still in his room, I showed him how to do one of the most powerful Eastern mind/body exercises. This exercise was designed to clear the mind, stimulate cognitive energy, and balance the endocrine system.

He did the exercise—and his life changed.

This single exercise had a profound effect upon him. It almost immediately relieved an onerous mental sensation that he said had been "smothering" him. For several years, he said—as his life had become increasingly stressful, owing to his business involvement—he had experienced a growing sense of mental dissociation. He described it as a "thin veil" that seemed to separate him from the world.

But when he did the exercise, he said, the veil lifted. His mind felt free, uncluttered, and energetic. He said the exercise helped to make him "feel like myself again."

He had me teach him more mind/body exercises. Each of them slightly increased his inner sense of wholeness and connection to the world—though none had quite the same dramatic effect as the first exercise.

When I next spoke to him, he had been doing the mind/body exercises for several months. They were still having a powerful effect upon his psyche.

Because the mind/body exercises were helping him to feel so much better, he redoubled his efforts in the other elements of his brain fitness program. He began eating a lighter, more vegetarian-oriented diet, and he started taking some additional supplements that I recommended (including a peptide-rich, green-algae type product). He also began meditating regularly. In addition, he cut back his involvement with his business affairs.

The net result was that his brain began to function as well as it ever had. He no longer experienced the feeling of chronic dissociation. His lapses of memory became quite rare. He again had the crystalline clarity of thought that allowed him to pluck details from the remote recesses of his brain. He also regained the ability to "lose himself" in thought, and to cruise from medicine to business without becoming confused.

He had restored the optimal function of his brain.

What struck me as most interesting about D.G. was that his improvement hadn't really begun until he'd engaged in a *complete* brain longevity program, including the mind/body exercises. All of his supplements, careful eating, and aerobic exercise had probably kept him from declining precipitously. But only a *complete* program had reversed his course—from one of degeneration to regeneration.

D.G.'s case strongly reinforced my belief that the various elements of a brain longevity program are synergistic. With a brain longevity program, one plus one equals three.

4

Results of
Three Patients

Because my brain longevity programs are empirically and rationally based, they are not "miraculous." But they do sometimes work miracles in the lives of patients.

So let's talk about patients. Let me tell you what happened to the first three patients whose stories I have told.

As you'll recall, one was a middle-aged Beltway attorney with moderate age-associated memory impairment. Another was a sixty-four-year-old woman who wanted to feel better mentally and emotionally, but who lacked the willpower to help herself. The third was an elderly former associate of President Kennedy, who was in the early stages of Alzheimer's.

All three responded remarkably well to the brain longevity programs I devised for them. This positive response was achieved even though each patient had very different symptoms, and a unique case history. The success of all three was possible, of course, because my brain longevity programs include a wide variety of therapeutic measures. They were all on relatively similar programs, but each appeared to respond primarily to different aspects of his or her program.

The Case of the Beltway Attorney

I expected the attorney's recovery to be the most expeditious of these three patients, because patients with the least neurological damage generally respond most quickly. They also usually achieve the most complete recovery.

This underscores an important point: Patients suffering from age-associated cognitive decline should address their problems *as early as possible,* because neurological degeneration is much easier to prevent than to repair.

Based on the attorney's medical history, I suspected that he might have a mild metabolic disorder that limited his ability to assimilate or transport B vitamins. This was indicated by some of his behavioral symptoms—particularly his daily downswings of mood and energy. B vitamins help provide mental endurance, stable physical energy, and a steady positive mood. The attorney lacked all three characteristics.

His fifteen-year-old daughter—whom I also began treating—had a similar lack of these same three attributes. She had enough intelligence to be a very good student, and enough physical ability to be an accomplished athlete, but she was performing poorly in school, and also in her favorite sport, swimming. Like her dad, she was ambitious to get as much as possible out of life, but she just didn't have the physical and mental stamina she needed to achieve her goals. She "ran out of gas" practically every afternoon, just as her father did. Because of the similarities in their symptomatologies, I suspected that they both might have a genetic predisposition to the same metabolic disorder.

At the outset of the attorney's therapy, I placed him on a high dosage of vitamin B complex. He took 100 mg of a multiple-B formula three times daily. This was, of course, a megadose of the nutrient. He responded almost immediately. His mood swings and irritability declined practically overnight, and within five days he was functioning better than he had in several months.

I had not reversed the apparent disorder that had inhibited his utilization of B vitamins, but I had effectively compensated for it by vastly increasing his intake of B vitamins.

Of course, the B vitamins were only one element of his brain longevity program, so it's possible that another aspect of his program was just as important in his recovery. There was no way to be certain, though. And, frankly, I was much more concerned about simply helping him than about ascertaining exactly *how* I was helping him.

The other aspects of his program included dietary therapy, stress management, cardiovascular exercises, mind/body exercises, and administration of natural medicinal tonics.

He responded so well to the naturalistic aspects of the program that I did not prescribe any pharmaceutical medication for him. As I've mentioned, when possible, I prefer not to use prescription medications. My therapeutic goal for most patients is to encourage their bodies, through enhanced nutrition, stress management, and exercise, to provide the primary impetus for healing.

The attorney had to make only minor modifications to his diet. He had already been eating a healthy, well-balanced diet. I simply recommended he eat less red meat and more of a few high-protein, nutrient-dense, nonmeat foodstuffs.

In addition to a wide range of vitamins and minerals, his nutritional program also included regular ingestion of a number of natural medicinal tonics, including *Ginkgo biloba;* a high-quality Chinese ginseng product, *Ching Chun Bao;* a full-spectrum "green-juice" product; and high dosages of vitamin C (up to 7 grams daily).

According to the Western interpretation of nutritional therapy, these medications provided the optimal biochemical milieu for his cognitive function. According to the Eastern interpretation, these medications "tonified" his basic life energy (*chi*), making it "hard" instead of "soft," and bringing it "up" to his brain. Both interpretations, I think, are as accurate as they are different.

Stress reduction was also an important part of his program, because he was badly entangled in the stress/degeneration downward spiral: The more his mental powers declined, the more stressed out he became; and the more stressed out he became, the more his mental powers declined. For years he had compensated for his gradual cognitive degeneration by working longer hours and pushing himself harder. Unfortunately, this had caused him to chronically oversecrete cortisol, which had exacerbated his mental and emotional problems.

There was also clinical evidence that he had begun to suffer from the decline of his ability to biochemically "turn off" the cortisol-producing stress response. This phenomenon can make it very difficult for people to escape the downward spiral of brain degeneration.

To combat his stress, he embarked upon a regular regimen of meditation. Although he was a hidebound rationalist, he was eager to try any proven stress-management technique. In fact, he told me, he had for many years been casually performing various forms of meditation—without labeling his efforts as such. As far as he was concerned, he had simply been "trying to relax" and to "turn off my worries."

When he began a concerted, consistent program of meditation, however, he quickly enhanced his ability to deal with stress. By employing meditative practices similar to the "relaxation response," he began to have a less pronounced physical response to stressors. He became less of a "hot reactor" to troublesome situations, and his blood pressure lowered.

Soon he became much less prone to make poorly reasoned decisions during periods of elevated stress.

In Western terms, he had learned to better control his physical stress response. In Eastern parlance, he had learned to shift his focus from the finite to the infinite, and had thereby become less vulnerable to the vicissitudes of the material, temporal world.

By both definitions, he was a much happier man.

In coordination with his meditation, he also began doing a series of mind/body exercises. He meditated at the same time he did the exercises, and this synergistically increased the power of both modalities. Combining mind/body exercises and meditation has a fascinating physical effect, in that it simultaneously enhances both alertness and relaxation. This condition is not only pleasant, but also facilitates physical healing.

The attorney's mind/body exercises included the "basic spinal energy series," which involves about thirty minutes of breathing, movement, and meditation. It does not require difficult yogic positions—the so-called "pretzel exercises." Instead, it's composed of simple exercises that flex the spine. The flexing exercises work sequentially from the lower spine (where a substantial amount of tension is stored) to the middle parts of the spine, then to the neck, and finally to the head.

From the Western perspective, this exercise releases muscular tension in the lumbar plexus, the solar plexus, and the cervical muscles, where "locked-in" stress impinges upon breathing and nerve conduction. It also releases stimulating catecholamine neurotransmitters, which enhance cognitive function. It increases oxygen delivery to the brain, and aids neurological glucose metabolism. It also stimulates circulation of cerebrospinal fluid from the spinal canal to the brain.

From the Eastern standpoint, the exercise channels basic life energy from the lower energy centers, or *chakras,* to the highest physical energy centers, which are in the brain. Then, according to Eastern thought, this energy is directed from the brain to the cosmos, linking the individual's energy to the energy of the universe.

From both Eastern and Western perspectives, this spinal energy series creates greater flexibility. In the Eastern medical tradition, however, flexibility is relatively more prized than it is in the West. In fact, many Eastern practitioners measure aging in terms not so much of chronology as of flexibility. I don't completely agree with this measurement of aging, but I think it offers a valuable metaphor: Flexibility—in life, as well as in muscles—helps us retain our youthfulness. If we can learn to "bend without breaking," we will be healthier and happier, and feel more youthful.

The attorney responded quite positively to these exercises. When he did not have time to perform them, he experienced a noticeable decline in his overall mental energy. Virtually every time he did perform them, he received a burst of cognitive energy.

I doubt that the attorney felt that these exercises had enabled him to tap into the "power of the universe." According to *his* belief system, he had simply tapped into the power of his own body. But it made no difference which interpretation he employed; the end result was the same.

After five weeks on his program, he had an experience that showed him how much he had progressed. In an important meeting with his associates and a client, he felt extraordinarily focused and mentally fresh. He experienced almost none of the stress or mental lapses that had recently hampered him in these situations. He told me that he "controlled the meeting," and that he surprised and impressed his colleagues with his new mental vigor.

After a year on the program, the attorney was a profoundly different man. He no longer experienced the mental lassitude that had once clamped down on him almost every afternoon. His mind stayed clear and focused throughout the day, and his mood swings were completely gone. He was a much more potent force at work, and got along with his family better. He was no longer frequently irritable with his wife and kids.

Also, without employing any kind of mnemonic device or memory gimmick, his memory had become as powerful as it was during his childhood. He had excellent recall of important information, and he could easily remember minor events that he had not consciously consolidated into his memory—such as where he'd put his car keys. He had developed the proper brain biochemistry needed to lay down new memories, and to retrieve existing memories efficiently.

The attorney told me that he felt he had been "reborn." Of course, he hadn't been reborn. His brain had merely been revitalized.

Three years later, when I was in Washington to speak at a medical conference, we met again. He looked ten years younger.

Clearly, he was on a course of regeneration.

The Case of the Woman with No Willpower

As I mentioned, the attorney's recovery was quicker than that of the sixty-four-year-old woman whose willpower had been sapped. She responded more slowly because she had suffered more neurological damage, and also because she was not as conscientious as the attorney about adhering to her program.

For example, she was reluctant to make significant changes in her diet. While she was consulting with me in Tucson, during the first week of her program, she should have been maximizing her dietary therapy, because the earliest stages of a brain longevity program generally require the most rigorous participation. I advised her to switch temporarily to a vegetarian diet, in order to reduce her serum cholesterol and thereby increase her cerebral blood flow, but she kept eating a relatively high-fat diet. She did want to improve her cognitive function, but she simply was not a very disciplined person.

Similarly, she was reluctant to engage wholeheartedly in any form of exercise. At the beginning of her program, she half-heartedly performed the mind/body exercises, but derived only a modest benefit from them.

Because she had significant cognitive decline, with accompanying endocrinological dysfunction, you'd think she would have been extremely motivated to improve her condition. Unfortunately, though, she was in a catch-22: Her physical problems had virtually destroyed her willpower, but to solve her physical problems, she desperately needed the power of her will.

To intervene in this self-perpetuating spiral of decline, I prescribed two powerful pharmaceutical medications, deprenyl and DHEA. I believed that these medications would help revive her willpower.

Deprenyl, which was developed about thirty years ago as an antidepressant, stimulates the brain to produce more of the neurotransmitter *dopamine*. Extreme dopamine depletion causes Parkinson's disease, and moderate depletion causes depression, lethargy, cognitive dysfunction, and decreased sex drive.

Dopamine is an *adrenergic,* or energizing, neurotransmitter, and a lack of it can cause an almost paralyzing sense of torpor and apathy.

Deprenyl, however, restores dopamine to its proper levels. It helps repair damaged brain cells, and stimulates learning ability, strength, and mobility. In animal tests, it has increased lifespan by up to 40 percent. In human tests, it has improved memory, concentration, and language ability. The sixty-four-year-old woman's response to deprenyl was swift and encouraging. She showed renewed vigor and energy.

Her reaction to the other pharmaceutical medication, DHEA, was just as positive. DHEA is a form of a steroid hormone that commonly declines with age. Because it acts as a so-called neuroprotective growth factor in the nervous system, DHEA also shields brain cells from metabolic damage. A shortage of DHEA often results in memory loss. In fact, DHEA content in the brain peaks at about age twenty-five to thirty—the same approximate age when memory powers are at their height.

DHEA, however, generally exists in an inverse proportion to levels of cortisol, because the two compounds are both used in similar biochemical processes. Thus, as cortisol increases, DHEA declines.

When I prescribe DHEA, I administer dosages that return blood levels to those of a person of about twenty-five to thirty years of age. When DHEA is restored to this level, it commonly elicits a "re-youthing" effect, characterized by enhanced memory, increased sex drive, greater mobility in the joints, increased energy, and improved concentration.

When the woman with weakened willpower first consulted with me, her energy level was so depleted that she literally had to prop her hand under her chin to hold up her head. She'd had a hard time focusing on what I was telling her, and showed little enthusiasm. Early in her therapy, I tried to give her "pep talks," but she barely seemed to hear them.

In addition, when I first met her, her skin was puffy and pasty white. Chronic stress, which she'd endured for years, releases an antidiuretic hormone, which was probably causing her to retain water. Her sallow complexion, I presumed, was primarily a result of poor circulation to her extremities, including her head and face.

Administration of deprenyl and DHEA, however, quickly brought an end to these most obvious *physical* manifestations of her decline. In less than a month, her cheeks began to glow with the ruddy hint of improved circulation, and her face lost its bloat. She no longer had to hold up her head with her hand. Instead, she began to look at me straight on, head high, with a far more animated expression.

Her "aura" brightened and sharpened. A practitioner of traditional Chinese medicine would have said that her *chi* had become much more concentrated, and that it was "circulating" better.

Her mood and mental outlook also improved dramatically. Her depression lifted, and her mental focus became much more acute.

Within a couple of months her short-term memory improved significantly. It appeared as if the root cause of her memory problems had been a mixture of depression and attention deficit disorder. This often creates a syndrome that mimics severe memory disorder. People with this problem are simply unable to focus long enough to lay down new memories.

The DHEA and the deprenyl had helped to alleviate her depression, and to improve her ability to concentrate. Both medications had also given her a great deal more energy.

As her energy returned, so did her willpower. As I had suspected, she did not lack the *desire* to improve her situation; she had merely lacked the vital energy necessary to implement her desires.

With the return of her willpower, she began to participate much more vigorously in her brain longevity program. She improved her diet, and began to consistently use natural medicinal tonics, such as *Ginkgo biloba*. She gradually replaced the pharmaceutical medications she was taking with these natural medicinal tonics. She requested that I reduce her dosage of deprenyl, because as her natural energy returned, the deprenyl began to make her feel overstimulated.

In less than a year she had achieved a remarkable recovery. She had become vivacious and astute, and had recaptured the "substance" of her life: the particular perspective and style that made her unique. She started an exciting new romantic relationship, and began a challenging schedule of work with at-risk teenagers.

Her life, once again, became her own.

To me, this woman's recovery illustrates an important point: Often a new, improved attitude requires a new, improved biochemistry. It's currently very much in vogue to believe that a positive attitude can spur miraculous physical healing. Often that can be true. But, too often, practitioners of this approach carry it to an illogical extreme. They claim that a positive attitude is *always* the first step to physical healing. Sometimes *physical healing is the first step to a positive attitude.*

Attitude and biochemistry create each other. I believe that doctors and patients should be very pragmatic and flexible about their philosophies of healing. They should not become "addicted" to any limited, isolated philosophy, but should accept healing wherever they find it.

The Case of JFK's Aide

Now I'll tell you about the patient whose response warmed my heart the most. It was the elderly gentleman who had once advised John F. Kennedy. He was such a fighter! And his struggle was all uphill.

When he came to see me, he was reportedly already in approximately stage three of Alzheimer's. His doctor's prognosis, he said, was that he would decline precipitously over the next seven to eight years, losing virtually his entire identity, as Alzheimer's destroyed his brain.

During our initial consultation, he listened intently to my

recommendations, even though his powers of concentration had diminished.

Then, however, an unexpected incident occurred. His daughter, who was a nursing student, voiced concern about the complementary medicine aspects of my therapeutic protocol. As a student of conventional Western medicine, she was skeptical about the healing power of such modalities as nutritional therapy or naturalistic medications.

She urged her father to return to the therapy of his primary physician.

The elderly man did not have the heart to oppose his daughter's wishes, so he discontinued our consultations.

Some months later, however, I contacted him, to see how he was doing. He sounded better! On his own, working with his son—who was much more receptive to my medical philosophies—he had begun to follow a brain longevity program that was very similar to what I had proposed for him.

He had modified his diet considerably, limiting his intake of high-fat, circulation-impeding foods. He was eating a nutrient-dense diet, rich in protein and complex carbohydrates. It was, essentially, a "health food" diet.

In addition, he was supplementing his diet with several important natural medicinal tonics, including ginseng and *Ginkgo biloba*. He was also taking high amounts of the important memory-enhancing nutrient lecithin, which, as noted earlier, is the nutritional precursor of the neurotransmitter acetylcholine, the primary chemical carrier of memory.

He was getting some exercise, staying mentally active, and trying to keep his stress under control.

His daughter, he said, was still hesitant about him trying complementary medicine, so he preferred to continue his own self-managed program. I respected this wish, since it would have been harmful to create discord within the family.

Besides, the man's son was already helping him implement a comprehensive, coordinated brain longevity program. The son was a principal in one of the most successful American startup companies of the 1980s, and was quite capable of guiding his father's program.

About a year and a half after my first consultation with the elderly man, I got in touch with him again, and was delighted with his condition. He was still in considerably better mental and physical health than he'd been when I'd first met him. And he was still enthusiastically participating in his brain longevity program.

Theoretically, by this time, he should have declined further. By standard medical reckoning, he should have been approaching a later state of Alzheimer's in which short-term memory would be decimated, and long-term memories would increasingly disappear. However, he had not only halted progression of the disease, but actually improved.

It's difficult to predict whether he will be able to live the rest of his life without further decline. Nonetheless, it does appear very possible that he can at least slow the progression of his Alzheimer's. And that, of course, is of primary importance, because if he can live his full life before Alzheimer's destroys his mind, he will have effectively "beaten" the disease.

This man's courageous fight against Alzheimer's taught me an important lesson about brain longevity programs: They can be effective even in the absence of a physician's vigilance.

After all, these are *lifestyle programs,* designed to be implemented by the patients themselves.

With enough motivation, and sufficient knowledge, virtually anyone can take control of the "care and feeding" of his or her own brain, with wonderfully positive results.

Already, we're at the end of Part One. By now, you have a full introduction to brain longevity. You know the fundamentals of my program.

In the next chapter—which begins Part Two—you'll start to learn what you will need to know to begin your *own* brain longevity program: the five basic principles of brain longevity. In the rest of Part Two, you'll learn how the brain works, how memories are formed, and why the brain generally deteriorates over time.

Then, in Part Three, you'll learn exactly *how you can achieve brain longevity.*

A Case in Point

It's Never Too Early and It's Never Too Late

M.B. was the daughter of the Beltway attorney. When I first talked to her, this girl, who was in her early teens, was struggling to excel in school, and to achieve excellence in her favorite sport, swimming. But she was constantly falling short of her goals. Like her father, she often had considerable lapses in her mental energy, especially in the late afternoon. When these downswings hit, she couldn't concentrate well, and she couldn't muster the energy to swim well.

Unfortunately, she was so young that she was beginning to believe that her problems were an innate aspect of her personality. She just couldn't imagine life without them. As a result, she was starting to see herself as a mediocre student and a poor athlete. She just didn't see herself as a winner.

The brain longevity program I placed her on was similar to her father's. With his help and encouragement, she began to conscientiously follow her program.

M.B.'s response was fast and exciting. She completely overcame her periodic mental lassitude. Her grades improved dramatically, and so did her performance as a swimmer.

In a matter of months, she had an entirely new self-image. She saw herself, quite simply, as a winner. Because she was one.

Luckily, M.B. had begun her brain longevity program early in life.

Now I'll tell you about a patient who began her program very late in life.

P.L. was the mother of the female patient who had weak willpower. After this weak-willed patient began to respond to her program, she became so enthusiastic about it that she sent her mother to see me.

P.L. was ninety-one years old, and was on the verge of entering a nursing home. She had a debilitating degree of cognitive dysfunction. She often "blanked out" in the middle of a sentence, and forgot what she was talking about. She also had begun to be very absentminded about little things around the house, like leaving her stove on. This kind of minor oversight can be dangerous to an elderly person living alone. Both she and her daughter had decided that she needed an assisted-care living situation. But neither of them wanted it.

One of the first things I did for this ninety-one-year-old woman was to place her on the medication called pregnenolone. Pregnenolone is a precursor to several hormones, including the hormone DHEA (which had helped the elderly woman's daughter considerably). I could have prescribed DHEA to the ninety-one-year-old woman, but very elderly people, in my clinical practice, have responded better to pregnenolone than to DHEA.

The elderly woman responded wonderfully well. The medication powerfully stimulated her cognitive function, and her forgetfulness disappeared.

She soon began taking deprenyl, which improved her mental function even more.

Within a few months she had begun to do active volunteer work. She held a Ph.D. in psychology, and was soon leading workshops at her church.

She became such a "star patient" of mine that she has been interviewed in television news segments about my work, and has been videotaped while leading her workshops.

What's my point with these two patients? The obvious: It's never too early, and never too late, to begin a program of brain longevity.

Optimal mental function—*at any age*—is one of the most precious experiences that any person can enjoy.

PART TWO

How the Brain Works

5

The Five Principles
of Brain Longevity

Come! Come with me, and we'll travel together on one of the most fascinating journeys of your life: a journey deep into the core of your own brain. So *much* is there—far more than you now know. Your brain holds a rich vault of knowledge and wisdom that, at this moment, may be partially inaccessible to you—because your memory and cognitive powers may be starved, battered, and underdeveloped.

But that wealth of understanding is definitely there, very much alive, physically encoded—virtually immortal—waiting for you to reach it.

When you do reach it, you will probably feel like a new person. You will no longer feel as you do now—like your old self. But you won't be a *new* self. You'll be your *real* self—the self that has been within you since the day you were born. That self has been beaten and bruised by stress, exhaustion, neurological toxins, and your own fear and anger. Nonetheless, after all of this punishment, it's still there, waiting.

You've probably already glimpsed your own rich vein of awareness—your real self—in fleeting moments of total lucidity. Those moments probably seemed almost mystical to you when you experienced them, because they were so powerful and so unusual.

But there is really nothing mystical about feeling like your real self. To me, the greater mystery is why we humans spend so much of our lives shrouded in a fog of ignorance about the one subject we should understand best: ourselves.

Perhaps it was as a child that you sometimes felt the full power of your mind—because children often possess wondrous cognitive strengths that are eventually weakened by the ravages of time and by the struggle to survive and succeed. One in every ten children, for example, has the amazing capacity for eidetic, or photographic, memory—a gift that carries over into adulthood in only about 10 percent of those born with it. Further, the only people who can commonly learn to speak a new language without an accent are kids eighteen or younger.

Another time that you may have experienced the full potential of your mind might have been during a moment of meditation—either during a formal session of yogic meditation, or during a spontaneous meditative experience, such as while watching a hypnotically lovely sunset, when heaven and earth merge. During these moments, your brain may have surged with the power of *theta waves*—bioelectric currents that afford near-transcendent powers of perception.

You may also have experienced the full miracle of your mind during a particularly momentous challenge. Perhaps this happened during a professional crisis, or maybe while you were participating in an athletic event that was important to you. You probably prepared unstintingly for this challenge, visualized your success, focused the full force of your being on it, dispelled your fears and doubts, and then sailed through the challenge with crystalline clarity of mind and a perfect concert of intellect and emotion. During that situation, time may have "stopped" for you. If you've ever experienced this—even once—you may sometimes find yourself daydreaming nostalgically about it, and savoring not its triumphant outcome, but the *feeling* you had while achieving the victory.

If you've had any of these experiences, then you already know there's a vast storehouse of strength and understanding within you. What you need now is *access* to that storehouse. As you begin to apply the principles of brain longevity, you will start to have *daily* access to elevated cognitive function and inner awareness. With effort and application, you will begin to experience moments of full brain power virtually every day. Such periods of peak mental experience may be relatively long in duration, or relatively short—but their length will not matter to you, because during them you will experience an inspiring sense of timelessness.

When your day ends, it will be those periods of elevated cognitive power that will stand out as times when you enjoyed your greatest abilities to solve problems and make decisions. During such times, your memory will be as sharp and clear as it was during your childhood.

Additionally, each day that you participate in your brain longevity program, you will ensure many *future* days of enhanced mental power. Just as there is a biological degenerative spiral that haunts all living creatures, there is also a regenerative upward spiral that intelligent beings can tap into.

Success builds on success. Strength builds on strength.

It is now time for you to start building.

It's time for you to begin applying the principles of brain longevity to your own life.

You will be guided by five primary principles, the keys that will unlock the door to your elevated cognitive power.

1. Your Brain Is "Flesh and Blood"

Every piece of knowledge you possess, and every memory you've ever had, exists as a *physical* entity. If there were a powerful enough microscope, you would be able to *see* your thoughts and memories. You would see biochemical structures, alterations in your cells' DNA codes, and bioelectric currents of energy.

Because your mind, memory, and thoughts are "flesh and blood," they are vulnerable to physical abuses. Obviously, you can damage your brain with chemical substances such as alcohol and mind-altering drugs. Less obviously, you can also damage it with stress, poor nutrition, lack of physical and mental exercise, and various toxins.

You can also, however, *protect and repair* your brain with a wide variety of physical, biochemical approaches. Throughout this book, I will offer you a panoply of simple but highly effective physical measures that you can take to improve your cognitive function and memory.

I guarantee you that these *physical methods* of improving your memory will be more beneficial to you than learning a number of mnemonic devices and memory tricks. Although the memory gimmicks that you can learn in other books may indeed help you occasionally to "jog" your memory, they're essentially designed to make the most of a poor memory. My goal is to help you *physically change* your poor memory into a good memory.

It may seem odd to conceive of your thoughts and memories as being made of flesh and blood, but they are. One of the most dramatic illustrations of the physical existence of memories comes from experiments done with a primitive type of worm called planaria. In a fascinating experiment, scientists kept a group of planaria in a dark box, then flashed a light at them. Each time they flashed the light, they administered an electric shock to the worms. The worms gradually learned to roll into a ball when they saw the flash of light, because they anticipated a shock. Then the scientists ground up these worms and fed them to a new group of worms. A light was flashed at the new group of worms. The worms rolled into balls! They had apparently "learned" by "eating a memory."

This experiment illustrates the physical existence of the type of memory commonly referred to as "instinct." We were all born with many innate instinctual "memories." Those instincts are just as much a part of our genetic coding as the color of our eyes.

From a therapeutic perspective, it's profoundly significant that the mind and memory are physical entities. It means, of course, that we can intervene in the mind and memory on a physical level. We can put "matter over mind." And we can also put "mind over matter."

2. The Powers of Your Brain Are Virtually Limitless

Your brain is the most complex and capable entity in the universe, far more chemically intricate and variegated than any star, and vastly more capable of fact storage and random information access than the world's most sophisticated computer. In fact, the brain is so complex that mankind will, in all probability, never fully understand it. It's been said that if the brain were simple enough to be understood, we would be so simple that we couldn't.

As incredibly powerful as our brains are, their full capacity remains untapped. Until the 1980s it was believed that people used only parts of their brains. But that's not true. Recent technological breakthroughs, such as advanced imaging techniques, have shown that we do, indeed, use all of our brains. However, we do not use them with peak efficiency.

Many of my patients on brain longevity programs, though, have increased their brain's efficiency. They have remarked that they can now "think faster" and "soak up information better."

Another relatively common reaction among brain longevity patients is that they can better perceive and remember the *full range* of their environments—the sights and sounds, smells and textures of their daily experiences.

Part of these patients' enhanced perceptual abilities, I believe, stems from their generally heightened levels of relaxation. All brain longevity patients devise strategies that help them to relax, because this helps them to avoid the brain-damaging effects of cortisol. Their increased sense of calm lends itself psychologically to a fuller awareness of daily life.

But there is an even more fascinating explanation about why many of my patients are better able to "take in" more of the world around them: in effect, they develop better brains. Most of them experience a notable rejuvenation of the important part of the brain called the limbic system. The limbic system is the area of the brain that is most responsible for emotion, and for memory, and it is also the part of the brain that appears to be most damaged by cortisol. The limbic rejuvenation my patients experience offers them tremendous advantages. It certainly improves their memories. It also enhances their sense of emotional well-being.

Limbic rejuvenation also appears to increase slightly some patients' capacity for an ability called *synesthesia,* one of the most interesting phenomena known to neurology.

Synesthesia is, basically, the blending and coordinating of the senses. You probably enjoy a mild degree of synesthesia yourself, because a modest degree of it is very common. For example, your senses of taste and smell are closely linked. If something smells bad to you, it probably tastes bad, too. Also, for most people, high-pitched sounds evoke images of bright colors, and low-pitched sounds suggest dark colors.

But people with profound synesthesia—which occurs in one out of every 100,000 people—are able to literally "see" sounds and "taste" colors. This may sound like a disturbing trait—akin to schizophrenic hallucination—but it is not a pathological condition, and causes no distress to the otherwise normal people who experience it. In fact, people with synesthesia usually love the condition, because it offers them such a rich and sensual experience of the world. When a person's synesthesia fades, as it sometimes does, he or she usually regrets the loss very deeply.

Synesthesia tends to be more heightened in creative people. The writer Vladimir Nabokov had "colored hearing," and the painter Georgia O'Keeffe was able to "see" music. Jerry Garcia once noted that "musical notes, for me, have shape, and form, and color."

One of the unique advantages of elevated synesthesia is that it offers incredible powers of memory. For example, one famous synesthete, a Russian named Shereshevskii (who was studied by the prominent psychologist A. R. Luria), was able to remember lists of hundreds of numbers, poetry in languages he did not know, and seemingly endless strings of letters. He could repeat this material backward, and could remember it for many years. In fact, his greatest problem was finding a way to *forget* information. (He solved the problem by imagining himself writing facts on a blackboard, and then erasing the board.)

No one is sure why synesthesia aids memory. It probably does, though, simply because it allows people to make *more associations* with each memory—in much the same way that looking at a number, then saying it out loud, helps you remember it. For example, you would be more apt to remember a walk on a freezing cold, gorgeous day, with beautiful music playing, than you would a walk on a nondescript day—because each of your senses would be experiencing something memorable.

None of my patients has achieved profound synesthesia, nor do any aspire to. But many have "fine-tuned" their mental "instruments," and this has enabled them to experience their surroundings in a way that is richer, more textured, more fulfilling—and more memorable.

Even people who have no accentuated degree of synesthesia, however, can still have virtually perfect memories. One noted memory expert, Professor A. C. Aitken of Edinburgh University, could perform almost supernatural feats of memory. Once he memorized a list of twenty-five words, along with a passage of literature; then, *twenty-seven years later,* he was able to repeat the list, in order, and to recite the passage without error.

This level of recall undoubtedly seems utterly beyond your own capability. Astonishingly, it probably is not. If an electrode were placed directly upon the temporal lobe of your brain (which holds most long-term memory), you would probably be able to recall past events with almost "photographic" perfection. This procedure has been performed a number of times, and it almost always evokes the same effect: an "experiential response" that feels almost exactly like reliving the actual event. People who have done this are able to remember verbatim conversations and minute details about long-since "forgotten" episodes.

In short, most of what once went into your long-term memory is probably still there, waiting for you to develop the power to retrieve it.

Even if you do not have a good memory now, you almost certainly have a much greater potential than you realize for developing a sharp memory. For example, in the last years of his life, the philosopher William James became concerned about his memory. So, in a powerful display of will, he sat down and memorized all of John Milton's twelve-volume *Paradise Lost*. It took one month, and was, he said, a "supremely inspirational" experience.

But you do not have to be a "great thinker" to develop an extraordinary memory. Napoleon could greet many thousands of his soldiers by name. The businessman Charles Schwab knew the names of all eight thousand of his employees. The politician James Farley was able to call about fifty thousand people by their first names. General George Marshal was able to recall virtually every single event of World War II. The conductor Arturo Toscanini could remember every note of every instrument for one hundred operas and two hundred and fifty symphonies.

Make no mistake—the powers of the mind and memory are virtually limitless.

Regardless of your current level of power, your brain can be physically enabled to operate with much greater efficiency.

3. Your Brain Is Capable of Infinite Joy and Pleasure

At this point in your life, if you have been laboring for years to be as productive as possible, you may have almost forgotten how to find daily joy and pleasure in life. You may even have damaged your biological ability to feel pleasure.

But this ability can be recaptured.

And—if you want to achieve your peak intellectual power—it *should* be recaptured. One of the best things you can do to regenerate your full intellectual power is to learn once again to take as much pleasure as possible from life, as you did when you were a child, with a steel-trap mind.

For many years you may have been pushing yourself through one stressful day after another, and this has probably physically damaged both your memory and your "fluid intelligence," or brain power. When you endure stress on a regular basis, you chronically oversecrete brain-destroying cortisol. When this happens, brain function deteriorates.

Unfortunately, when cognitive function declines, people tend to push themselves even harder, to compensate for the decline. Thus a degenerative cycle is created.

The *psychological* result of this degenerative cycle is a general loss of joy. Life becomes too difficult to be pleasurable.

But this vicious cycle also takes a *biological* toll on your ability to feel joy. It damages the biological functions and structures in the brain that contribute to feelings of well-being, happiness, and excitement.

One important brain chemical that is depleted by chronic stress is the stimulating neurotransmitter norepinephrine, which not only helps "cement" memory, but is also vital in helping you to maintain a positive, happy mood. It is an essential ingredient in your brain's "pleasure pathway."

There is another biological phenomenon, though, that is even more destructive to happiness. If the biochemistry of the brain becomes too disrupted for too long a period, this disruption can lead to a physical condition called *anhedonia*, the inability to feel pleasure. With anhedonia, you're no longer biochemically capable of being excited, happy, or joyful. The condition is commonly seen in people who have chronically abused a highly stimulating drug such as cocaine. In effect, these people have "used up" their "pleasure" chemicals, including norepinephrine and other stimulating catecholamine neurotransmitters.

You may have experienced a mild version of anhedonia at the end of a long, stressful period of work. When you finally finished, you knew you should feel happy about being done, but you couldn't really feel any pleasure. You just felt numb. That's anhedonia. Your brain's "happiness chemicals" were "burned up" by excessive stress.

Fortunately, this condition can usually be repaired. It generally goes away if you relax and allow your brain to replenish its chemical deficits. Patients on brain longevity programs overcome this condition relatively quickly, because such programs recondition the depleted biochemical milieu of the brain.

Many of my brain longevity patients, however, are not satisfied with just achieving "normal" levels of joy and pleasure. Just as they choose to pursue optimal intellectual function, they also choose to pursue the highest possible levels of happiness. Many of them become happier than they've ever been before.

The first step to achieving optimal function of the brain's "pleasure pathway" is to rebalance and replenish overall brain biochemistry. The second step is to help biochemically support the function of the limbic system's *amygdala,* which processes emotional input and is generally considered to be the "pleasure center" of the brain.

When people's amygdalas have been surgically removed—during brain-cancer surgery, for example—it devastates their ability to feel happiness. In fact, they lose the ability to feel virtually *any* emotion. They become so emotionally dead that they don't even *regret* loss of emotion.

The same thing happens when the amygdala of an animal is removed. The animal loses its capacity for fear and anger. It also withdraws from social relations with other animals.

But what occurs when the amygdala of an animal is *stimulated*? Of course: The opposite happens. The most dramatic evidence of this was seen when the amygdalas of animals were stimulated with mild electrical charges. In experiments, cats and monkeys were allowed to trigger the stimulation of their own amygdalas. When they were given this opportunity, they did it incessantly—up to ten thousand times per hour!

In a similar experiment, hungry rats refused to cross a floor for food, because the floor was wired with 60 microamperes of electricity. To them, the electric shock was worse than starvation. Then, instead of putting food on the other side of the electrified floor, researchers installed a device that could stimulate the rats' amygdalas. The rats *willingly* ran across the electrified floor to get the stimulation. Then the researchers increased the electricity from 60 microamps to 450. The shock was so powerful it knocked the rats unconscious. But as soon as they revived, they charged off again in pursuit of more stimulation of their amygdalas.

In yet another experiment, rats were given only one hour per day to either eat, or to stimulate their pleasure centers. The rats, as you might guess, starved to death.

My point here is a simple one: Your brain is capable of profound joy and pleasure, and there are many simple, physical ways of maximizing the happiness that lies within you.

As you engage in your own brain longevity program, you will learn how to nourish and rejuvenate your own pleasure pathway. You will also learn how to avoid the lifestyle elements—such as stress, toxins, lack of exercise, and poor nutrition—that harm your brain and reduce your physical capacity for pleasure and joy.

When you learn to avoid the things that damage your brain, you will be able to create a regenerative cycle. As your biochemical capacity for pleasure becomes enhanced, you will probably desire fewer happiness "crutches"—such as alcohol and caffeine—that ultimately *damage* your pleasure pathway. As you gradually use less of these substances, a positive, regenerative cycle will be created.

Additionally, the more pleasure you feel, the less you will physically react to stress. The less you react to stress, the less you will damage your brain with cortisol. You will boost not just your cognitive power, but also your "pleasure power." When this happens—and it *will*—your regenerative cycle will accelerate.

4. Your Brain Has "Plasticity," and Can Renew Itself

No matter how badly damaged your brain is, it can grow new cells, and get more "thinking power" out of existing cells.

Until the 1990s, it was universally accepted that the brain could *not* grow new cells. Virtually all researchers believed that brain cells, unlike almost all other cells in the body, did not increase in number after birth.

But that piece of conventional wisdom was abandoned when scientists finally solved the mystery of the "canary scam."

This was a common fraud perpetrated in the 1930s, in which female canaries, which are unable to sing, were injected by unscrupulous pet store owners with the male hormone testosterone. When these female birds were given the masculinizing hormone, they temporarily developed the ability to sing.

Researching this phenomenon in recent years, neurologists discovered that the hormonal injections to the canaries produced new brain cells, or neurons. The female canaries actually grew new neurons in the parts of the brain where song originates.

This proved that new brain cells *can* be created, throughout life.

Currently there is no accepted clinical technique for stimulating growth of new brain cells in humans. Nonetheless, the philosophical implications of this discovery are profound. It means that people are not limited to just the brain cells they were born with.

I believe that new brain cells are most likely to grow when the biological environment of the brain is optimized. However, this has not been proven.

We do know, however, that it is definitely possible to renew the brain by *improving existing brain cells*. How? By increasing the connections among brain cells. All brain cells have branches, or *dendrites,* that reach out and connect with other brain cells; it is *through these connections that thoughts travel.* The more connections you have, the better your brain works. However, these dendritic connections to other brain cells are easily damaged, and are often destroyed. Alzheimer's patients, for example, have a terrible lack of dendritic connections. Their brain cells look like trees that have been severely pruned.

Until recently it was believed that once a connection was broken, it was broken forever. But now we know that's not true. When one connection dies, it can be replaced by another. Brain cells can grow new dendritic branches. That is why people are able to recover from brain damage caused by stroke or head injury. When you hear that someone "learned to walk all over again," it means that person grew new brain cell branches, and forged new thought pathways.

Very recently we've learned that new connections can be formed at virtually *any age*. We have also learned that the brain's memory center, the hippocampus, is exceptionally resilient, even in elderly people. The hippocampus is wonderfully adept at creating new dendritic branches and making new connections.

One effective way to create new connections is *simply to think*. Virtually every time you have a thought, your brain sprouts a few new connections to help carry that thought. Because of this, I counsel my patients to remain mentally active: Use it or lose it. Mentally active people tend to exhibit slower progression of Alzheimer's and age-associated memory impairment than do people who are not mentally active.

Another way to keep connections from dying, and to replace the ones that do die, is to furnish the brain with a properly balanced biological environment. If the brain is chronically abused by poor nutrition, high stress, and faulty circulation, no amount of "mental exercise" will keep connections from withering.

Brain plasticity is utterly invaluable to anyone on a brain longevity program.

It's never too late to regenerate your brain.

5. Much About the Brain Remains a Mystery

As you read this book, you may be astonished to learn that some of the most basic elements of cognition are matters of theory rather than fact. For example, no one is even certain how a memory is formed. There are several leading theories, but there is no absolute consensus. Furthermore, in the area of brain research, "facts" are constantly being disproven.

Also, many of the most critically important findings about the brain were discovered very, very recently. For example, we weren't certain that the amygdala was the "emotional center" of the brain until as recently as 1990. We didn't even know that the brain had three major divisions (brain stem, cerebellum, and cerebrum) until about 1975—and now that seems like a kindergarten-level fact. In many ways, brain research is still in its infancy.

Some clinicians, of course, cite the mysterious quality of the brain as a rationale for a passive therapeutic approach. They believe doctors should act only when they understand exactly why a certain treatment might work. This is good science; however, it's not always good for patients. I believe that sometimes doctors facing a mysterious problem should use a "mysterious" treatment—such as an Eastern medical technique—*if* there's a body of evidence suggesting that this treatment has worked for other patients with similar problems. For example, I think it is entirely appropriate to use acupuncture for migraine headaches, even though no researcher can fully explain why migraines occur, or why acupuncture sometimes stops them.

As I've mentioned, I'm a pragmatist. I'll employ any reasonable modality that provides evidence of effectiveness. This approach, I believe, accounts for much of the success of my brain longevity programs. Does it mean I *know* more about the brain than other doctors? Emphatically, no!

Furthermore, some doctors, in my opinion, are too quick to "play God," pretending to understand more than they really do. I don't do that. Like most doctors, I just try to help people, and some of the things that seem to help most are somewhat mysterious to me. I *think* I know why they work, but I can't be certain why.

Moreover, as a clinician, I *embrace* mystery—for a simple and logical reason. I believe that the best medical therapy is almost always a multimodality treatment. I don't think that single-modality, "magic bullet" treatments are very effective. In any multimodality treatment program, however, it is impossible to isolate exactly which component or components worked, and which didn't. Therefore, there is always an element of mystery in a multimodality program.

Despite my rigorous scientific training, I hold no emotional antipathy for mystery. In fact, I glory in it. It's the mystery of life that awakens our awe and inspires our reverence.

And in the presence of the human brain, awe and reverence are the only appropriate attitudes to have.

*   *   *

The above five principles are fact, but they are also philosophy. The philosophy they underscore is this: You can improve your life by physically improving your brain.

You have that power.

Your only limitations are those you choose to impose. Of course, one of the primary limitations you must overcome is lack of basic knowledge about your brain.

Let's remedy that.

The next chapter will give you the latest scientific findings about how the brain works. It will be your "Neurology 101" course.

The next chapter may not change your life. But it may tell you what you'll need to *know* to change your life.

A Case in Point

Your Brain Has Plasticity, and Can Renew Itself

K.D., forty-nine years old, was a woman badly in need of neurological renewal.

It was not unusual for someone of K.D.'s age to need brain regeneration. Many people at this stage of life need a "brain boost" to propel them into an energetic and satisfying middle age.

What was unusual about K.D.'s situation was that her daughters also were badly in need of neurological restoration.

The two girls were only teenagers, far too young to be suffering from neurological degeneration. In fact, their peak biological years of learning and memory were still about a decade away. Nonetheless, both girls were performing below their capabilities in school, were chronically fatigued and apathetic, and were frequently irritable. The older daughter commonly fell asleep as early as 6:00 P.M.

K.D. herself, however, had a set of symptoms that were relatively common for a person approaching age fifty. She frequently found her memory to be unreliable, and couldn't focus intensely for as long as she once had. She had difficulty doing two things at once, and found that she often became upset more easily than she had in her younger years. Most distressingly, she was beginning to lose her zest for life; many of the things that had formerly given her great pleasure now seemed as if they were boring, or just too much trouble.

Stress certainly seemed to be contributing to her neurological decline. Several years earlier her husband had died of cancer, leaving her to raise her children alone. She'd inherited a small business from him, as well as a portfolio of investments, and both the business and the investments required her constant attention. She worked long hours, traveled frequently, and had to make crucial decisions by herself. Exceptionally generous with her time and energy, she spent a great deal of time with her daughters, and was also very helpful to her friends. One friend was starting a business, and K.D. was giving a considerable amount of her time to that project.

Partly as a result of all of these demands, she was experiencing "accelerated aging." Her cognitive function was declining faster than that of most people her age. Also, she was in chronic endocrine distress, and just didn't have much physical energy. Although she was still very attractive, her appearance was marred by stress. Her eyes were shadowed by dark rings, she looked exhausted, and her complexion was sallow.

When K.D. began her brain longevity program, her response was not as dramatic as I'd hoped it would be. She reported that she felt much better, but objective testing indicated that she still had significant problems with memory and concentration.

Shortly after K.D. began her program, I started trying to help her two daughters. Their responses, too, were encouraging, but by no means satisfactory.

I began searching for clues that would explain why all three family members, separated widely by age and experience, would be suffering from cognitive decline. One possible explanation was that all three shared a genetic trait that was somehow related to their problems. But if that were the case, why hadn't K.D. shown symptoms earlier in her life?

It was also possible that all three family members had a genetic predisposition to cognitive dysfunction that had been triggered by *stress.* Perhaps their common loss of K.D.'s husband had paved the way for the onset of their disorders.

Another possibility was that their problems were being caused by something all three were being exposed to—such as a poor diet or a toxin.

But after they'd consulted with me, their diet had improved considerably, without causing a dramatic improvement in cognitive function.

I began to suspect that an environmental toxin might be the source of their maladies.

Soon, I helped to discover exactly what the problem was. My clue had been the relative severity of the older daughter's condition. Of the three, she seemed to be suffering most. She sometimes experienced dizziness and even blackouts. Therefore, as part of an effort to understand why she was being hit hardest, I scrutinized her room, and noticed that it had very poor air circulation. The room had no vents.

K.D. called in a contractor to improve the circulation, and he detected the real source of the family's problem: carbon monoxide poisoning. Improper combustion in the home's furnace was allowing carbon monoxide to build up in the house. The gas was most concentrated in the older daughter's bedroom, because of its lack of ventilation, and because it was located closest to the furnace. It created a dangerously toxic environment.

All three family members were suffering from chronic, low-level carbon monoxide intoxication. Symptoms of that disorder include headache, nausea, confusion, difficulty in concentrating, fatigue, and pallor.

The furnace was fixed immediately, and K.D. and her two daughters began to improve at a much faster rate. Previously, their responses to their brain longevity programs had been characterized by a "two steps forward, one step back" progression. But after the furnace was fixed, their progress became much more evenly paced. Their improvement quickly began to gain momentum.

K.D. showed an even greater burst of improvement when I placed her on deprenyl, an extremely impressive stimulator of brain plasticity.

I did not feel that the daughters required deprenyl. Because their brains were still young, the daughters enjoyed a somewhat greater degree of natural brain plasticity than did their mother.

Within a year, all three were functioning at an inordinately higher level. K.D.'s memory improved greatly, her concentration became knife-sharp, and she became able to easily do a number of things at once. Her general mood improved substantially, partly because she was more biochemically stable, and partly because she was so pleased with her renewed ability to function with excellence.

Both daughters began to achieve much more in school, and one became a straight-A student. The older daughter no longer fell asleep at six in the evening, and both began to experience the robust sense of energy that is typical of children in that age group.

The response of this family was very gratifying to me. It indicated that even after severe damage from a powerful and dangerous environmental toxin—and even after a tragically stressful experience—the brain, one of the body's most renewable vital organs, can still bounce back.

6

A Brief Tour of Your Brain: Putting Mind Over Matter and Matter Over Mind

It's time for you to learn some nuts-and-bolts information about your own brain.

By the end of this chapter, you'll have a basic, ground-level understanding of neurology. You'll know the fundamentals of how your brain works. This will enable you to appreciate fully why things like good nutrition, exercise, certain pharmaceutical drugs, resistance to stress, and natural medicinal tonics are so important to your intellect and emotions.

After reading this chapter, you'll know even more about many important aspects of neurology than most *neurologists* knew in, say, the 1960s—because so much of what we now know about the brain comes from recent discoveries. Imagine! In many ways, you'll be a better neurologist than the preeminent brain surgeon of the sixties: Ben Casey.

In this chapter you'll also learn about the all-important endocrine system, the network of hormone-producing glands that works closely with the brain. The endocrine system has a profound influence on how good you feel and how efficiently your brain functions. All your life, you probably assumed that your thoughts controlled your emotions. Actually, your thoughts control your endocrine system, and your endocrine system controls your emotions. The endocrine system releases the hormones that excite or depress you, and make you happy, sad, or angry.

The therapeutic implications of this simple fact are monumental. It means that you can control your *body*—via the endocrine system—by controlling your *thoughts*. You can put mind over matter!

Not only that, but you can control your emotions by *physically* controlling your endocrine system. Which means you can put matter over mind!

A Guided Tour of Your Brain

To really understand how to put your mind over matter, and matter over mind, you'll need to know the basics of neurology. So let's take a brief tour of your brain, from the neck up.

We'll be making three stops, at the three major divisions of your brain: the *brain stem,* the *cerebellum,* and the *cerebrum.*

First stop: the brain stem. Your brain stem sits atop your spinal column, and it was the first part of your brain to be formed in the womb. It was also one of the first brain types to evolve. Two hundred eighty million years ago, the first animals to walk the earth, reptiles, had *only* a brain stem. These reptiles had a brain stem that was very much like yours today. That's why we often call the human brain stem the "reptilian brain."

The brain stem relays information from the senses, and controls basic things such as breathing and heartbeat. But it doesn't do any *thinking* or *feeling.* That's why lizards don't make very good pets. Your lizard will never love you, and it will never learn its name.

Let's move on to the second division of your brain, the cerebellum. It has more interesting capabilities than the brain stem. The cerebellum lies just behind the brain stem, and helps your body to move. It governs coordination of your muscles. The cere-

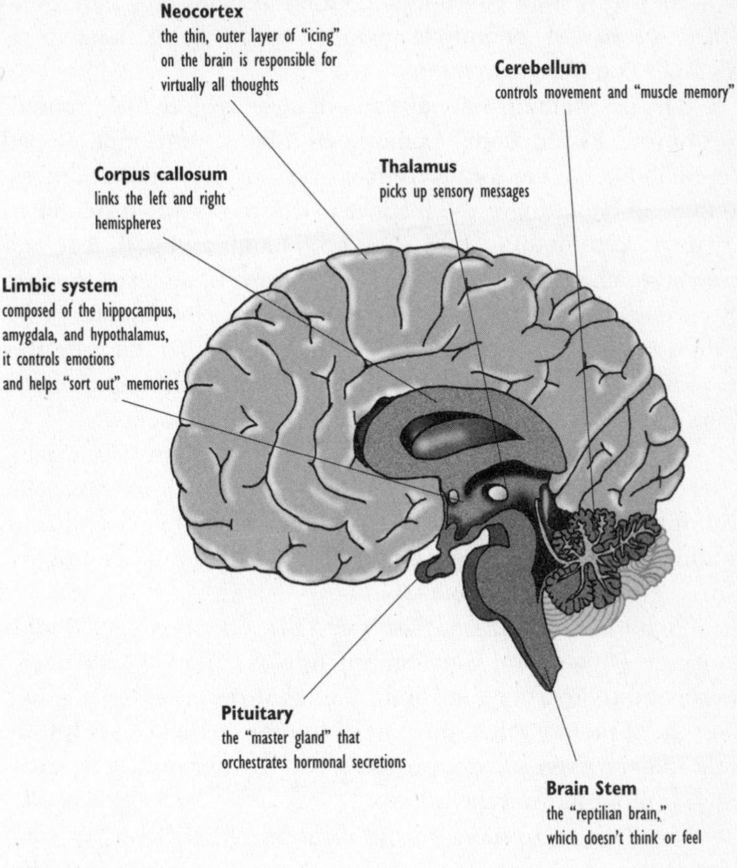

Neocortex
the thin, outer layer of "icing"
on the brain is responsible for
virtually all thoughts

Cerebellum
controls movement and "muscle memory"

Corpus callosum
links the left and right
hemispheres

Thalamus
picks up sensory messages

Limbic system
composed of the hippocampus,
amygdala, and hypothalamus,
it controls emotions
and helps "sort out" memories

Pituitary
the "master gland" that
orchestrates hormonal secretions

Brain Stem
the "reptilian brain,"
which doesn't think or feel

Figure 2
Because the brain is just flesh and blood, it can be physically regenerated.

bellum also holds some *memory* for movement. Most good athletes and good dancers have very well-developed cerebellums—that's why they're so well coordinated. Good athletes also have good *kinesthetic memory,* or muscle memory, which helps them to remember complex movements.

The cerebellum, as we age and mature, is gradually "trained" to improve its functions. As newborn infants, with undeveloped cerebellums, we have little control over our movements. For example, all babies have the instinct to grasp, but when newborns try to grasp something, they close both hands and both feet, and even scrunch up their midsections. As we grow, we learn to grasp by closing only one hand. But we never gain *complete* mastery over even a simple, fundamental task like grasping. To illustrate this lack of control to yourself, try to touch your little finger to the palm of your hand—without moving your other fingers.

Frustrating, isn't it? It makes you feel as clumsy as a baby. There are probably only two fingers you can touch to your palm without moving the others. They are your index finger and your thumb, which you've used much more than the other fingers. Give them a try at the same task.

That was much easier, wasn't it? This is because your thumb and index fingers are your "smart" fingers. They've "practiced" more, and the part of your brain that controls them has a better kinesthetic memory than the part of your brain that controls your little fingers. Even so, you probably had to concentrate to move them without moving the others.

Now let's go upstairs, to the third and final "layer" of your brain, your cerebrum. That's where the real action is: thought, emotion, and memory.

Your cerebrum was the most recent part of your brain to develop, and it's by far the most complex division. It was also the final stage of brain development in evolution. Cerebrums didn't exist until about 80 million years ago, when certain species of animals became our warm-blooded ancestors: the mammals. That's why the cerebrum is sometimes called the "mammalian brain." The only reason your dog is friendlier and smarter than your pet lizard is that it has a cerebrum.

The cerebrum is the part that we usually visualize when we think of "the brain." It looks like two halves of a walnut, joined together to form a sphere. It's covered with a thin layer of "icing," so to speak, that is only about one to two millimeters thick. This is your *neocortex*—your thinking brain. More than any other part of your body, this layer of neocortex is "you." Without it, you'd exist only in a vegetative condition. It is beige in color, but for some reason, everyone calls it "gray matter."

Your neocortex covers about two and a half square feet, but only about one-third of it is visible; the rest is hidden in a number of grooves and fissures. For the most part, the more grooves and fissures a species has, the smarter it is—because there's more room for the neocortex.

For example, a cat has a very smooth brain, with very few grooves. That means there isn't much area available for the cat's neocortex. Compared to humans, even such intelligent animals as monkeys have an absolute dearth of neocortex. In experiments, the entire neocortex was suctioned away from a group of monkeys, and their behavior remained almost identical to what it had been before the operation.

Birds have almost no neocortex at all (which is why the epithet "bird brain" is an insult). Nonetheless, in one recent experiment, a group of pigeons was trained to distinguish between Picasso paintings and Monet paintings. This showed the power of even the most primitive neocortex.

Beneath the icing of neocortex is a dense "cake" of whitish matter, which does a great deal of biochemical work—the "housekeeping" work that your body requires to stay alive. But this white matter does no real thinking or feeling.

The cerebrum is divided into four areas, or lobes: the frontal lobe (which does most of your abstract problem-solving); the parietal lobe (which helps process information from your senses); the occipital lobe (which governs vision); and the temporal lobe (which controls memory, hearing, and language). The frontal lobe, as its name implies, sits at the front of your brain; the parietal lobe sits behind it; and the much smaller occipital lobe sits at the base of your brain. Your tem-

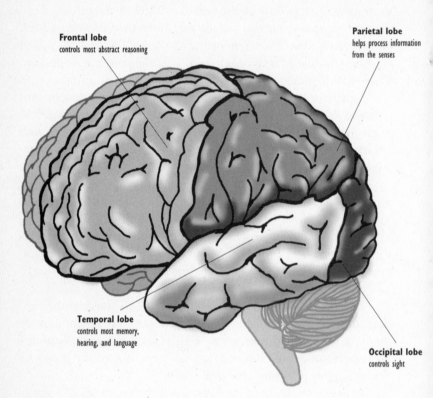

Frontal lobe
controls most abstract reasoning

Parietal lobe
helps process information
from the senses

Temporal lobe
controls most memory,
hearing, and language

Occipital lobe
controls sight

Figure 3
The four lobes of the brain work in perfect concert with each other when optimal
brain function is achieved.

poral lobe is located on each side of your brain, in the areas near your temples.

As you can see, different general areas of the brain tend to handle different elements of cognitive function. In the very early years of brain research, researchers thought that each area functioned independently. For example, they thought there was just one area of the brain that held knowledge about animals, and another that held all of a person's religious beliefs. But this archaic idea has been replaced by the concept that each memory and thought requires the functioning of several areas of the brain, often in different lobes. This relatively new idea, proven to be true by advanced imaging techniques, is called "multiple mapping."

According to the concept of multiple mapping, a thought such as "my red car" might be in a dozen different places in your brain. It might be in a small network of neurons that holds thoughts about cars, and also in an area that remembers red-colored things, and also in an area that remembers things in your garage.

Each of those areas, if triggered to consciousness, would help you to remember things about your red car. If you could see your brain, by means of a PET scan, you'd see that each time you thought about your red car, several tiny areas would "light up" with electrochemical activity.

To people on brain longevity programs, the phenomenon of multiple mapping has two important ramifications. First, it means that because memories must "travel" all around the brain to be complete, your brain's "transportation system" of neurotransmitters *must be maintained properly*. Second, it means that it's relatively hard to completely "kill" a memory, because parts of the memory exist in many widely separated areas. Even if a memory has been partly destroyed, it's still possible to preserve most of it by nurturing the remaining healthy areas of the brain.

The total weight of all three layers of the adult human brain is just under three pounds. That doesn't stack up very impressively against the weight of a whale's brain: twenty pounds. But the whale's brain constitutes a much smaller *percentage* of its entire body weight than a human's brain does. When total body weight is accounted for, human brains "outweigh" whale brains by a ratio of 250 to 1.

Among humans, though, the relative size of the brain doesn't seem to make much difference. Two "big thinkers"—Jonathan Swift and Ivan Turgenev—had massive brains weighing 4.4 pounds each. But Anatole France, who won the Nobel Prize for literature, had a brain that weighed only 2.2 pounds. Albert Einstein had a normal-sized brain. Women have brains that are usually about 10 percent smaller than men's, because women's bodies are generally smaller; but there is no apparent difference in intelligence between males and females.

The fact is, it's not the size of the brain that mostly determines intelligence, but the number of connections between neurons. These connections are among the major areas of focus in my brain longevity programs. The connections are *physical entities,* and can therefore be nurtured and stimulated with various physical measures.

The cerebrum's left and right hemispheres, as you probably know, have somewhat different functions. The left half of the cerebrum is relatively more involved in analytical thought: language, and sorting out time and sequence. The right side of the brain is rather more involved with creative, imaginative functions: music, recognizing faces, spatial organization, and visualizing images.

Males generally have thicker, more developed right hemispheres, and females often have thicker, more developed left hemispheres, which is probably why females often learn to speak earlier than males, are usually more adept at language than men are, and are generally better able than men to repeat "tongue twisters." Females are also better at fine motor control, which probably accounts for their generally superior penmanship. I have also noticed, during my many years in operating rooms, that females are often outstanding surgeons. Males, though, are usually better at spatial tasks, such as reading a map or working through a maze.

The brain's left and right hemispheres are connected, as

noted previously, by a band of nerve fibers called the corpus callosum, which coordinates the functions of one side with the other. This extremely sophisticated communication system tends to be larger in females, enabling them to have relatively better communication between the two sides of their brains.

Females have a larger corpus callosum for an interesting reason. As children grow, their two hemispheres become increasingly specialized, each more interested in "doing its own thing." As this specialization increases, the corpus callosum gets thinner and weaker. At puberty, though, the thinning stops. Females, however, usually reach puberty *before males do.* Therefore, the thinning of their corpus callosums stops before a male's does, so females end up with thicker corpus callosums.

Thus, men tend to have brains that are more *specialized,* with relatively less communication between the two hemispheres. Several things result from this. One is that men are more vulnerable to problems like dyslexia and hyperactivity, which are exacerbated by a lack of hemispheric coordination. Another is that men tend to have more difficulty recovering from strokes or brain injuries, because the injured parts of their brains are less able to "hand over" their functions to the remaining healthy parts. Yet another result is "feminine intuition"—the ability to coordinate logic with emotion, and make decisions that are "emotionally intelligent."

Men's increased hemispheric specialization, however, probably accounts for their frequent superiority in mathematics, mechanics, and engineering. Also, because men's thinking is generally more "compartmentalized," men may generally be better at isolating specific problems in their attempts to solve them.

In my opinion, though, too much has been made of the differences between the "logical left brain" and the "emotional right brain." I think the left-right distinction has become an intellectual fad. In fact, the two hemispheres are vastly more similar than different. That's not to say, though, that there is not a functional distinction in the brain between logic and emotion. I believe, however, that the basic dichotomy between logic and emotion does not exist because of differences between the left brain and right brain. Instead, it exists because of differences between the neocortex and the limbic system.

The Intelligence of Your "Emotional Brain"

The neocortex and the limbic system are both in the cerebrum, and are both part of the cortex—but they have very different functions. Essentially, the neocortex is the "thinking brain" and the limbic system is the "feeling brain."

I love the limbic system. I think it's long been the most underrated part of the brain. It has astonishing capabilities, and is the nexus of the mind/body connection.

The limbic system has an enormous influence not just on your emotions, but also on your memory—because your hippocampus, which is your brain's primary memory center, is part of your limbic system.

In evolution, the limbic system was the first part of the cerebrum to develop; it's about 150 million years old. The advent of animals with limbic systems marked the beginning of social cooperation, because before limbic systems were developed, animals had absolutely no feelings for one another. That's why reptiles, lacking limbic systems, often eat their own young.

The limbic system is similar in shape to a doughnut, with one bite taken from it. In fact, the word *limbic* is derived from the Latin word *limbus,* which means "ring." The limbic system rests upon the top of the brain stem.

The primary parts of the limbic system are the *hippocampus,* the *amygdala,* the *hypothalamus,* the *thalamus,* and the *pituitary gland.* To understand your own emotions and memory, you'll need to know at least a smattering of detail about each of these parts. So here's a quick description of the various parts. Note how beautifully they knit together the mind/body connection.

Hippocampus. As the brain's memory center, the hippocampus stores some short-term and a few long-term memories. But it "ships" most long-term memories to the neocortex.

The hippocampus especially governs the storage of dry, unemotional facts. Therefore it's the part of your brain that processes most "book learning," or *semantic memory*.

The hippocampus doesn't fully develop until a person is about one and one-half to two years old, and many researchers think that the reason we can't remember our infant years is that we didn't have a hippocampus then that was able to "ship" memories to "long-term storage."

In Alzheimer's patients, the hippocampus is among the first areas of the brain to be damaged. That's why Alzheimer's patients lose their short-term memories before they lose their long-term memories; most of their long-term memories are already safely stored in long-term memory banks, in the neocortex.

The hippocampus appears to be particularly vulnerable to damage caused by cortisol.

Amygdala. Recent research indicates that the amygdala is the main processing area for *emotional* memories.

The amygdala helps the hippocampus to sort out and store memories, but focuses mostly on information that has an emotional impact. Your memory of your first kiss, for example, was probably processed by your amygdala.

Working with the "thinking" neocortex, the amygdala decides how much emotional impact each thought carries. The more emotion a thought carries, the more likely it is to be shipped to long-term storage by the amygdala.

If your amygdala were to be surgically removed, you would be bereft of emotion—you'd be no more emotional than a lizard.

Your amygdala, working in conjunction with your hippocampus, tells your body and your "thinking" neocortex how to react emotionally to every situation.

However, your "thinking" neocortex also feeds *intellectual* information to your amygdala and hippocampus. This gives them the data they need to make "intelligent" choices about emotional responses.

Hypothalamus. The hypothalamus is closely connected to the amygdala, and helps to tell the body how to respond to various situations. But it does this only *after* the hippocampus, amygdala, and neocortex have decided how *important* the situation is.

The hypothalamus gives its messages to the pituitary gland, which relays the messages to the rest of the body (through its own hormones, and through "releasing factors," which trigger other hormones).

The hypothalamus also controls body temperature, thirst, hunger, and sexual function.

If you're in a crisis, it's your hypothalamus that first sends out orders for more adrenaline.

Thalamus. Incoming! Incoming! Your thalamus is primarily responsible for making sense of your body's constant sensory bombardment. It picks up all incoming sensory messages (except smell) and relays them to the appropriate processing centers in the brain.

Thus, your thalamus is basically a relay station.

Pituitary. Your pea-sized pituitary is your master endocrine gland. It tells your other glands what to do. It receives messages from the hypothalamus, then helps your body to produce the hormones it needs to respond to various situations.

Controlling Your Own Mind/Body Connection

As you can see, the limbic system is where *mind meets body.* It's where the endocrine system directly interfaces with the brain.

It's also where *thought meets emotion.* As mentioned previously, the limbic system does not produce its emotions in a vacuum. Instead, it produces emotions—and the body's physical responses to emotions—in close coordination with the thinking brain, the neocortex. Before the limbic system "decides" to get excited or depressed about an event, it consults the neocortex, to gain as much information as possible. The limbic system and the neocortex work in tandem—to form your thoughts and emotions, and to determine your body's physical responses to those thoughts and emotions.

For example, let's say you step on a snake. Your senses gather information about the snake and give it to your limbic system. Your limbic system organizes this information, and passes it to your analytical neocortex. Your neocortex then tells your limbic system, "This is a snake, and it might be dangerous." Your limbic system becomes alarmed. It sends out a jolt of adrenaline, via your endocrine system, and you jump. But your senses continue to monitor the snake. Let's say they notice the snake is made of plastic. When your neocortex finds out the snake is plastic, it tells your limbic system, "Relax, no problem." So your limbic system tells your body to calm down. No more adrenaline. End of crisis.

But if you were a bird, without a neocortex, you would remain alarmed by the plastic snake. You'd be too much of a "bird-brain" to realize that plastic snakes don't bite.

However, if you stepped on a snake and it *rattled,* your neocortex would tell your limbic system that it was a rattlesnake. It would tell your limbic system, "Be afraid. Be very afraid."

At that point your limbic system would unleash a flood of stimulating chemicals that would give you the power to escape from the snake. The primary stimulating chemical would be norepinephrine.

Norepinephrine empowers the memory, just as it empowers the muscles. Therefore the experience of stepping on the rattlesnake would dramatically activate your memory. Your brain would be so loaded with norepinephrine that the snake would be "burned into" your memory.

The flood of norepinephrine that's released in an emotional crisis accounts for our clear memories of emotionally upsetting events. That's why people remember the Kennedy assassination so clearly. We remember it not so much because it was important to the nation's fiscal policy or foreign policy, but because it was important to *us,* personally. It was the emotional impact it had on us, as *feeling* individuals, that caused the release of the chemicals that created our vivid memories of the assassination. If, for some reason, you'd been under the influence of an adrenal-inhibiting drug at the time, such as one of the group known as beta blockers, you would not remember the event nearly as well.

Ironically, it's possible that the people who were most affected by that assassination—such as members of the President's family—do not remember it as vividly as the rest of us. How come?

Because their emotional reactions were probably *too* strong. Too much norepinephrine is just as bad for memories as none at all. Limbic stimulation can easily become limbic overload, if the stress of an event is too severe. The chemicals needed to create memories can be squelched and scattered by a severe trauma. That's why we sometimes have amnesia about devastating personal events. It's also why, in a very stressful situation, we sometimes succumb to the "panic effect" and act irrationally. It's why, as a student, your mind sometimes "went blank" just before an important exam; you were unable to regain focus until you'd "settled your nerves" and stabilized your brain biochemistry.

When you go on your own brain longevity program, you must remember how important your limbic system is to your memory. To attain an enhanced memory, your limbic system should be alert, activated, and even excited. But it should not be *overwhelmed*. If your limbic system is overwhelmed by anxiety or fear, your memory will suffer. Also, if your limbic system is dulled by boredom, your memory will suffer. Even sensory overload (such as that produced by noises and distractions) will interfere with your limbic system and hurt your memory.

Further, if your limbic system lacks the physical nurturing it needs (such as good nutrition and good circulation), your memory will suffer.

However, many aspects of your brain longevity program will stimulate the physical health of your limbic system.

As you stimulate the physical health of your limbic system, you will function better intellectually and feel better emotionally. As your limbic system becomes fine-tuned, your mood will improve noticeably. This emotional boost may eventually be even more satisfying to you than your intellectual boost.

In addition, as your limbic function improves, you will experience an improvement in your physical well-being. Why? Because your limbic system is the primary nexus between your mind and your body. Your immunity, energy, sex drive, stamina, and ability to control your weight will all probably improve.

This will be possible because of the effect of your brain upon your endocrine system—and the effect of your endocrine system upon your brain. You will learn ways to put mind over matter, and matter over mind.

The endocrine system is an absolute miracle of mind/body coordination. So let's continue our tour of the brain by considering your amazing endocrine glands, which work in close association with your brain. It's your endocrine glands that enable your mind and body to function as one.

How Your Endocrine System Affects Your Emotions

The limbic system's hypothalamus, hippocampus, amygdala, and pituitary gland are so important that they are sometimes called the "second brain." This interlocking neurological network is so incredibly adept at maintaining stability in the human body and brain that it sometimes seems to have "a mind of its own." This limbic network links the brain to the endocrine system, which, in turn, controls the body.

Your endocrine system is your series of glands that secrete hormones. Hormones are the "signaling chemicals" that activate many other organs throughout your body, and that also influence your brain.

Endocrine gland secretions don't travel through their own system of vessels. Instead, the endocrine glands secrete hormones directly into the bloodstream. As those hormones travel throughout the body and brain, they find "target cells" on the organs that they are intended to influence. They enter the organs through the target cells, and then stimulate various physical actions. In the brain, hormones trigger emotions.

There are eight endocrine glands (plus the liver and kidneys, which also secrete hormones). Some of those glands have a relatively limited function; for example, the thymus gland just secretes hormones used by the immune system.

Other endocrine glands have more dramatic functions, and are more closely tied to how we think and feel. Those that most affect cognitive function and the emotions are the adrenal

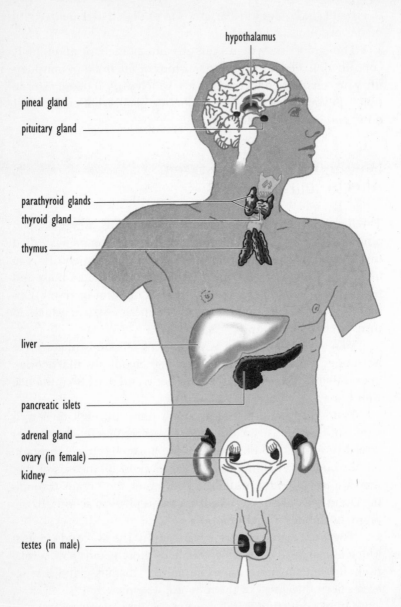

Figure 4
The glands of the endocrine system, working in conjunction with the brain, are partly responsible for declines in mood, energy, and sex drive during aging. But this decline can be stopped.

glands, the gonads, and the pineal and pituitary glands. Some hormonal secretions, such as the hormone DHEA, also help maintain brain cell function.

The gonads, located in the male and female sex organs, release the sex hormones testosterone, estrogen, and progesterone. These hormones influence, among other things, sex drive and secondary sexual characteristics, including the ratio of muscle to body fat. One of the reasons men tend to gain weight as they age is that their declining testosterone levels allow fat storage to increase, and lean muscle mass to decrease. This decline of testosterone appears to be reversible, however.

Sex hormones also have a powerful influence on the mind. They influence how efficiently we think, how well we remember, how well we perform physical tasks, and how good we feel emotionally.

Females are prone to heightened emotion when their hormonal levels fluctuate prior to ovulation and menstruation. Their intellectual and physical abilities are also affected. Before ovulation, when a woman's estrogen levels are high, she generally enjoys improved verbal ability and improved muscular coordination. When her estrogen levels are low, at the beginning of her menstrual cycle, she often has improved ability for tasks involving spatial relationships.

Sex hormones appear to play some role in memory. Estrogen replacement therapy in aging females appears to slow progression of some memory disorders, including Alzheimer's.

Now let's consider the function of another important endocrine gland, the pineal gland. The pineal secretes *melatonin,* a hormone that regulates sleep, and is involved in a wide range of other biological activities, including immune function. Melatonin is valuable as a sleep aid, especially among older people, who produce far less of the hormone than young people. Conventional wisdom has long held that older people need less sleep than younger people, simply because they generally *get* less sleep. I believe, however, that older people need as much sleep as younger people, if they wish to maintain a "longevity level" of physical and mental fitness. I believe older people sleep less merely because it's harder for them to sleep, owing to their underproduction of melatonin.

Just as the brain chemical *serotonin* promotes well-being during our *waking* hours, melatonin creates calmness at *night*. I recommend the biochemical stimulation of serotonin during the daytime hours, and melatonin during the evening hours. Hence, my aphorism: Serotonin by day, melatonin by night.

The reason melatonin declines as people age is that the pineal gland gradually withers and calcifies as we grow old. Doctors believed for many years that this was unavoidable, but I no longer believe that this calcification is inevitable. Empirical evidence from Eastern medicine, as well as recent technological evidence from Western medicine, indicates that the pineal can sometimes function properly in elderly people.

Eastern medical practitioners actively strive to support pineal function in the elderly, using advanced mind/body exercises and natural medicinal tonics. In fact, the Eastern concept of the "crown chakra" (the highest energy center) is generally believed to represent the pineal gland. Supporting the pineal gland, I believe, is preferable to taking melatonin supplements because it marshals the body's own natural forces. Also, there has been some speculation recently that long-term melatonin supplementation might possibly have some negative side effects. While these side effects remain unproven, it's still wise to be very cautious when using any medication.

Now let's look at the pituitary. This gland secretes a number of hormones, some of which have direct effects upon various organs, and some of which activate other endocrine glands. The pituitary is called the master gland because of its ability to "turn on" other glands.

The pituitary receives its messages straight from the brain's hypothalamus. Therefore, more than any other single site, it's the "meeting place" of body and mind. In Eastern cosmology, the pituitary is considered the "third eye," and is believed to be involved in intuition. In fact, yogic masters believe that intuition can be heightened by mind/body exercises that stimulate the pituitary.

The glands that the pituitary stimulates are the adrenals, the thyroid, the gonads, and the mammaries. The pituitary also secretes human growth hormone, which, as its name indicates, triggers growth, and which may be a factor in a variety of other biological functions, including weight gain and brain function.

The Stress Response and Brain Degeneration

Now we'll examine the endocrine glands you are probably most aware of—your adrenal glands. You're probably most aware of them if you choose to stimulate release of their hormones each morning, when you drink a cup of coffee. In fact, if you're the type of person who sometimes worries that you have "too much blood in your caffeine system," you may be *very* well acquainted with your adrenals.

Adrenaline (which is also called epinephrine, and which is very closely related to norepinephrine) raises blood sugar levels, causes the blood vessels to constrict, influences sexual characteristics, helps control your balance of salt and water, and helps govern your fat and protein metabolism.

The primary function of adrenaline, however, is to drive the "fight-or-flight response," which is also called the "stress response." The stress response was created, through millions of years of evolution, to enable us to move away from things that scare us. In fact, the word "emotion" is based on the Latin word *motere,* which means "to move."

The physical effects of the stress response are far-reaching and profound. The first step occurs when one or more of your senses, such as your sight or hearing, perceive a change in your environment. Your senses pour their input into your thalamus, which organizes the raw sensory data. Then the thalamus feeds the information to your "thinking" neocortex and to your "feeling" limbic system (in particular, to your hippocampus and amygdala). Your neocortex and limbic system then have a "dialogue" about the information. If the information looks threatening enough, your neocortex will tell your limbic system that it should be afraid.

If your limbic system registers fear, it channels an alarm to your hypothalamus, which relays the alarm to your pituitary. Then your pituitary secretes an adrenal-activating hormone. This activating hormone "wakes up" your adrenal glands.

The activated adrenal glands then give your body a major jolt by secreting several adrenal hormones. Among the first things the adrenal hormones do is travel to your heart, and raise your heart rate. As a result, you have more blood to move your muscles and activate your brain. Your adrenal hormones also cause your blood vessels to constrict, which helps speed blood flow. This constriction can also chill you, especially in your extremities. You'll get fear-induced "cold feet."

Adrenal hormones cause your muscles to become rigid momentarily, which fixes a look on your face that we identify as fear. It may also make you temporarily immobile—you'll "freeze in your tracks" (a survival mechanism that made your ancestors less visible to predatory animals). This "freezing" mechanism also helps ensure survival in another way: It gives your rational neocortex another second or two to think, enabling it to overrule the irrational instincts of your limbic system.

Next, adrenaline causes blood sugar to pour out of your liver, fat, and muscles, which gives you more energy to meet your immediate physical needs.

Adrenal hormones also cause some of your nonessential metabolic functions to slow down or cease. Your digestion will be grossly inhibited, as blood leaves your stomach. This may cause a feeling of "butterflies" in your stomach, and may kill your appetite. Your appetite may stay away until the stress is gone.

Adrenal hormones will also activate your cognitive function. Your brain, flooded with norepinephrine, will be working so efficiently, and recording memories so adeptly, that you will become acutely aware of all ongoing, subtle changes in your environment. That's why things may seem to happen in "slow motion."

Also, the memories you will be creating will be stored very efficiently by the norepinephrine in your brain—unless, of course, you fall victim to panic. If that happens, you may develop amnesia about the stressful event.

Another nonessential function that will be short-circuited is your sex drive. Similarly, your fertility will be impaired. If the stressful event persists, your immunity to disease will also nosedive.

The stress response may well solve your immediate problem. As you can see, it's a beautifully constructed biological mechanism, powerful, far-reaching, and fast. Unfortunately, though, the stress response has some potentially devastating side effects, in that it can wreak havoc upon your heart and circulatory system. That's why stress is implicated in cardiovascular disease.

The stress response can also literally poison the brain—because it causes excessive secretion of the adrenal hormone cortisol. Cortisol is released at about the same time adrenaline is. However, it stays in your system much longer than adrenaline does, and that creates a terrible problem. Cortisol gives your hippocampus, as well as other parts of your brain, a highly destructive "toxic bath." It can be so destructive that your brain may never again recover absolutely all of its cognitive function.

If you experience the stress response day after day, year after year, its toxic effects will gradually injure and kill billions of your brain cells. Over the course of a very stressful lifetime, this assault will be disastrous to your brain.

The stress response is a wonderful tool, but only for overcoming *short-term* problems. It's probably already saved your life once or twice, enabling you to jump away from a speeding car, or to avoid breaking your neck during a vigorous sports event. It may also have helped you to "save your career," enabling you to "do the impossible" during a job crisis.

Unfortunately, though, the stress response was created many thousands of years ago, when virtually all threats were physical ones that required a strong physical response. These days, most threats are not physical, and our physical reaction to them can hurt us more than help us. In our life today, the threats that trigger the stress response are usually psychological in nature, such as upsetting phone calls, bad credit ratings, losses in the stock market, traffic jams, and other manifestations of mechanized, modern life.

When we have these intangible, nonphysical problems, though, we can't "burn off" our stress response with a vigorous physical reaction—such as a half-mile sprint away from a tiger.

Also, in today's fast-paced, high-tech world, we're almost sure to be assaulted by *repeated* stressful events. Modern stress—because of the complexity of our industrial society—tends to be chronic, the kind we face day after day, year after year. And enduring the chronic stress response, day after day, year after year, is a killer. It kills our hearts and our brains.

In a brain longevity program, it's vitally important to shut off the chronic stress response. The most obvious way to do this is to avoid stressors, by trying to keep your life as relaxed as possible. When problems do arise, try not to overreact. Let your logical neocortex "talk sense" to your emotional limbic system.

In other words, try to "put mind over matter."

But you can also avoid the chronic stress response by putting *matter over mind*. How? By biochemically manipulating your endocrine system and your brain. Here's an obvious example: Drink less coffee. If your adrenals aren't in a constant uproar from caffeine, you won't trigger the stress response every time you have a minor problem. Another simple example: If you're nervous, go ahead and follow your natural instinct to pace the floor. Your body wants to use up its adrenal hormones, and it's better to pace them away than to let them "cook" your brain.

Of course, there are a host of other techniques you can employ to keep your brain and endocrine system from suffering the effects of the chronic stress response, some of which are considerably more sophisticated than just pacing, or drinking less coffee. Many involve nurturing and carefully manipulating the chemicals that "operate" your brain.

And that will be our final stop on our tour of the brain: a quick peek at the amazing—almost magical—neurological chemicals that make your brain the most incredible thinking machine in the universe.

Your Thought Chemistry

The cartoonist's image of a thought as a light bulb going on isn't too far from reality. Brain cells do, indeed, run on electricity. In fact, your brain has enough electric current running through it at this moment to light a twenty-five-watt bulb.

Thoughts travel through your brain cells on electrical currents. Long strings of brain cells "light up" with electrical energy to form complete thoughts and memories. If part of this chain reaction of bioelectric current is interrupted, the memory or thought becomes incomplete, or gets destroyed.

Brain cells are uniquely capable of building these memory chains (which are known as *memory traces*) because of their shapes. Unlike many other types of cells, most brain cells are elongated. In fact, they are shaped rather like trees, with a "branch" system at one end and a "root" system at the other. Of course, they're unimaginably small "trees"—twenty thousand of them would fit on the head of a pin.

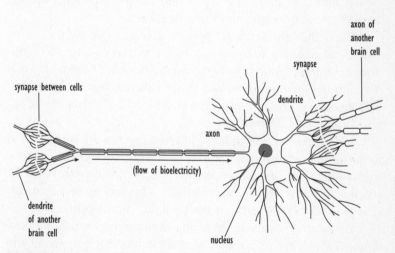

Figure 5

Long chains of brain cells, connected by neurotransmitters, form complete thoughts and memories. To preserve memories, the brain cells and neurotransmitters must remain both healthy and abundant.

The "roots" of the neuron are called *axons*. Information flows into axons from the dendritic "branches" of adjacent neurons. Then, in the form of an electrical impulse, this information travels up the "trunk" of the neuron, which is the *cell body*. Finally it reaches the "branches," or *dendrites*. From the dendrites, the nerve impulse travels to the axons of another neuron. Eventually this forms a complete, chainlike thought or memory.

Because dendrites make the connections that allow thoughts and memories to occur, dendrites are of tremendous importance in brain function. They're often the focus of my brain longevity programs. For the most part, the more dendrites, and connections, you have—and the healthier the dendrites are—the smarter you are.

In Alzheimer's patients, billions of dendrites gradually wither and die. More than anything else, it's probably this lack of dendrites that destroys the brains of Alzheimer's patients.

In recent years, though, researchers have proven that new dendritic branches can be stimulated to grow. Many of the therapeutic measures undertaken by brain longevity patients are intended to optimize growth of new dendrites.

Even though dendrite branches reach out to the axon "roots" of adjacent neurons—in order to carry along thoughts and memories—brain cells never actually touch. There is always a tiny gap between neurons, and this is called a *synapse*. Thoughts and memories bridge these gaps by "swimming" across them on chemicals called neurotransmitters.

When an electrical thought impulse reaches the very tip of a dendrite, it is transformed into a neurotransmitter. This neurotransmitter then floods into the gap between the cells. When it reaches the next cell, it attaches itself. This sets up an electrical charge in that cell—and thus the thought continues to travel.

There are probably at least one hundred neurotransmitters, many of which are referred to as *neuropeptides*. But only six major ones are involved in most cognitive processes. One of the most fascinating things in all of the neurosciences, I think, is that each of these neurotransmitters (or neuropeptides) has a different function, and conveys different moods and feelings. For example, one causes excitement, another causes relaxation, and still another carries most of our memories. We can help control our moods, and vastly improve our memories, just by stimulating release of various neurotransmitters. Thus, once again, we have an extremely powerful mechanism for putting matter over mind.

Here are your "Big Six" neurotransmitters. When you understand their functions, you'll have another key to unlock the door to your own intellectual power and emotional wisdom.

ACETYLCHOLINE

This is the "superstar" neurotransmitter of memory and thought. If you have a poor memory, but are not old enough to be suffering from age-associated memory impairment, there is an excellent chance that you simply have a deficit of acetylcholine.

Another symptom of acetylcholine shortage is poor ability to concentrate. Many millions of Americans could almost immediately improve their concentration just by ingesting appropriate amounts of the nutrients that support production of acetylcholine. These nutrients are lecithin, the B vitamins, vitamin C, and certain minerals. Of these nutrients, lecithin is by far the most important.

Acetylcholine is the most abundant neurotransmitter in the brain. As you might imagine, it is particularly concentrated in the brain's memory center, the hippocampus. But acetylcholine also helps perform many functions outside the brain. For example, it helps nerve cells in the muscles to trigger muscle action.

Acetylcholine is produced within neurons by a complicated chemical process that requires oxygen, glucose, and choline (which is a primary ingredient of lecithin). The mind/body exercises that I recommend appear to be very helpful in delivering oxygen and glucose to the brain, and thus in aiding manufacture of acetylcholine. Also, the Brain Longevity Diet provides a wealth of the nutrients that create acetylcholine.

NOREPINEPHRINE

As you may remember from our discussion of stress, norepinephrine is a hormone that also functions as a neurotransmitter. Norepinephrine (also called *noradrenaline*) is "excitatory"; it causes the brain to be more alert. Norepinephrine is absolutely vital in helping to carry memories from short-term storage in the hippocampus to long-term storage in the neocortex. Norepinephrine is the chemical that allows us to remember exciting or stressful events for all of our lives. As mentioned earlier, however, too much norepinephrine can prevent the laying down of new memories, and can interfere with rational thought and decision making.

Norepinephrine also helps govern our sleep patterns; with too much norepinephrine in the system, it's almost impossible to fall asleep. In addition, norepinephrine helps regulate sex drive; when levels are low, the sexual urge diminishes dramatically.

Excessive norepinephrine kills the appetite; that's why stimulating "diet pills" keep you from feeling hungry. Norepinephrine also helps to stimulate the rate of your metabolism.

Another crucial function of norepinephrine is to help you maintain a positive mood. Low levels of norepinephrine is one of the classic causes of depression. The power of norepinephrine to elevate mood is particularly evident when people use a powerful stimulant, such as cocaine. A cocaine abuser might be in the throes of a desperate and depressing existence—with no job, no money, and no love—but for the few minutes when he or she is riding a norepinephrine high (caused by cocaine's effect upon brain chemistry), the user will be in a buoyant mood. A similar, but less dramatic, effect comes from drinking coffee. Your first cup in the morning not only increases your cognitive power, but also elevates your mood.

The nutritional building material for norepinephrine consists primarily of two amino acids, or partial proteins: *L-phenylalanine* and *L-tyrosine*. To make norepinephrine, though, these amino acids need to be combined with vitamins C, B_3, and B_6, and copper. My Brain Longevity Diet and supplement program provides an abundance of these nutrients. Other elements of the program, such as exercise, also significantly increase norepinephrine production.

DOPAMINE

The primary function of dopamine is to help control physical movement. Dopamine generally decreases with age, as do many other neurotransmitters and hormones. If levels get too low, the result is Parkinson's disease, which is characterized by loss of muscular control.

If your dopamine levels can be maintained throughout your life at a high level, it can help you achieve physical longevity and brain longevity. As mentioned previously, one of the drugs I frequently prescribe, deprenyl, helps the body to maintain high levels of dopamine.

High levels of dopamine also improve mood, sex drive, and retrieval of memory. Dopamine is also important in maintaining proper function of the immune system.

Furthermore, dopamine stimulates the pituitary gland to secrete growth hormone, which burns fat, builds muscle, and improves mobility.

SEROTONIN

This is your brain's primary "feel good" neurotransmitter. The only other neurotransmitter that's more important to the overall function of your brain is acetylcholine.

The drug Prozac works by increasing your brain's amount of available serotonin. The wide popularity of this drug, as well as that of similar antidepressants, shows how common serotonin deficiency is in our current population.

Serotonin also helps initiate sleep, and control pain.

Serotonin is derived from the amino acid L-tryptophan, which is in abundant supply in the Brain Longevity Diet.

In brain longevity programs, patients attempt to optimize their levels of serotonin with nutritional therapy (and with mind/body exercises). You probably recall my adage: Serotonin by day, melatonin by night.

L-GLUTAMATE

This neurotransmitter is not as well understood as many others, but we do now know that it is of vital importance to memory.

L-glutamate is critical to both the laying down of new memories and the recall of existing memories. Furthermore, L-glutamate can be especially helpful in brain longevity programs because it inhibits the chronic stress response and, consequently, oversecretion of cortisol.

Low levels of L-glutamate in the brain generally indicate decreased cognitive function.

GABA

This calming neurotransmitter (gamma-aminobutyric acid) is absolutely necessary for relaxation and sleep. Without GABA, our minds would become increasingly overstimulated, and we would collapse from nervous exhaustion. GABA is vital in our battle against the "mega-information syndrome," which bombards our nervous systems with an avalanche of sensory input.

Many pharmaceutical sedatives activate the brain's GABA receptors. Valium, for example, attaches to GABA-type receptors in the brain.

One of the more reliable predictors of alcoholism is a chronic undersecretion of GABA. People who don't have enough GABA almost invariably experience high levels of tension and anxiety. They then often attempt to self-medicate with alcohol.

A major pharmaceutical company is now testing on Alzheimer's patients a drug which affects the GABA system. This is another indicator of GABA's importance.

Endorphins

These brain chemicals are technically not neurotransmitters, but their effects are similar.

You've probably heard that endorphins cause the well-known "runner's high." Actually, they do much more than that. Endorphins are released in response to virtually any kind of significant physical or emotional stress. Very commonly, they relieve both pain and anxiety.

One practical purpose of endorphins is to encourage you to continue what you're doing; endorphins stimulate interest, focus, and concentration. Another function of endorphins is to shield you from the psychological and physical effects of extreme stress. As stress mounts, your endorphins counteract some of the effects of the stress response. Still another effect of endorphins is to protect you from pain. When someone has a delayed reaction to a painful wound, it's because endorphins are flooding the brain, temporarily blocking the pain.

Production of endorphins can, of course, be physically stimulated. Obviously, you can increase your endorphin output by stressing your body with exercise. You can also increase it with acupuncture; in Eastern medicine, acupuncture is used very effectively as an anesthetic procedure during surgeries. Endorphin production can also be stimulated with the mind/body exercises.

Production of endorphins probably accounts for the common effectiveness of placebos in killing pain. In experiments, it's been shown that approximately 30 percent of pain patients who are given placebos experience relief. For those patients, the *belief* that they will experience relief appears to trigger an output of endorphins. This is a classic example of "mind over matter."

As you can see, all of your neurotransmitters have a profoundly important impact upon your life. If your neurotransmitters are not furnished with the proper biochemical environment, your intellect, memory, and emotions will suffer.

Nonetheless, problems with your neurotransmitters can often be remedied quite quickly—in some cases, almost immediately. This is possible because your neurotransmitters are merely "free floating" chemicals rather than permanent neurological structures, which can take years to rehabilitate.

Therefore, when neurotransmitter problems are the primary cause of cognitive deficiency, as they often are, brain longevity programs elicit an almost magically quick response. One relatively young patient of mine, for example, began his program because he was experiencing a serious deficit of concentration and short-term memory. But after only about two weeks on his program, he experienced a remarkable recovery.

To me, his recovery was relatively predictable and not out of the ordinary.

But, to this man, his healing was truly a miracle.

So—was the healing of this man's brain a miracle? Or was it the predictable application of science?

It was, of course, both.

A Case in Point

Much About the Brain Remains a Mystery

During my initial consultation with him, J.L. appeared to be an extremely challenging case. To many doctors he would have seemed a hopeless case, because his symptomatology was profound and baffling. But I do not believe in the concept of hopelessness. I believe we all have an obligation to try to solve problems—no matter how baffling—and that as long as we're still trying, there's always hope.

J.L.'s doctor had made a diagnosis of dementia, but not of the Alzheimer's type. J.L. had memory loss, and a decline in his reasoning skills. But he also had more deep-seated and disturbing symptoms, which in many ways mimicked those of Alzheimer's. It was as if he had been picked up and dropped into late-stage Alzheimer's, without going through the normal progression of the disease.

For example, J.L. was quite delusional, especially late at night. He suffered from "sundowner's syndrome," a phenomenon characterized by gross exaggeration of symptoms in the nighttime hours. At around 2:00 A.M., he would suddenly awaken in a delusional condition. He would believe it was morning, and insist on getting dressed and going for a walk.

Sometimes he would empty his closet, and not recognize his clothes. He believed that people were putting strange clothes into his closet.

This behavior was causing his wife great distress. For one thing, it was keeping her from being able to sleep at night.

J.L. was totally dependent upon his wife, and would defer virtually all decisions to her. Of course, his wife's role, like that of all caregivers for Alzheimer's patients, was terribly stressful. In fact, when researchers study stress, they often choose Alzheimer's caregivers as their subjects, because these people have one of the most stressful roles in our society.

J.L. had long been known for his sharp sense of humor, but he had become unable to master the complexity of wit. He still frequently tried to make jokes, but they didn't make any sense. He had become a sad caricature of his former witty self. When he made a joke, though, his eyes still sparkled with humor, even though he was the only person who understood his jokes.

He also had an unsteady gait, and seemed unsure of himself when he walked.

During his intake testing, he barely seemed to know where he was.

One aspect of his medical history that stood out was his habitual use of the drug phenylpropanolamine, a drug that's often used in over-the-counter appetite suppressants. The drug was prescribed to raise blood pressure.

The drug had successfully elevated his blood pressure, but it seemed to me to be a poor choice of medication. Phenylpropanolamine is not intended for constant daily use, because it has several potential side effects during long-term use. One of the possible side effects is cognitive dysfunction, which may have gone undetected.

As J.L. began his program, I contacted his doctor, and suggested that she replace the phenylpropanolamine with another drug. She agreed to do so.

After J.L. began his program, however, his blood pressure stabilized, and he showed no need for a replacement medication.

J.L. began taking a full spectrum of supplements, altered his diet, and used a number of natural medicinal tonics (including *Ginkgo biloba* and ginseng). I also placed him on the pharmaceutical drug deprenyl.

Shortly after he began his program, my wife, Kirti—who works with me—began calling him to monitor his progress. When she would call, he would not recognize her name, or know who she was. He would not feel competent enough to talk to her, and would mumble, "Let me get my wife." Then his wife would update Kirti on his progress.

Then one day, after we had not heard from him for a few months, Kirti called, and he answered the phone.

This time it wasn't "I'll get my wife." Instead he said, "Hi, how are you?"

"Do you know who I am?" Kirti asked.

"You're the doctor's wife," he said.

"Do you know why I'm calling?" she asked.

"Either to check on me," he said, "or to *get* a check." Kirti laughed.

"This is really you, isn't it?" Kirti said.

"It better be—or my wife's in trouble," he said.

I got on the phone, and was astonished at how coherent, buoyant— and funny—he was. He had markedly fewer signs of cognitive decline.

J.L. had fought for his life, and he had won it back.

How? I am not certain. Perhaps taking him off the phenyl-propanolamine had made the critical difference. Maybe the deprenyl had been the key factor. Maybe one of the supplements or tonics had been instrumental in helping him to recover. Or maybe the entire multimodality program, working synergistically, had spurred his recovery.

I will never know exactly what enabled J.L. to recover. I am just glad he *did* recover.

The fact that his recovery was somewhat mysterious does not bother me. Much about the brain remains a mystery—precisely because the brain is so powerful and complex.

As a man who respects science, I accept that mystery as a challenge. And as a man who loves God, I accept it as a blessing.

7

How Memory
Works

Now it's time to take a quick look at how memories are formed.
Once you understand this, you'll know how you can form memories with greater efficiency.

Memories, as previously mentioned, do not reside in single
brain cells, but in vast chains of brain cells called memory traces.
Each brain cell holds only a small portion of an entire memory.

It is not known, however, exactly *how* each brain cell holds on
to its small portion of the complete memory trace. The current
leading theory, though, is that these individual "bits" of a memory
trace are created when a thought, or a fragment of sensory input,
physically alters the structure of a brain cell's RNA, or ribonucleic
acid.

Just as your brain is your body's "memory bank," your RNA
appears to be the memory bank of each of your brain cells.

RNA is found in a cell's nucleus, and also in the jellylike *cytoplasm* that surrounds the nucleus. The nucleus and cytoplasm
are the sites where all genetic codes are stored. Those areas of a
cell are its "information centers."

RNA also helps the body to synthesize the proteins that it needs. It is theorized, therefore, that memories are stored in the RNA as "coded" proteins.

To be encoded as a memory by brain cells, information must first, of course, *enter the brain*. There are three main ways information can do this: from seeing, from hearing, and from doing (such as learning a dance step). Those three types of memory are called *auditory memory, visual memory,* and *kinesthetic memory*. Virtually every memory that you now have is one of these three types. So let's take a quick look at the three main ways that information enters your brain.

The Three Types of Memory

Most auditory memories are stored in the left side of the brain's neocortex, and most visual memories are stored in the right side. Most kinesthetic memories are stored outside the neocortex, in the cerebellum.

Most people are relatively more adept at laying down one of the three types of memory than the other two. About 65 percent of us are most oriented toward visual memory. About 20 percent of us are best at auditory memory. About 15 percent are most adept at kinesthetic memory.

Sometimes it's possible, just by listening to the way a person describes things, to tell which type of memory he or she is most skilled at laying down. If people use rich visual imagery, they're often primarily visual learners. If they are particularly skilled at recalling conversations, they're probably good auditory learners. If they describe an experience mostly in terms of how it *felt*, they may be oriented mostly toward kinesthetic memory.

Some people are equally adroit at all three memory styles. When they have this characteristic, they tend to be excellent learners, with powerful memories. Why? Because they are able to strongly encode each memory in three different ways, each of which triggers recollection of the other two. As noted earlier, the durability of a memory depends not just on how emotionally charged (and adrenally "cemented") the memory is, but also on how richly encoded the memory is. If it is encoded visually, auditorially, *and* kinesthetically, it will exist in a maximum number of brain cells.

Good teachers often try to tailor their lessons to the learning style preferred by each of their students. The legendary basketball coach and teacher Tex Winter always tried to determine which of his players were primarily visual learners, which were auditory learners, and which were kinesthetic learners. For example, when Winter was with the Chicago Bulls, he noted that his player Horace Grant had a primarily kinesthetic memory, and learned basketball plays best by performing them. The cerebral John Paxson, on the other hand, was an "X and O" player—a visual learner who liked to learn plays from diagrams. One player on the team, though, was equally proficient at all three memory styles. That player was Michael Jordan. Winter believed that a significant amount of Jordan's extraordinary ability stemmed from his elevated cognitive powers.

In general, visual learners learn more quickly than auditory and kinesthetic learners, and are usually more confident about remembering the material they've learned. Often, however, they tend to focus too much on the "big picture," without understanding its separate elements. They also tend to learn too much irrelevant information, because it's difficult for them to ignore extraneous information in the "big picture." Because they aren't very good at compartmentalizing, they tend to confuse the order of things.

Auditory learners are generally better at compartmentalizing complex material, but they frequently lack confidence in their memories, even when their memories are correct. Visual and auditory learners are essentially equal in their memory capabilities, but visual learners are usually more sure of what they've learned—even when they haven't learned it any better than auditory learners.

Kinesthetic learning is not very effective for most types of academic subjects, but it is by far the most enduring type of memory. Kinesthetic memory endures well partly because the cerebellum (where most kinesthetic memory resides) is relatively less vulnerable to degenerative damage than the neocortex and the hippocampus, which process most visual and auditory learning. The "steel trap" nature of kinesthetic memory accounts for the adage, "Once you learn to ride a bike, you never forget how." Alzheimer's patients don't lose their kinesthetic memories until the very last stages of the illness.

Kinesthetic memory may even contribute to one of the most unusual of neurological conditions, "savant syndrome," in which people who are intellectually and socially retarded possess extraordinary memory skills. A fictional character with this syndrome was portrayed by Dustin Hoffman in the film *Rain Man*. One theory holds that this condition is caused by an acutely active kinesthetic memory. Theoretically, autistic savants, like the character in *Rain Man,* process virtually all of their memories kinesthetically, rather than visually or auditorially. Thus, for them, reading a page of the phone book produces a memory that is as indelible as the "skill memory" most people acquire while learning to ride a bike.

Another interesting aspect of kinesthetic memory is that it seems to be the only form of memory that functions best *without* the help of associated memories from other parts of the brain. In fact, the more you *think* about a skill memory, such as playing the piano or hitting a baseball, the less able you are to do it. That is why athletes playing in games often try to reach a mental "zone," much like a meditative state, that is devoid of reflective, neocortical thought. They attempt to simply "go with the flow" of their "muscle memory."

Locking In Long-term and Short-term Memories

Although kinesthetic memory is the type of memory that is most likely to endure, visual and auditory memories can also easily move to long-term storage—as long as the brain is physically healthy.

The primary area of the brain that "ships" short-term memories to long-term storage is the limbic system—and particularly the hippocampus and amygdala. As mentioned earlier, the limbic system is the "emotional brain," and one of its major jobs is to decide whether a memory is *worth* keeping. When the limbic system is presented with information, it has a "dialogue" with the neocortex to determine whether a memory is important enough to send to long-term storage in the neocortex.

The hippocampus makes this decision about most unemotional information, and the amygdala makes this decision about most emotional information. If it weren't for the "sorting and shipping" abilities of the limbic system's hippocampus and amygdala, virtually no new information could be sent to long-term storage. This, in fact, is exactly what happens to Alzheimer's patients and (to a lesser extent) to people with age-associated memory impairment. Their hippocampi lose the biological ability to send memories to long-term storage. The hippocampus, as you know, is particularly vulnerable to biological assault—especially the assault of cortisol. When this assault does serious damage over a long period, the hippocampus gradually stops shipping memories efficiently to the neocortex. After degeneration of the hippocampus has become severe, the hippocampus even begins to lose its ability to store its own *short-term* memories (within the hippocampus itself).

Thus, the first stages of memory loss are almost always characterized by an inability to create new memories. That is why older people are often able to remember things that happened many years ago, but are unable to remember what happened yesterday.

Not all short-term memories are held in the hippocampus, though. Many short-term memories are temporarily stored in the prefrontal lobe of the neocortex. This is an especially common temporary storage area for *very* short-term memory, which is generally called "working memory." Working memories are memories that the brain decides are trivial, such as phone numbers that you need to remember only long enough to dial them.

The very shortest working memories are your "sensory memories"—the afterimages that your brain holds immediately after you see or hear something. Actually, because of these afterimages, you could truthfully claim that you have a 100-percent accurate photographic memory. The only problem is, your perfect photographic memory only lasts one-tenth of a second.

I'll give you an example. Visual sensory memory, called *iconic memory*, is employed by circus knife-throwers as they try to convince their audiences that they're actually throwing knives. In fact, of course, the knives they "throw"—which barely miss the person strapped to the target—are actually punched through the target from behind. However, when the audience watches a knife "leave" the thrower's hand, they swivel their heads toward the target. Because of the phenomenon of "afterimage," it looks as if the knife is actually flying through the air. In reality, all they see is the iconic afterimage of the knife. The knife appears to sail toward the target only because the audience's *eyes* move toward the target.

You can test this "persistence of vision" phenomenon by spreading your fingers and moving them back and forth in front of your eyes. The faster you do it, the more your vision of each finger is blurred. Your brain simply can't keep up its efforts to process the image of each individual finger. The hand is not "quicker than the eye." It's quicker than the *brain*.

Sensory memory that originates from hearing lasts somewhat longer than visual memory's one-tenth of a second, so it tends to be relatively more dependable than visual memory. For example, if I were to show you a list of ten numbers, you wouldn't be able to remember them as well as if I recited the list. That's why you often vocally repeat a phone number to yourself before you dial it; you instinctively know that your auditory, *echoic memory* is more dependable than your visual, iconic memory. Of course, you also remember the number better simply because you have doubly encoded the memory, storing it in two different places, each of which can trigger the other.

Any type of working memory, though, is laid down very superficially, and can easily be destroyed. For example, if you look at a phone number, then say the Pledge of Allegiance, you'll probably forget the phone number. In very much the same way, stress hampers working memory. If the limbic system is preoccupied with stressful concerns, it will subtly bombard the prefrontal areas—where most working memories are stored—with electrochemical "static." In this way, stress prevents working memories from becoming short-term memories (and then, possibly, long-term memories). Technically, this is not memory "loss," because you can't lose what you never had. But the net result is the same, in that you don't retain the memory.

Even under ideal biochemical circumstances, working memory is quite limited. People are generally able to retain only about seven bits of information at a time in their working memories. For example, the average person can usually remember a series of only about seven numbers. To demonstrate this "digit span" phenomenon to yourself, read one of the following lines of numbers, then look away and repeat it. If you are able to remember the lines that have nine or more numbers, you have a good working memory. Having a good working memory is often a sign that your brain biochemisty is functioning well, because working memory—unlike short-term and long-term memory—is hard to bolster with memory tricks. You either have it or you don't.

```
8 9 3 2
1 4 6 7 8
9 3 2 6 4 1
5 2 8 3 6 4 2
7 4 9 8 3 7 4 2
2 4 6 1 4 0 0 1 2
3 0 9 7 3 4 7 5 4 5
```

Because most people can only remember up to seven digits, seven has become a popular and somewhat "magical" number. For example, phone numbers have seven digits, because more digits would make them much harder to remember. In Australia, the language of the aborigines has only eight words for numbers: one, two, three, four, five, six, seven, and "many." There are seven days in a week, seven wonders of the world, seven deadly sins, and so on.

If you *were* able to remember a nine-digit series of numbers in the preceding exercise, you probably did it by using a strategy called "chunking": You probably grouped the nine-digit number into three "chunks" of three numerals each. Similarly, you may have grouped two numbers into one "chunk," remembering "1 9" as "nineteen" instead of as "one nine."

A similar "chunking" strategy can be applied to letters. For example, it might be hard for you to remember the letter sequence "AMTCTI." But if you "chunked" these letters into "ATT-MCI," it would be easy to remember, because you would have reduced six meaningless memory bits to two meaningful ones, which already have many memory associations in your brain. We use this strategy every time we use acronyms, such as M.A.D.D. (Mothers Against Drunk Driving).

There are a number of memory tricks like this that we all use constantly, and I'll mention them in this book. But they're certainly not my primary interest. My main interest is in helping you learn how to *biologically* create a good memory, not how to make the best of a bad one.

I mention the "chunking" strategy mostly to make a simple point: Working memory, and even most short-term memory, is terribly vulnerable to disruption, and often needs "tricks" to bolster it. After you've begun your own brain longevity program, you won't have to rely so much on these tricks. Still, there's nothing wrong with them; even the memory expert A. C. Aitken—the professor who could remember virtually everything—used the "chunking" strategy.

Memories are shipped to long-term storage by the limbic system in two basic ways.

One way occurs when your emotional limbic system becomes excited or stimulated about an event or a fact. When this happens, you naturally secrete excitatory catecholamine neurotransmitters, such as norepinephrine, that powerfully engrave memories upon the brain. Norepinephrine not only acts as a neurotransmitter, but also causes the body to deliver an extra supply of oxygen and glucose to the brain, which helps the brain lay down memories. As I've noted, the Kennedy assassination is still a vivid memory for most of us because it was an extremely emotional event.

The other primary way that you send messages to long-term storage is by repeating them to yourself. Even the most boring facts can be memorized through repetition.

Often these two methods work together. This happens naturally during any exciting event. First you cement your memory of the event by pouring out loads of norepinephrine. Then, because the event was important to you, you think about it again and again. By the end of the day, you may have "replayed" the event in your mind ten or twenty times. By then, because of this repetition, the memory is virtually indelible.

One important biological mechanism that supports learning by repetition is called *long-term potentiation*. Discovered in 1973, this phenomenon is great news for anyone who wants to biologically develop a good memory.

Because of long-term potentiation, or LTP, every time you see or think about a particular piece of information, it becomes *biologically easier* to remember it the next time you're exposed to it. Each exposure doesn't just add to your memory—it adds *exponentially*. In other words, if you see the same information five times, you won't be five times more likely to remember it—you'll be about *twenty* times more likely to remember it.

This happens because the memory trace that was created by the information becomes, in effect, an "often-traveled road." The path of the memory is, so to speak, "beaten down," making the path easier for neurotransmitters to travel.

Here's how this works in biochemical terms: When a memory is created for the first time, it temporarily changes the biochemical makeup of the synapses between certain brain cells. One of the changes is an influx of calcium into the synapse, accompanied by the neurotransmitter glutamate. Another chemical that is released is an excitatory amino acid called NMDA (N-methyl-D-aspartate). When these three chemicals are present, the synapse is easier for a thought to cross. After about the tenth time you've thought the same thought—activating the same synapses—it literally "sails" across these synapses.

This condition is not permanent, but it can last for days or weeks. The stronger the initial stimulation, the longer the condition will last. If the initial stimulation was relatively weak, the condition of LTP might last for only a few minutes.

LTP occurs most frequently in the hippocampus, the primary

"shipping yard" for long-term memories. But it can also occur in other parts of the brain.

The phenomenon of LTP is responsible for the huge learning boost most people get when they review information repeatedly. As most students know, the best way to learn something is to read it thoroughly once, and then to skim it several more times over an extended period. This method "locks in" memories by activating LTP.

Unfortunately, LTP tends to deteriorate as people age. The biological assault of cortisol and free radicals—especially upon the hippocampus—disrupts the stable biochemical environment that LTP requires.

Brain longevity patients, however, are less vulnerable to disruption of LTP, because the enhanced biochemical milieu of their brains provides adequate amounts of the chemicals that LTP requires. Also, brain longevity programs help control output of cortisol, which hampers LTP.

Though long-term memory, as you can see, can be difficult to create, accessing it can be even more difficult. The current leading memory theorists believe, however, that virtually all of your long-term memories still exist—though perhaps deeply buried.

There is, though, a grave threat to these memories: the biological ravages of time.

In the next chapter we'll look at the toll that time—and aging—can take upon the brain. And we'll look also at ways to *reverse* that toll—enabling you to overcome the tyranny of time.

A Case in Point

A Spiritual Journey

A.I., sixty-four, was a successful man, by the standard measures of success. He was the head of a major corporation, he had a nice family, and he was highly regarded as a philanthropist. But he was not a happy man.

He came to me because he could feel his cognitive function beginning to slip. He ran a company that earned hundreds of millions of dollars annually, and the demands on him were high. His job performance was hurt by even minor declines in his brain power. His memory, however, was no longer razor-sharp. In fact, my intake testing revealed that he was suffering from moderate age-associated memory impairment. In addition, he often found it almost impossible to focus for long periods of time. In midafternoon he would usually run out of energy and have to either take a nap, or perform only easy tasks. He was puffy with weight gain, and his forehead was furrowed with worry-wrinkles.

His personal life was also beginning to suffer. He was becoming increasingly short-tempered with his wife and daughters. He had a pervasive sense of malaise; he just didn't feel content with his life anymore.

He had recently been to a prominent medical clinic, but he told me the doctors there had not been able to help him. They reportedly confirmed that he was suffering from age-associated memory impairment, but had not offered him a course of drug therapy.

When I did his intake testing, his laboratory tests revealed that his kidney function was mildly impaired. Sometimes, when the kidneys aren't functioning adequately, this dysfunction will contribute to high blood pressure. A.I. did have high blood pressure, which was probably contributing to some of his cognitive decline.

From the Eastern perspective, however, his lack of adequate kidney function was somewhat more ominous. In traditional Chinese medicine, "kidney yang energy" is considered to be the wellspring of the entire body's energy flow, and is also closely related to mental function.

According to this model, his lack of kidney yang energy was responsible for his low energy, unstable mood, and sense of malaise. Because the kidneys and adrenals are adjacent to one another, traditional Chinese medicine practitioners consider both to be part of the same energy system. In Western medicine, however, this proximity is believed to be nothing more than an anatomical coincidence. Most Western doctors don't believe there's any relationship between kidney function and adrenal function (even though it's generally believed that stress is bad for the kidneys).

As I explained his brain longevity program to A.I., he looked at me with an expression of basic indifference. "You know," he said, in a rather smug tone, "it really doesn't matter much if I get better. I've already done everything there is to do. I've been around the world, I've been married three times, and I've made millions of dollars. What have I missed out on?"

At that moment I had a flash of intuition—one that gave me more insight into him than all of my scientific tests. I looked him in the eye and said, "*I* think you've missed out on something. I think you've missed out on the most important relationship you could ever have: the one with your own soul."

He sat in silence and looked at me. I didn't know whether he was going to stand up and leave, or start crying, or punch me in the nose.

Then he sat on the edge of his chair, and began to nod slowly.

"I think," he said softly, "that's the *real* reason I came to see you. I just have this *longing* for a spiritual renewal."

The next day he began his program, and threw himself into it wholeheartedly. He drastically changed his dietary habits, and began eating a mostly vegetarian diet. He began taking vitamins and natural medicinal tonics, as well as deprenyl. He incorporated the mind/body exercises into his daily routine, and started to counteract the stress in his life with various stress-management techniques, including meditation.

Within twelve weeks he had experienced a virtually complete turnaround. He lost about twenty pounds, and became fit and taut. His blood pressure normalized. His kidney function improved significantly, and his adrenals began to provide him with much more energy and buoyancy.

His cognitive function also improved dramatically. His memory grew strong again, and he no longer had trouble concentrating. He stopped feeling chronically irritable, and stopped losing his temper with his family. His energy improved, and he no longer became fatigued in the afternoon. Even the deep furrows in his forehead began to fade, as his life became less stressful.

He used his renewed energy to complete a summer camp for kids who had cancer. I was very proud of him for using his physical and mental regeneration to help others.

After he had been on his program for about a year, I felt that, in a very essential way, he had become enlightened. By this, I don't mean that he sat around all day in the lotus position, spouting wisdom. I mean that he had apparently connected with what I think of as his own "best self," or his "true identity." It had been inside him all along—but now he could *feel* it, every day. He had found the physical energy and the mental power to touch the depths of his inner self.

His journey through life was, in a sense, complete—but his spiritual journey had just begun. After a supposedly full life, he had finally begun to explore his most important relationship: the one with his own soul.

His spiritual journey was just starting, but he had already "arrived." He was, at long last, a happy man.

8

Optimal Function of the Age-Forty-five-Plus Brain: Overthrowing the Tyranny of Time

One of the terrible ironies of our modern era is that millions of people are being punished for achieving longevity. Most of those people have worked hard to avoid the risk factors associated with cancer and cardiovascular disease, the maladies that kill approximately three out of four people, but still—precisely because they are living longer than the average person—millions of them are losing their most precious possessions: their own minds.

The brain—over a period of decades—is a dreadfully vulnerable organ. In a great many elderly people, the brain fails before the heart or the lungs or the kidneys. In fact, most gerontological researchers say that up to 90 percent of persons in nursing homes suffer from moderate to serious loss of cognitive function. And, as you know, up to half of all people eighty-five or older have Alzheimer's.

Contrary to popular myth, this loss of intellect, memory, and creative problem-solving does not happen *suddenly* when a person reaches old age. It is a slow, insidious process, one that is often so gradual that it goes unnoticed.

Some researchers believe, however, that even by the time most of us have reached young adulthood, we have lost approximately one-half of our synaptic connections. Most of those connections have been grossly underutilized, and have withered from lack of use. This does not mean that we are only half as intelligent as we once were, but it does imply a certain degree of cognitive decline—and lost opportunity. It also points out how easily damaged the brain is, even in the presence of a *youthful* biochemistry.

During our twenties, most of us reached the peak of our mental capabilities. Those were our best years for laying down long-term memories and for engaging in protracted, complex thought processes. One indication of this heightened cognitive power is the fact that most people in their fifties and sixties remember their twenties better than they remember their more recent thirties and forties. Of course, a person's twenties are often filled with change, turmoil, and excitement, and this, too, aids the biological consolidation of memory.

At about thirty, though, our brains—already beset by significant neuronal loss—begin to shrink measurably. The degree of shrinkage does not, however, correspond exactly to the same degree of cognitive decline. In other words, if your brain shrinks by 10 percent, you won't necessarily suffer a 10-percent decline in intelligence. Instead, you might suffer only a 1-percent decline in cognitive ability, because the plasticity of your brain allows you to make new synaptic connections. Nonetheless, as shrinkage increases, so does cognitive decline.

For unknown reasons, men lose brain tissue significantly faster than woman. Recent examinations with CAT and PET scans indicate that men may lose brain cells as much as three times faster than women. By midlife, the brains of males—which are larger than female brains early in life—generally shrink to about the same size as female brains, though an increase in metabolic activity apparently compensates for some of the decline in size. Some researchers think this phenomenon may be one reason females live longer than males.

After about age forty to fifty, there is at least a 2-percent decrease in overall brain weight every decade. This may not sound

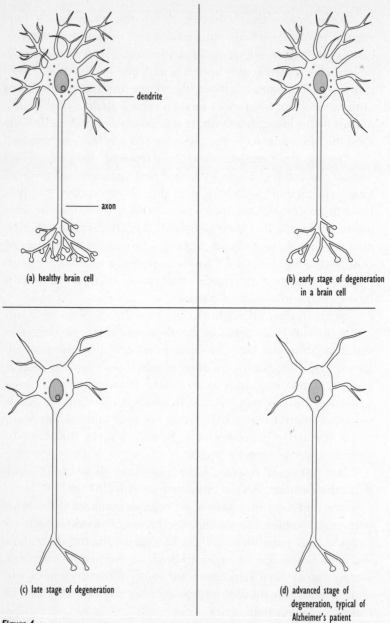

(a) healthy brain cell

dendrite

axon

(b) early stage of degeneration in a brain cell

(c) late stage of degeneration

(d) advanced stage of degeneration, typical of Alzheimer's patient

Figure 6
As the years pass, the brain cells of Alzheimer's patients wither and die. The number of dendrites declines drastically, resulting in degeneration of the brain cell.

particularly dire, but the areas of the brain that are most closely associated with memory are hit hardest. The limbic system's hippocampus and amygdala, for example, commonly shrink by about 20 to 25 percent by the time a person reaches sixty to seventy. Also, the myelin sheath, which "insulates" neurons, appears to decline more in the limbic areas than in other parts of the nervous system.

As memory declines, there is also often a decline in creativity. This may be because creativity is closely bound to memory. The current most prominent theory about creativity is that it consists of the brain "taking inventory" of everything it knows about a subject, and then stringing together disparate elements of that knowledge in a novel, inventive way. To do this well, a person must have mastery over his or her ability to *recall* memories, and must be able to *focus* intently on those memories.

Studies on creativity indicate that many creative people, including novelists and mathematicians, do their most creative work in their twenties. Similarly, chess players, who rely on creativity as well as logic, generally begin to decline in skill during their forties. Studies indicate that younger chess players are better able than older players to consider a larger number of potential moves. Younger players can do this simply because they have a larger neural network of memory traces than older players.

By the time most people reach their sixties, they have begun to suffer from a noticeable decline in cognitive ability. Most people, by this time, have lost a significant degree of their ability to memorize facts, and to focus intensely. This cognitive decline is often characterized by a decreased ability to match names and faces, recall phone numbers, or learn new material.

In addition, most people of this age suffer from a decline in *fluid intelligence*, the measure of intelligence that's based on current processing skills, instead of knowledge.

Also, most people who are sixty or older aren't as capable of doing complex tasks as quickly as younger people, partly because the overall speed of their entire nervous system has begun to slow down.

Often, at around age fifty to sixty, people become less able to do two things at once (in the current age of "multitasking," this can be a serious problem), and they begin to have more problems than young people at learning complex new mental skills. This may account for the adage, "You can't teach an old dog new tricks."

As you can see, it is not just memory that generally begins to decline as we age, but overall cognitive function. In fact, approaching Alzheimer's is usually indicated more by a decline in cognitive function than a decline in memory.

Of course, memory, too, does often begin to deteriorate noticeably at about age fifty. Both visual and auditory memory may begin to decline at that age, while kinesthetic memory remains mostly intact. Auditory memory declines slightly faster than visual memory until about age eighty. At about eighty, though, the loss of visual memory exceeds the loss of auditory memory.

One recent study indicated that, in a cross-section of generally healthy people, memory declined by an average of 25 percent between the ages of twenty-five to eighty.

Over this same period, the decline of many brain-related endocrine functions is even more precipitous. These include maintenance of energy, stability of sex drive, ability to sleep, and ability to maintain muscle mass. Similarly, endocrine-related mood disorders generally increase during the aging process. These mood disorders may be subtle, evidenced merely as a loss of zest for life.

One apparent reason for memory loss in many elderly people is that they generally are less able to encode their memories as richly as young people do, with various "versions" of each memory. This interferes with recall, because there are fewer associations to support each memory. Many older people, though, also show elevated memory loss even when they are given associations, in the form of "cues," that would normally trigger memories. Thus they have not only a reduced ability to lay down multiple versions of new memories, but a reduced ability to retrieve existing memories.

Clearly, then, the brains of most people deteriorate as they age, but this deterioration does not happen to everyone. Nearly one-third of all people enjoy steady lucidity as they age. In one major study, approximately 25 to 30 percent of all eighty-year-olds performed as well on cognitive function tests as young people did. In this study, some people in their eighties and nineties performed *better* than the vast majority of young people.

Thus, cognitive deterioration during aging *is not inevitable,* even though the phenomenon can be relatively hard to escape. It's my belief, of course, that a person can most effectively escape brain aging by beginning a brain longevity program.

To better appreciate the value of such a program, let's look at *why* the brain deteriorates during aging. Then, once we understand why it happens, we'll look at biological strategies that can stop it from happening.

Why the Brain Deteriorates with Age

Why does the brain deteriorate? Simple answer: Because it's flesh and blood. That's the bad news. But it's also the good news—because any flesh-and-blood organ can, with the right maintenance and rejuvenation program, be encouraged to function properly throughout a person's entire life.

One of the primary causes of age-associated cognitive deterioration is the significant decline of neurotransmitters in aging people. Probably the most important neurotransmitter deficiency is a decrease in acetylcholine. As you may remember, acetylcholine is the primary carrier of memory. Almost all people with Alzheimer's show a marked deficit of acetylcholine; this shortage is especially severe in the memory circuits of the temporal lobe, where many long-term memories are stored.

An acetylcholine shortage means that even if part of a memory trace is still intact within a neuron, it may be unable to connect with other parts of the memory in other neurons, because its "transportation system" is not working properly. This phenomenon also accounts for the fragmentary memories that often characterize age-associated memory impairment. Many of my patients have such "holes" in their memories—the condition I call "Swiss cheese" memory.

Acetylcholine is not the only neurotransmitter that declines in people with age-associated memory impairment. Other important neurotransmitters that become depleted include serotonin, dopamine, and norepinephrine. There is also often a decline in certain neuropeptides, such as endorphins. Endorphin decline not only affects our moods, but also harms immunity. Though we generally think of endorphins as just being good for mood, they're also a vital link between the mind and the immune system.

Because serotonin and norepinephrine are important to the maintenance of good mood, it's probable that a lack of these neurotransmitters contributes to the frequent negative moods and depression that many older people suffer from. Thus, it's quite likely that the clichés of "grumpy old men" and "crotchety old women" have a biological root.

It's also clear that clinical, biological depression tends to increase during the aging process. More than 6 million of the current 40 million Americans age sixty-five and older will experience depression. A recent survey indicated that more than half of all older Americans consider depression a natural part of aging.

However, the neurotransmitter shortages that cause depression and other mood disorders can usually be overcome rather quickly, through a number of nutritional and pharmacological approaches. Frequently my patients show dramatic, almost instantaneous reversals in cognitive decline and mood disorders shortly after their programs begin.

One fifty-five-year-old patient of mine, for example, improved significantly within *one hour* after I administered specific concentrated nutrients (phosphatidyl choline, phosphatidyl serine, and acetyl L-carnitine), which restored his neurotransmitter function. This patient was, of course, amazed and overjoyed at the speed of the response.

Another factor that badly injures the aging brain is impaired circulation. Decreased blood flow in elderly people hurts the function of virtually all of their major organs—including their brains. Because the brain uses about 25 percent of all blood pumped by the heart, it is particularly vulnerable to any deficiencies of the circulatory system.

About 20 percent of *all cases* of serious cognitive decline in the elderly result from poor circulation. Very often, people who think they have Alzheimer's are actually victims of a series of minor strokes that have severely impaired the brain.

Even more common than minor strokes is a general mental lassitude caused by decreased blood flow to the brain, which also contributes to the slow degeneration of the brain, by allowing millions of neurons to die gradually.

Patients on brain longevity programs are generally much less susceptible than most people to brain damage from impaired circulation. Many aspects of my brain longevity program address circulation; these include nutritional therapy; administration of natural medicinal tonics and of certain pharmaceutical medications and food supplements; and exercise (especially the mind/body exercises). Even stress reduction helps circulation, by helping lower high blood pressure.

As I've said before, what's good for the heart is good for the head.

Another major contributor to the decline of the aging brain is cortisol.

As noted in chapter 2, cortisol damages the brain in three primary ways.

First, it interferes with the brain's supply of glucose, the "fuel" that powers the brain. When this happens, new memories are hard to lay down, and existing memories are hard to retrieve.

Second, it interferes with the function of neurotransmitters.

Third, it causes an excessive influx of calcium into brain cells, and this calcium—over a long period—creates free-radical molecules that cause dysfunction of the brain cells, and eventually kill brain cells. Billions of neurons die from this phenomenon, and billions more are badly damaged.

When the brains of Alzheimer's patients are examined at autopsy, there is virtually always evidence of a great deal of calcium buildup in brain cells.

Neuronal death from excessive cortisol is especially apparent in the hippocampus and the amygdala. Because these are the primary "sorting and shipping" areas for memories, memory is particularly damaged by cortisol during the aging process.

Memory is not the only cognitive function that is hurt by excessive cortisol. People whose brains have been damaged by cortisol also have difficulty focusing their attention for extended periods. This, of course, prevents adequate storage of memory, and also interferes with general intellectual function. It hurts high-speed cognitive processing, and it hurts creativity.

Excessive cortisol production also severely interferes with the phenomenon of long-term potentiation—the ability of a brain cell to process a memory with greater ease during repeated exposures. Excessive cortisol suppresses long-term potentiation by interfering with the neuronal receptors that "catch" memories as they cross synapses. Because of this, people with excessive cortisol production *lose the ability* to absorb information easily by quickly reviewing it. Each time that people suffering from cortisol overproduction review information, it's as hard for them to process as it was the first time they saw it. This makes learning much more difficult.

Cortisol's damage to memory, learning, and general cognitive function was proven recently in a joint study by the University of Montreal and McGill University. The study was funded by the American Alzheimer's Association and the National Institutes of Health. In this study, directed by Dr. Sonia Lupien, researchers studied a group of elderly patients over a four-year period. They found that increases in these patients' cortisol levels accurately predicted *decreases* in memory and cognitive function. They also found that patients with low cortisol levels performed as well on cognitive tests as young people.

I believe it's extremely encouraging that elderly people with low cortisol levels can equal the mental function of younger people. This clearly indicates that deterioration of the brain during aging is *not* inevitable.

The subjects in the study with healthy brains had apparently found ways to control their cortisol levels. Unfortunately, this can be very difficult for people as they age—because of a destructive phenomenon called the "feedforward mechanism," one of the worst problems that afflicts aging brains.

Normally, when too much cortisol is secreted, the brain

senses the oversecretion, and stops further production of cortisol. This is the brain's normal "feedback mechanism." Many years of damage by cortisol ruins the feedback mechanism, transforming it into the harmful feedforward mechanism.

Here's how that happens, in biological terms:

Normally, in response to stress, the hypothalamus secretes a substance called *corticotropin-releasing factor,* which then causes the pituitary gland to secrete a hormone called *corticotropin* (or ACTH). ACTH then causes the adrenals to secrete cortisol. When levels of cortisol rise to a certain degree—a "setpoint"—several areas of the brain tell the hypothalamus to turn off the cortisol-producing mechanism. This is the proper "feedback" response.

However, one of the areas of the brain that is most responsible for telling the hypothalamus to turn off cortisol production is the hippocampus. And the hippocampus, as we've seen, is the area that is most damaged by cortisol. The hippocampus is often so damaged in older people—who may have lost about 20 to 25 percent of their hippocampus cells—that it is unable to give the proper feedback to the hypothalamus.

When that happens, the hypothalamus keeps pumping out the chemicals that cause cortisol oversecretion.

This, in turn, causes even more damage to the hippocampus. And this, of course, causes *even more cortisol production.*

Thus, a catch-22, "degenerative cascade" begins. And this cascade can be *very* difficult to stop.

The net result is that many middle-aged and older people simply can't control their production of cortisol. Even when they are not under stress, they secrete high amounts of the hormone.

The effects of this degenerative cascade can be anxiety, irritability, inability to relax, and difficulty in sleeping—as well as memory and concentration impairment.

An interesting study was done recently that illustrates how the feedforward mechanism makes it especially hard for some older people to shut off their biological response to stress. In the study, two groups of men—one older group and one younger group—were monitored for stress while they played miniature golf. Miniature golf was chosen as a stress test because it is an exacting procedure that requires a great deal of concentration and self-control. The players in the study played in casual practice rounds, and then in relatively intense competition rounds. The researchers found that the older players played as well as the younger players during the practice rounds, but that their performance deteriorated during the stressful competition rounds.

It was noted that, during competition, when younger players focused on an upcoming shot, their heart rates would fall, then speed up again after the shot. The lowered heart rate before the shot indicated concentration, and the ability to "tune out" stress. When the older players focused on their upcoming shots, however, their heart rates did *not* fall. This indicated that their concentration was not as strong, and that they were unable to force themselves to calm down, and "tune out" stress.

It's interesting to note that among professional golfers, the first skill to erode during the aging process is generally putting. One might assume, of course, that the first skill to deteriorate would be a golfer's driving, since it requires strength and flexibility, but putting—which requires calmness and focus—almost always deteriorates before driving. I believe this happens because of the feedforward mechanism. Older pro golfers, most of whom have been under considerable stress almost all of their lives, just don't have as much biological ability as younger pro golfers to turn off stress.

The severity of chronic stress that a person has suffered generally determines how much he or she will suffer from the feedforward mechanism. For examples, studies of Vietnam War veterans who suffer from post-traumatic stress disorder indicate that these men have terrible difficulty in shutting off their biological response to stress. One study showed that they produced 40 percent less of the chemicals that automatically turn off the feedforward mechanism. In the vernacular, these former soldiers' "nerves are shot."

It's likely, I believe, that the feedforward mechanism is a primary culprit in the very existence of post-traumatic stress disorder. Obviously, persons with post-traumatic stress disorder have memories that haunt them—but the *biological* presence of the feedforward mechanism "locks in" those painful memories. Then the stress-producing memories perpetuate the feedforward mechanism. Thus another degenerative spiral is created.

My brain longevity programs can intervene in this spiral, by addressing not only the psychological elements of the spiral, but also the biological elements.

I'll give you one example of how the stress-induced feedforward mechanism can be avoided. The great cortisol researcher Dr. Robert Sapolsky found that if he petted laboratory rats for fifteen minutes each day during the first few weeks of the rats' lives, it prevented the rats from later suffering from the feedforward mechanism. This one simple act of nurturing was all it took to protect the animals from this insidious problem.

Humans are obviously much more complex creatures than lab rats, and need a much more sophisticated system of nurturing, but the fact remains that psychological nurturing can greatly inhibit the feedforward mechanism (by quelling the stress that perpetuates it).

Of course, my brain longevity programs address more than just psychological nurturing. They cover the gamut of psychological *and* biological nurturing.

Because of this, many of my patients are able to avoid, or to remedy, the feedforward mechanism.

How Free Radicals Cause Brain Aging

As you know, I believe that our incredibly stressful lifestyles, which create neurotoxic cortisol, contribute to accelerated brain aging. But I certainly don't think stress is the *only* factor that causes brain degeneration.

As you'll recall, cortisol doesn't *directly* kill brain cells. It kills them by creating free-radical molecules—and it's those free radicals that directly kill brain cells. Thus, anything that creates free radicals in the brain causes neurological degeneration.

Free radicals can be created by a number of factors. Even oxygen creates them as a by-product of the natural process of oxidation. Therefore, there's no possible way to avoid at least some damage from free radicals. Actually, a certain degree of free-radical formation is healthy and necessary. For example, free radicals play an important role in the function of the immune system. One element of immunity is the production of free radicals that kill foreign microbes.

The brain isn't the only part of the body that is hurt by free radicals. Every cell in the body is vulnerable. Free radicals, for example, often contribute to the formation of cancer cells. One popular theory of aging states that it is the gradual toll taken by free radicals that causes the aging process.

A free radical is any atom that has an "unpaired" electron. Normally, all electrons are present in pairs—which is the natural and healthy condition. These pairs can be "broken up," however, by a number of factors, including cortisol, such environmental toxins as pesticides, and even excessive intake of fat. When the electrons are "broken apart," both unpaired electrons search for other electrons, so that they can once again form pairs, and maintain the biological "health" of the atom. Soon the unpaired electrons find new "mates," and steal them from other atoms. Then the atoms that were "stolen from" find still more atoms to "rob." In this way a chain reaction of destruction is caused.

In each of the body's cells, an area that's especially vulnerable to destruction from free radicals is the energy-producing area called the *mitochondria*. When enough damage is done to the mitochondria, the cell can become so badly damaged that it dies. Every day, this happens to many millions of your cells—including your brain cells. Over a long period, this destruction of cells by free radicals causes the skin to harden and wrinkle, the bones to soften and shrink, the muscles to weaken, and the brain to degenerate.

However, there are therapeutic measures—utilized by brain longevity patients—that can neutralize free radicals. The most effective is nutritional therapy with "free-radical scavengers," which are also called *antioxidants*.

Some of the most effective antioxidants are vitamins C and E, the nutrient coenzyme Q-10, and the minerals zinc and selenium.

The peptide *glutathione* is an effective antioxidant, as are the amino acids *L-methionine* and *L-taurine*.

Later we'll examine in more detail the incredible restorative powers of antioxidants.

If all of the factors occur together, with sufficient severity, and if nothing is done to remedy them, the eventual result will be age-associated memory impairment—or even Alzheimer's disease.

In the next chapter we'll look at Alzheimer's disease. We'll see what causes it, how it develops, and what we can do to avoid it.

A Case in Point

The Mind and Body Are One

B.J., sixty-seven years old, had the look of someone who had been ravaged by alcohol for many years. He was gray, gaunt, and exhausted, and his skin, which had lost its elasticity, hung on him like a thick plastic bag. I believed, however, that he did not abuse alcohol. He told me that many years earlier he'd had a drinking problem, but he had overcome it. He hadn't had any alcohol for fifteen years. He'd also stopped smoking.

In addition to a general lack of vigor, he suffered from age-associated memory impairment. He still retained an excellent vocabulary, because he had long been a very articulate intellectual, but he now had a "Swiss cheese" memory.

The normal progression of his condition would probably have resulted in major cognitive dysfunction within about five to ten years. Without aggressive intervention, it was possible that within ten years he would have cognitive symptoms similar to those of early-stage Alzheimer's. Based on his symptoms and case history, though, I did not believe he had classic Alzheimer's.

His condition would probably not threaten his life, as would classic Alzheimer's, but the possibility of the worsening of his symptoms filled B.J. with dread. He was proud of his fine mind.

In addition, he suffered somewhat from a mood disorder in which he became easily frustrated, and had little patience. He also exhibited an unsteady gait, which disturbed him very much. He said that being wobbly on his feet made him "feel like an old man."

Initially, I was perplexed by B.J.'s cluster of symptoms. His marked pallor, as well as the loss of turgor (elasticity) in his skin, were not common among patients whose primary complaint was age-associated memory impairment. During intake testing, though, I discovered the probable root of many of his problems. B.J., much to his surprise, was diabetic. I do not know how this problem had gone undetected, but apparently it had.

When I first tested his blood sugar, it was extremely high. After an overnight fast, it remained high, indicating probable diabetes. His condition proved to be so severe that I was afraid he might at any moment lapse into the diabetic condition of ketoacidosis, and go into a coma.

I considered hospitalizing him, but was able to control the diabetes on an outpatient basis, with dietary change and exercise. As B.J.'s diabetes stabilized, he began his brain longevity program. He modified his diet a great deal; this wasn't very hard for him to do, because he no longer craved sweets (as do most untreated diabetics). He began doing mind/body exercises and started taking deprenyl and a number of nutritional supplements and natural medicinal tonics.

He experienced a dramatic shift in cognitive function. On his way home from consulting with me, he endured a long wait in the Dallas airport without becoming emotionally upset. Normally, he told me, a frustrating experience like that would have "driven him crazy."

His memory improved almost immediately, and his ability to concentrate became considerably enhanced. Within a short time, his color was much more normal, and his skin regained some of its natural elasticity. Gradually he overcame his unsteady gait. I believe that the impressive, sudden benefits B.J. experienced stemmed less from his brain longevity program than from the proper treatment of his diabetes.

It's very important to realize that serious physical ailments, including diabetes, can have a profound effect upon cognition. Diabetes, for example, starves the brain of glucose, its only source of energy. This starvation disturbs cognitive function, as well as mood. If B.J. had adhered closely to his brain longevity program, but not treated his diabetes, his decline would almost certainly have continued.

I fear to think what would have happened to B.J. if he had sought treatment for his cognitive problems from a narrowly focused specialist. If, for example, he had been treated by a neurologist who had not noticed the diabetes, the consequences might have been disastrous.

In B.J., I saw evidence, once again, of an important phenomenon: *The body can control the brain,* just as the brain can control the body. If the body is suffering from a serious illness, the brain may very well be affected as well. Thus, to nurture the brain effectively, you must nurture the body, too.

Brain longevity programs are much more than just programs designed to enhance the longevity of the brain; they are also *body longevity programs.* The mind and body are one.

9

Avoiding the Tragedy of Alzheimer's Disease

Alzheimer's disease was first noted clinically in 1907 by a German physician named Alois Alzheimer. Dr. Alzheimer discovered the disease in a relatively young person, but it soon became apparent that the disease was far more common among elderly people.

Currently, the formal medical term for Alzheimer's disease is "senile dementia/Alzheimer's type," or SDAT. In most developed nations, Alzheimer's is the third-most-common cause of death by disease, after cardiovascular disease and cancer. When a patient is diagnosed with Alzheimer's, his or her life expectancy decreases by about one-third, compared to that of a healthy person the same age.

Although memory loss is the most widely known symptom of Alzheimer's, the disease impairs many other elements of cognitive function. For example, the ability for abstract thought declines, and so does judgment. Emotional and behavioral changes are also common. Often the first sign of approaching Alzheimer's is not memory loss, but difficulty in carrying out complex thought processes.

In the later stages of Alzheimer's, dysfunction of the brain becomes profound and extensive. Patients often lose not just all of their memories, but also their personalities, and even their ability to effectively move their own bodies.

By the time Alzheimer's patients die, their brains have generally suffered from two disturbing biological changes. One is the widespread development of abnormal fibers in the brain cells' cytoplasm, the jellylike substance that surrounds the nucleus. These abnormal fibers look like a tangle of threads, so they're called *neurofibrillary tangles*. The tangles hurt the function of brain cells, and eventually kill them. The tangles are composed of tiny tubes and filaments that normally run in smooth, symmetrical lines through brain cells. These tubes and filaments, when healthy, provide structural support, and help move nutrients through the cells. In Alzheimer's patients, though, they become terribly disorganized, and knot themselves into the tangles that eventually destroy the entire cell. They occur most frequently in the hippocampus, the brain's primary memory center. Therefore, the hippocampus is the brain area most likely to suffer damage from Alzheimer's.

The other deadly change that occurs in the brain cells of Alzheimer's patients is the accumulation of clots of dead cellular material. These clots of debris, which are about the size of BBs, are called *senile plaques*. The senile plaques accumulate around a core of a partial protein called *amyloid*. Senile plaques, like neurofibrillary tangles, interfere with the function of brain cells, and eventually kill them.

Tangles and plaques are especially harmful to the delicate dendrites of brain cells; in Alzheimer's patients, billions of dendrites wither and die. Both senile plaques and neurofibrillary tangles can eventually infest most of the brain, but they are *not* widely found in one notable area: the cerebellum. The cerebellum, you will recall, governs movement of the body. Memories about movement, therefore, are almost always the very last to be destroyed by Alzheimer's. "Motor memories" do not begin to fade until the areas surrounding the cerebellum are devastated.

Besides plaques and tangles, the other most noticeable change that occurs in the brains of Alzheimer's patients is a decrease in the amount of the neurotransmitter acetylcholine. Acetylcholine, the primary carrier of memory, can diminish by more than 90 percent in Alzheimer's patients. When it reaches this very low level, the patient is largely unable to form new memories, or to effectively gain access to existing memories.

As brain cells die in the Alzheimer's patient, his or her brain shrinks, and changes shape. The brain of even a relatively young Alzheimer's patient shrinks to the size of a very elderly person's brain. As the brain decreases in size, its inner "open" spaces (or ventricles) increase in size, while the outer layer of neocortex becomes thinner, and less dense with cells.

Researchers still do not agree on *why* all these changes occur. One reason they may occur is genetic predisposition. In the mid-1990s, researchers discovered that a certain gene, *apo E* (apolipoprotein E), is linked to incidence of Alzheimer's. Apo E comes in three varieties: E-2, E-3, and E-4. E-2 *protects* people from Alzheimer's. E-4 makes Alzheimer's onset much more likely. E-3, which is the most common apo-E gene, is linked to possible risk of Alzheimer's.

Because you inherited two copies of all of your genes—one from each of your parents—you have one of six possible combinations of these three apo E genes.

The worst genetic fate you can have is to carry two E-4 genes, as does 2 to 3 percent of the population. If you do, you may have up to a 90-percent chance of having Alzheimer's by age eighty. However, I believe you can reduce these odds by engaging in a brain longevity program.

The best genetic fate you could have is to carry two E-2 genes. Although this condition is uncommon, it provides great protection against Alzheimer's.

If you have one or two E-3 genes, your likelihood of having Alzheimer's falls somewhere in a mid-range category. This is the most common genetic condition.

Regardless of genetic predisposition, however, many researchers believe that onset of Alzheimer's is influenced by exposure of the brain to a variety of negative forces that are believed to kill neurons directly, and to create free-radical molecules, which subvert normal cellular function in the brain. As this occurs, neurofibrillary tangles grow, and dead cellular plaque accumulates.

What exactly are these forces?

Until recently, exposure to aluminum was considered by some researchers to be a negative force that contributed to neuronal death and damage. In fact, based on autopsy results, there does seem to be an excess of aluminum in the brains of almost all Alzheimer's patients. The excess, however, is extremely small—so small that testing for it cannot be done with regular glass beakers, because enough aluminum can leach out of the glass to ruin the test results.

Another negative force that some researchers have linked to Alzheimer's is the presence of a special type of "slow" virus that can lie dormant in the body for many years. Some researchers believe this virus eventually becomes activated in a person's elderly years, and attacks the genetic coding of brain cells.

Some physicians and researchers believe that the same general toxins that harm other organs in the body also harm the brain. These include pesticides and herbicides, various environmental pollutants, and a number of industrial chemicals.

Other experts on the disease believe that damage is done by the body's own immune system; they theorize that the immune system mistakenly produces antibodies that attack brain cells.

Yet another theory is that brain cells die because they do not receive proper amounts of certain hormones, such as the one called *nerve growth factor.*

A number of researchers think that genetic mutations in the mitochondrial "power plants" of neurons may cause Alzheimer's. Dr. Douglas Wallace of Emory University believes that as mitochondrial mutations increase with age, the possibility of Alzheimer's increases.

It has also been hypothesized that brain injuries, such as concussions, might later influence onset of Alzheimer's in some patients. Other general risk factors include cardiovascular disease, Down's syndrome, and, in late-onset cases, a history of depression more than ten years before.

Of course, another theory states that excessive cortisol production, caused by chronic stress, contributes to onset of the disease. This theory, which I obviously endorse, is quickly gaining adherents. While I favor the cortisol theory, I do not reject all the other theories. I believe that any or all of them may play at least a partial role in the onset of the disease. I further believe that the degree of damage done by each of these factors may differ greatly from patient to patient.

Just as I do not believe that there will ever be a single, isolated "magic bullet" cure for most degenerative diseases (including Alzheimer's), I also do not believe there is a single, isolated cause of most degenerative diseases. Every degenerative disease—including cardiovascular disease, cancer, and Alzheimer's—exists in a tangled, complex web that involves each person's unique biochemistry, genetic makeup, immunity, psyche, health, habits, and environment.

Because of this belief, I am certain that the most effective therapy for most degenerative diseases, including Alzheimer's, is a broad-based, multifaceted therapeutic program that includes nutritional therapy, stress management, exercise, lifestyle alteration, and pharmacology. Only this type of program will attack the disease on every conceivable level.

Therefore, my brain longevity programs address *all* of the reasonable theories of Alzheimer's causation. The programs do not rejuvenate only brains damaged by excessive cortisol; they also rejuvenate those damaged by any number of causes. How? Quite simply, by restoring health instead of just trying to fight disease. My programs are, in the final analysis, not "anti-Alzheimer's" programs; they are "pro-brain" programs.

Diagnosing Alzheimer's

The only absolutely accurate way to diagnose Alzheimer's is to examine the brain tissue of a deceased Alzheimer's patient. But the disease *can* be diagnosed with about 95-percent accuracy through cognitive function tests, and with advanced imaging techniques.

The technological progress now being made on advanced imaging techniques is extremely promising. In fact, researchers at the University of Arizona have developed a brain scan that may be able to detect the onset of Alzheimer's at its inception, even before symptoms arise.

For many patients, however, relatively simple cognitive function tests can reveal probable Alzheimer's. When I see new patients who are suffering from apparent cognitive impairment, I give them a number of tests. Some determine the severity of the impairment, while others help determine its cause.

It's important to remember that only half of all patients with severe cognitive impairment are suffering from Alzheimer's. Most of the rest are suffering from cognitive decline caused by multiple minor strokes, clinical depression, or lifestyle errors (such as excessive alcohol consumption or substandard nutrition).

When I first meet patients, I get their complete medical histories. Sometimes, if their memory loss is extensive, a family member will help them prepare and present the medical history. I also try to learn each patient's personal history; this can help me to determine how much stress they've been subjected to, and how they deal with stress. It also helps me understand other lifestyle factors, such as diet or chronic exposure to toxins, that may be contributing to their problem. In addition, it helps me to get to *know* the patients, and that's important to me because I don't treat diseases; I treat *people*.

I also give each patient a thorough physical exam. This not only determines possible loss of sensory and motor functions, but also sometimes helps me to uncover physical conditions that may be contributing to cognitive impairment. This phase of testing generally includes a complete blood count (which detects possible anemia, leukemia, and chronic infection), a urinalysis (which detects diabetes, and diseases of the kidneys and liver), and an electrolyte test (which can detect metabolic abnormalities). I also perform tests to determine the function of every major organ system. Other tests include an assay of cholesterol, high-density and low-density lipids, triglycerides, and the hormones DHEA and IGF-1 (a marker of growth hormone).

Probably the most helpful tests in determining the *extent* of cognitive dysfunction are the intellectual ability tests I administer. One is my cognitive function questionnaire, which I included in chapter

1 of this book. Mostly, though, I rely upon a short general screening test that determines overall cognitive function. This simple exam includes tests of orientation, attention, short-term recall, ability to do simple arithmetic, ability to follow three-stage commands, ability to identify common objects, and visual-spatial ability. I also pinpoint the patient's placement on the Global Deterioration Scale.

Another self-scored test I give patients is my Brain Longevity Stress Impact Index, which you'll find in chapter 14. As you'll see, this test is an adaptation of standard stress inventory tests, but it includes an important variation, in that it evaluates not only *how many* stressful events people have experienced, as do other stress inventory tests, but also how they have *perceived* these events. For example, losing a job may affect two people very differently. One person may have loved the job, and be very traumatized by losing it, while another may have hated the job, and be glad to be rid of it.

Other doctors use similar tests to determine cognitive function. Common tests include the Wechsler Adult Intelligence Test, and the Wechsler Memory Scale. The intelligence test consists of reasoning-skill questions such as, "If two buttons cost fifteen cents, what will be the cost of a dozen buttons?" The memory scale test includes subtracting by sevens, and also a test for memory of a simple story. Here's one such story:

"A man in Chicago got on an elevator on the eighth floor and rode to the tenth floor. On the tenth floor, the elevator got stuck, and a repairman came to let the man out. The man had to take the stairs, and was late for his appointment."

Patients are asked to repeat the story immediately, and then to repeat it again in fifteen minutes. They are given one point for remembering each of these details:

1. Chicago
2. elevator
3. eighth floor
4. tenth floor
5. stuck
6. repairman
7. stairs
8. late for appointment

Most cognitively healthy people remember five to eight details immediately after the story. The important element of the test, though, is how many details they can remember after fifteen minutes. Cognitively healthy people usually forget only one detail, or two at the most. People with early-stage Alzheimer's, though, may recall only one or two details.

In addition to cognitive-function tests, another diagnostic method that can be extremely valuable is the use of advanced imaging techniques. These include CAT scans (computerized axial tomograms), MRIs (magnetic resonance imaging), and PET scans (positron emission transaxial tomography).

A CAT scan is essentially a computer-enhanced X ray. It can detect shrinkage of the brain, thinning of the neocortex, expansion of the brain's "open spaces," and the presence of neurofibrillary tangles and senile plaques. A CAT scan can't provide a definitive diagnosis of Alzheimer's, but it can indicate a probability.

An MRI is more sensitive than a CAT scan; it can even detect tiny burst capillaries, which can harm cognitive function.

A PET scan provides a "moving picture" of the interior of the brain, and monitors how much glucose is being used by various parts of the brain. If an abnormally low amount of glucose is being used, it indicates impairment. The brains of Alzheimer's patients use much less glucose than do the brains of healthy patients, because so many brain cells are dead.

With this extensive battery of diagnostic measures, the presence of Alzheimer's can almost always be accurately identified.

The Stages and Symptoms of Alzheimer's

As you may remember from chapter 1, Alzheimer's is a disease that destroys the mind over an approximately ten-to-twenty-year period.

Before onset of frank Alzheimer's, a patient might experience up to seven years of cognitive decline, suffering from symptoms that are extremely similar to the symptoms of mild age-associated memory impairment.

Frequently symptoms wax and wane, but the progression to total failure of the brain has long been considered inexorable.

Of course, this dire assessment of Alzheimer's progression is based upon treatment of the disease with conventional protocols, which are notably unaggressive. I believe, based upon my clinical successes, and upon recent research in the field, that aggressive intervention can significantly retard progression.

Interestingly, the very earliest, mildest symptoms of Alzheimer's may actually be present up to *sixty years* before onset of frank Alzheimer's. This rather shocking piece of news surfaced in 1996, with the release of the well-known "Nun's Study." The "Nun's Study" was a long-term examination of a group of 104 nuns from the School Sisters of Notre Dame. The study included a postmortem examination of the brains of twenty-five nuns who died. Ten of them had Alzheimer's.

The study examined the language abilities of the nuns early in their lives, at an average age of twenty-two years, assessed by studying their early writings. Nine of the ten nuns who developed Alzheimer's had relatively poor language skills, even in their early twenties, whereas only 13 percent of the nuns who had *good* language skills in their twenties developed Alzheimer's. Researchers concluded that the disease might have been affecting the women even when they were in their twenties.

In most people, however, noticeable negative symptoms do not appear until well past middle age.

The symptomatic distinctions that divide so-called normal age-associated memory impairment from early Alzheimer's disease are essentially matters of degree. People with age-associated memory impairment, as well as people with early Alzheimer's, may have difficulty recalling certain words, or names of friends, or locations of objects (such as car keys). They may also suffer from concentration difficulties, and have trouble sustaining complex thought processes for extended periods. Their ability to retain information may decline, and they may frequently get lost when traveling to unfamiliar places. Often people with these symptoms suffer anxiety because of them, but are defensive about their cognitive problems.

These symptoms are not, however, considered indicative of early Alzheimer's until they become progressive, worsening from year to year.

Frequently a diagnosis of early Alzheimer's is withheld until the symptoms begin to interfere markedly with a person's life. When this occurs, the patient is no longer considered to have benign senescent forgetfulness, but instead is considered to have early-stage Alzheimer's.

As you can see, the symptomatic distinctions used to reach the diagnosis of Alzheimer's can be rather arbitrary. The diagnosis may depend in part upon the daily responsibilities of the patient. If he or she has no significant responsibilities, the condition of forgetfulness may be considered essentially benign, because it causes only minor annoyance. If, however, the patient has a demanding job, his or her memory lapses may have an extremely negative impact, which might elicit a diagnosis of early Alzheimer's.

As mentioned at the beginning of this section, a patient who eventually converts to dementia may live in the "gray area" between age-associated memory impairment and Alzheimer's for about seven years. After approximately that interval, though, frank Alzheimer's symptoms may begin to appear—especially if the patient remains therapeutically passive, and is not on a brain longevity program.

Detecting Early Alzheimer's

Patients in the early stage of frank Alzheimer's, which lasts about two years, generally are unable to perform relatively complex professional and personal tasks, such as managing personal finances, or planning business strategies.

The early stages of frank Alzheimer's are characterized by symptoms that are similar to those of severe age-associated memory impairment. This is, of course, often frightening for people with age-associated memory impairment, because they fear that they will soon begin suffering from frank Alzheimer's, but most people with age-associated memory impairment never develop full-blown Alzheimer's.

Most people who have Alzheimer's *did,* however, suffer from symptoms similar to those of age-associated memory impairment during their midlife years. Partly because of this phenomenon, and partly because the symptoms of early Alzheimer's are so similar to those of age-associated memory impairment, I believe that in many patients the two problems exist on a continuum.

Nevertheless, I must stress that age-associated memory impairment is not a definite predictor of Alzheimer's, even though a subpopulation of people with age-associated memory impairment will progress to Alzheimer's disease.

Patients with frank early Alzheimer's virtually always have difficulty creating new memories, because of damage to the hippocampus. They generally have a decreased ability to remember recent events in their own lives, and have difficulty recalling current public events. They also usually have problems with relatively simple cognitive processing skills, such as counting backward by sevens. Because of this, their ability to solve problems often decreases.

They may have difficulty traveling, even to familiar places. They may also begin to develop a few gaps in their recollections of their own personal histories. This indicates that their retrieval mechanisms are beginning to weaken, partly because of decreased levels of acetylcholine.

There is also often a decrease in emotional response, which doctors refer to as a "flattening of affect." This occurs mostly because of deterioration of the brain's limbic system, its "emotional center."

As noted, these early Alzheimer's symptoms generally persist at this level for about two years—if nothing is done to counteract them. And, usually, nothing *is* done. Unfortunately, the approach espoused by most doctors is simply to "wait and see" if symptoms worsen. Almost invariably, when no therapy is undertaken, symptoms do worsen.

This passive approach will probably soon change for two reasons: (1) the increasing acceptance of multimodality therapeutic programs, such as my brain longevity programs; and (2) the development of new drugs, which we can hope will be more effective than those in current use.

Unfortunately, though, many patients now accept a passive therapeutic approach, partly because they are in denial about their problem. Ironically, many of them are in denial precisely because they have been told that nothing can be done for them. If they were told that they could be helped, many patients would probably reconcile their denial, and face the problem squarely.

Detecting Moderate Alzheimer's

After about two years of early frank Alzheimer's symptoms, the patient generally progresses to a stage of "moderate Alzheimer's." This stage, which lasts about eighteen months to two years, is characterized by the increased inability of patients to remember significant and simple aspects about their current lives, such as their own addresses, or the names of some of their family members. They also begin to become somewhat disoriented about time, sometimes confusing the time of the day, the day of the week, or the season of the year. Their cognitive processing skills deteriorate significantly, to the point where it can be difficult for them even to decide which clothes to wear. Complex problems at work become virtually impossible to solve.

During this stage of the illness, patients lose not just current (hippocampus-processed) memories, but also remote memories from the distant past. Those memories, although well consolidated for many years, are no longer easily accessible. This is a result not only of neuronal death in the neocortex, but also extreme shortages of various neurotransmitters (particularly acetylcholine). People may forget the schools they attended, and other vital details about their pasts.

At this stage, most patients are unable to live without some assistance.

By the end of this stage, it has probably been about eleven years since onset of minor cognitive problems. Unfortunately, progression of the disease begins to accelerate at this point—in the absence of an aggressive therapeutic program.

At this stage, the disease will be very apparent to family members, though some patients may still be in denial about their symptoms.

Detecting Moderately Severe Alzheimer's

During the next stage, which lasts about two to three years, the patient loses most of his or her ability to lay down new memories, as function of the hippocampus and amygdala become grossly deficient. Patients are usually no longer able to remember events from one day to the next, and lose their ability to follow current events. Thus they begin to live in an "eternal present."

Also, as the neocortex becomes increasingly damaged by neuronal loss, and as neurotransmitter levels continue to decline, patients lose access to vast banks of previously processed memories. Often a patient becomes unable even to remember the name of his or her own spouse. One Alzheimer's patient of mine, a seventy-year-old man, carried a piece of paper in his pocket with his wife's name on it.

Emotional changes become much more pronounced at this point. The "emotional" limbic system and the "rational" neocortex are no longer able to have coherent "dialogues" about behavior. Increasingly, as the limbic system becomes isolated from the neocortex, patients engage in behavior that may seem emotionally satisfying to them at the time, but is actually quite irrational. Their behavior is sometimes rather similar to the behavior of people on drugs or alcohol, because these substances also often sever the "dialogue" between the neocortex and the limbic system.

Another cause of emotional turmoil is dysfunction of neurotransmitters and hormones that are involved with emotion. Emotional changes that may occur include increased impulsiveness, delusional thinking, paranoia, and obsession. Such emotional changes are often much more devastating to the patient than loss of memory. Not only is the emotional turmoil painful, but it also alienates family members and caregivers, upon whom the patient is now extremely dependent. Frequently, patients become very angry at family members, and make bizarre accusations against them.

By this time, cognitive processing skills have become terribly eroded. The patient may be unable to count backward from ten, by ones, and has virtually no creative problem-solving skills. The ability of the neocortex to make logical associations among related memory traces begins to vanish. The vocabulary shrinks drastically. Even routine living skills, such as brushing one's teeth, become difficult.

At this stage there is even degeneration of the cerebellum, which was previously spared from damage. Because the cerebellum governs movement of the body, there is a loss of coordination and a decrease in some motor skills. One symptom of this is urinary and fecal incontinence.

By the end of this stage of the disease, it may have been as long as thirteen or fourteen years since the onset of mild memory impairment. Nonetheless, the patient may remain alive for up to seven more years.

The long course of the disease often destroys family finances, and even family cohesion.

Obviously, Alzheimer's is a very slowly progressing disease. That's why any therapeutic program that can significantly retard this already slow progression can be extremely valuable. If a person does not begin to suffer from cognitive decline until he or she is sixty-five or seventy-five years old, any significant retardation of the disease can mean that the person will die of old age long before the worst symptoms strike.

Avoiding the worst symptoms, because of death, may seem an ironic victory. But, believe me, to families who face this crisis, such a victory can be of monumental benefit.

Detecting Severe Alzheimer's

The final stage of Alzheimer's is by far the most difficult and debilitating. Unhappily, this stage can last for as long as seven years.

If even this final stage of the disease could be avoided, the patient—and his or her family—could be spared terrible suffering.

During the first phase of the final stage, which lasts about a year, the vocabulary dwindles to about a dozen words. The hippocampus and amygdala are virtually nonfunctional, and the neocortex is in a state of utter deterioration. Only the cerebellum, governing bodily movement, retains a vestige of functional ability. But over the next year or two, even the cerebellum ceases to function.

When the cerebellum "crashes," the patient loses first the ability to walk, then the ability to sit upright. Many other motor skills also disappear. Over the next couple of years, as the patient descends into an essentially vegetative state, he or she loses virtually all control over the body.

As the neocortex ceases function, the vocabulary generally shrinks to just one or two words. As a rule, the last word that remains is *yes* or *no*. Sadly and touchingly, the final losses that frequently occur are loss of the ability to smile, and to hold up one's head. In a sense, the patient has regressed to the level of a newborn infant.

By this time, which may be up to twenty years after the onset of mild memory problems, the patient exists in a grim twilight between life and death. Even the human spirit is gone. The only spirit remaining in the patient, I believe, is the divine spirit. And yet, tragically, this divine spirit is caged in a body that is mostly devoid of life.

Still, even at this stage, people are able to feel pain. And still they cry out when pain strikes. Death most frequently occurs from pneumonia, or from infection. Sometimes there is no discernible cause.

Most people who contract frank Alzheimer's never reach this final stage of severe Alzheimer's. Since most people contract the illness very late in their lives, they die before the symptoms totally ravage the quality of their lives.

Based upon my clinical experiences, I believe that even the moderately severe stage of Alzheimer's can often be avoided, if a person begins a brain longevity program when symptoms of *early*

Alzheimer's begin to arise. Because of Alzheimer's slow progression, and because of its late onset, retarding the progress of the disease is an effective way of preventing destruction from it.

The slow-progressing nature of Alzheimer's is analogous to the slow progression of the most common form of prostate cancer. Almost all men in their eighties have a slow-growing malignancy in their prostate glands. But because this type of cancer progresses so slowly, and because its onset occurs so late in life, it rarely becomes a serious problem; men die from other causes before this cancer ever really hurts them.

I believe that destruction by Alzheimer's disease can be similarly avoided—if a person is willing to apply himself or herself diligently to a brain longevity program.

A Case in Point

Forty Days to a Better Brain

A.B., fifty-nine years of age, is an excellent example of a patient who responded remarkably well during his first forty days on a brain longevity program. In fact, the majority of my patients exhibit significant signs of recovery during approximately the first forty days of their programs. I describe this phenomenon in the final chapter of this book, "Forty Days to a Better Brain."

A.B. is a pastor in a Southwest city. His father had contracted Alzheimer's at about sixty-five, and his father's suffering had had a profound effect on A.B. It had saddened him, and had caused him considerable fear; he was afraid he, too, would contract Alzheimer's.

His fear of Alzheimer's grew worse when he reached his mid-fifties and began to suffer from age-associated memory impairment. His memory loss was accompanied by a notable decline in physical energy, and by chronic depression.

Even before he consulted with me, A.B. had sensed that his cognitive, emotional, and energy problems were related to stress. In his fifties he had experienced several devastating stressors. Both of his parents had been ill, and he had been very involved with their care. In addition, he had been nagged by professional burnout; his role as a pastor had seemed increasingly difficult, partly because of his diminished cognitive abilities. He hated the idea of aging, because he associated it with decline. He told me that he "dreaded the idea of falling apart, piece by piece." He said he believed that, "at sixty-five, it's all downhill."

The more he worried about the difficulties in his life, the worse his difficulties became. His memory declined to the point where he could no longer remember his day's schedule. He frequently missed appointments, and often misplaced his list of activities. He was also unable to focus well enough even to play simple card games, such as solitaire. In addition, he was unable to perform most tasks efficiently, and therefore felt chronically pressed for time.

When he began his program, he experienced several plateaus of improvement within the first few weeks. Almost immediately he noticed an increase in physical energy. Shortly after that, his depression began to lift, and his sense of well-being increased. Then his ability to focus began to improve. Soon his short-term memory became rejuvenated. Within one month he felt markedly better.

After another week to ten days he felt even better, physically as well as mentally. He had become much more efficient in his use of time. He noticed that there somehow seemed to be "more time to do the things I need to do."

He would later credit much of his success to the mind/body exercises, and to the various natural medicinal tonics he was taking.

He was skeptical about the mind/body exercises at first, because they were a very new concept to him, but he told me he got an "energy rush" from them, and felt a greater union between his mind and his body after doing them. They gave him considerably more physical energy, and he used some of this energy to play racquetball several times a week.

After his first forty days, however, A.B. ran out of his natural medicinal tonics, including ginseng and *Ginkgo biloba*. He also ran out of deprenyl. He was reluctant to buy more of these medications because he was living on a very limited income. He believed he could continue to improve without the medications, because his recently rediscovered abilities had begun to feel like an integral part of him.

But when he stopped taking the medications, he gradually began to lose his newfound zest and clarity. During the *next* forty days he declined. "Forty days to a better brain" had segued into "forty *more* days to the same *old* brain." He began to have less physical energy. Because he had less energy, he gradually stopped doing the mind/body exercises. When he stopped doing the mind/body exercises, he no longer had the energy for racquetball. His days again began to seem rushed and unsatisfying; his focus and memory were no longer sharp; his upward spiral of regeneration had again become a downward spiral of degeneration. But A.B. was an intelligent, intuitive man, and he could sense his own decline. He was not defensive about it.

Gradually, after we consulted again, he began to add all of the elements of his program back into his life. He again bought his medications, even though doing so was a financial sacrifice. He made himself exercise through sheer force of will. He again began to do the mind/body exercises, whether or not he was in the mood to do them.

Like a perennial flower emerging from winter, A.B.'s mental and emotional powers once again began to blossom.

When he recovered the full strength of his cognitive powers, A.B. did not make the same mistake again. He continued to engage in his brain longevity program—and is still doing it today.

10

More Good News: Treatable Problems That Mimic Alzheimer's

If you *are* developing cognitive problems, there is a very important, positive thing that you should know: About half of all serious cognitive problems are *not* caused by Alzheimer's, or even by age-associated memory impairment, but by other factors. And most of those factors can be avoided, or compensated for.

There are over sixty biological factors that can cause dementia, but most of them fall into one of three general categories: *clinical depression, multiple minor strokes,* and *lifestyle errors* (such as substandard nutrition, or excessive alcohol intake).

Depression accounts for about 10 percent of all cases of memory disorder and cognitive impairment; multiple minor strokes account for 20 percent; and lifestyle errors account for about another 20 percent.

Very frequently, these problems are misdiagnosed by physicians who mistakenly believe that the patient is suffering from early-stage Alzheimer's. When this happens, the patient may be institutionalized, generally in a nursing home, and the real problem is never successfully addressed.

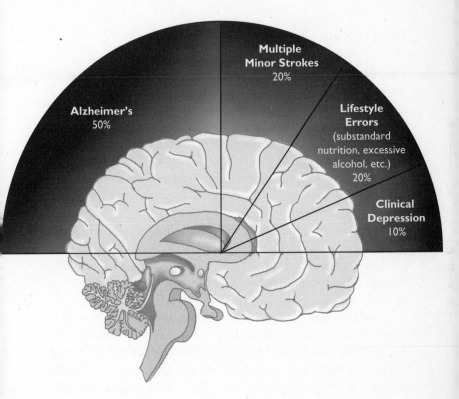

Figure 7
About half of all cases with Alzheimer's-like symptoms are actually Alzheimer's sufferers; the rest are suffering from other factors, most of which can be avoided or compensated for.

At this very moment there are probably hundreds of thousands of elderly people in nursing homes who have been labeled inaccurately as early-Alzheimer's patients. It is quite likely that many of those people will die before this misdiagnosis is corrected.

Depression

The symptoms of clinical depression often closely mimic the symptoms of early Alzheimer's, because depression severely impairs both memory and cognitive function.

Clinical depression is a biological phenomenon, characterized by changes in neurotransmitters and hormones. It is much different from simple sadness, which is caused by an unhappy experience or situation. Sadness usually decreases as time passes; clinical depression generally does not improve over time, unless it is properly treated.

A very sad experience, however, such as the death of a spouse, can trigger clinical depression, or exacerbate it. When this happens, a person must try to remedy not only his or her psychological sadness, but also the biological changes that this sadness triggers.

Older people tend to be particularly prone to depression, for three primary reasons: first, their brain biochemistries are often much more vulnerable than the neurochemistries of younger people; second, their stage of life often presents many difficulties; and, third, older people are more likely than younger people to be sedentary, and lack of exercise is a common contributor to depression.

As a result, 30 percent of all people over age sixty-five will suffer from a major clinical depression over the next three years. Unfortunately, this major depression, in itself, is a risk factor for Alzheimer's. There is a significantly increased risk of Alzheimer's ten years after onset of a major depression.

Depression mimics Alzheimer's in several ways. Clinical depression often slows down all thought processes, and all physical movements. People with clinical depression often speak very slowly, with long pauses, and have a vacant look in their eyes. Their movements are painfully slow and deliberate. This symptom, which is partly caused by a deficiency of the stimulating neurotransmitter norepinephrine, is often mistakenly considered to be a symptom of early Alzheimer's.

Memory loss is also a common symptom of clinical depression. As a rule, short-term memory suffers the most. Frequently this short-term memory impairment occurs because depressed people are inattentive to new information, as a result of which they fail to adequately lay down new memories. Their ability to lay down new memories is *also* impaired by their shortage of norepinephrine.

Women are particularly prone to memory loss from the pseudodementia of depression because they suffer from clinical depression about twice as often as men do. Some social factors play a role in the higher incidence of depression among females, but neurological factors are more frequently the cause.

Although depression often mimics early Alzheimer's, there are several ways to differentiate between the two problems.

One way is to note the pattern of progression. Depression usually is characterized by an uneven progression over a relatively short period, such as a number of weeks. Alzheimer's, however, shows a steady pattern of progression over a much more extended period, such as months or years.

Another revealing characteristic of clinical depression is that it is often worse in the morning, and then gradually improves throughout the day. In contrast, Alzheimer's symptoms are often more pronounced later in the day, because of fatigue.

Another way to tell the two diseases apart is to note how the patient *responds emotionally* to his or her memory loss. Depression sufferers tend to complain about their memory loss, while Alzheimer's victims generally tend to deny that any memory loss has occurred.

Also, people with depression are much more likely than Alzheimer's patients to try to self-medicate with alcohol or drugs.

Fortunately, clinical depression is very treatable pharmacologically. The most common treatment is administration of tricyclic antidepressants, which correct the neurotransmitter dysfunctions that cause clinical depression. Other adjunctive therapies—including counseling, meditation, increased exercise, and nutritional therapy—can also be of considerable value.

Any person who believes he or she may suffer from clinical depression should consult a physician as soon as possible. Relief may only be a few weeks away.

Multiple Minor Strokes

Another problem that is very often mistaken for early Alzheimer's is damage to the brain from a series of minor strokes. This accounts for about 20 percent of all cases of cognitive dysfunction in the elderly.

Strokes occur when the supply of blood to an area of the brain is shut off long enough to kill that area. Brain cells are very vulnerable to impaired circulation; they can survive for only one to two minutes without the oxygen and glucose that blood provides.

Blood circulation to various areas of the brain can be disrupted in two ways: Blood vessels may become blocked, or they may bleed into, or around, the brain (this usually happens when the blood vessels become hardened by atherosclerosis).

If either of these conditions occurs in a large artery, the effect is dramatic and devastating. It causes a "major stroke," which damages such a large area of the brain that the person dies, is partly paralyzed, or is left with severe cognitive impairment. But if it happens to a very small artery, the effect will be subtle, and possibly not even immediately noticeable. Nevertheless, a very small area of the brain will die, and cognitive function will be slightly impaired.

Unfortunately, in many elderly people, minor strokes occur repeatedly. Over months or years, an elderly person may be struck by a number of such strokes, or *infarctions*. If this happens too often, a person can develop *multi-infarct dementia*, which has many of the same symptoms as early Alzheimer's, in that it produces memory loss and cognitive impairment.

Although some advanced imaging techniques can reveal multiple minor infarctions, they are often difficult to detect. Thus, many people who have this problem are misdiagnosed as having Alzheimer's. Physicians are, however, becoming more aware of this diagnostic dilemma.

One major difference, though, between Alzheimer's and multi-infarct dementia is that Alzheimer's has a steadier rate of progression. Multi-infarct dementia is generally characterized by very sudden cognitive declines, which occur immediately after minor strokes. Then, as other areas of the brain begin to compensate for the damaged area, there is often a period of improvement. When another stroke hits, however, there is another immediate decline. Thus the progression of multi-infarct dementia tends to be "jerky."

A person can sometimes recover fully from a stroke, if enough of his or her brain remains sufficiently healthy to compensate for the damaged areas, but there is no medical cure for stroke.

Prevention of strokes is the best way to avoid damage from them. To prevent strokes, you should maintain proper blood pressure, refrain from eating high amounts of fat and from smoking, and get enough exercise. Of course, brain longevity programs help provide all of these stroke-prevention strategies.

Lifestyle Errors

Almost 20 percent of all cases of memory loss are caused by a wide variety of lifestyle factors, including inadequate nutrition, use of certain pharmaceutical drugs and of recreational drugs, cigarette smoking, exposure to environmental toxins, excessive intake of alcohol, and exposure to allergy-causing substances. Sometimes these factors cause only mild, transient cognitive impairment, but they may cause profound, irreparable harm.

Consuming excessive amounts of alcohol is one of the most damaging things a person can do to his or her brain. Chronic alcoholism commonly causes a deficiency of thiamine (vitamin B$_1$), which results in a debilitating neurological disease called *Korsakoff's psychosis*. This disease is characterized by extreme memory loss, and a decline of other cognitive functions.

Even limited intake of alcohol can cause some damage. Each time alcohol enters the bloodstream, it temporarily deactivates the protective mechanism called the *blood brain barrier.* This is a natural biochemical barrier that surrounds all of the capillaries in the brain, preventing them from "leaking" harmful substances from the bloodstream into the brain. When alcohol temporarily disengages this barrier, the brain is made much more vulnerable to toxic substances. Damage from these toxins can cause free-radical formation, which can result in death of neurons. Regular ingestion of relatively high amounts of alcohol partially destroys the myelin sheath that "insulates" nerve fibers. It can also cause shrinkage of internal areas of the brain.

Interestingly, even though small amounts of alcohol kill some neurons, it appears as if very moderate, long-term alcohol consumption is, on balance, relatively beneficial to cognitive function and memory. This conclusion was reached by researchers at the Indiana University School of Medicine, who performed a study on more than twelve thousand elderly twins. The group of twins who drank moderately fared slightly better than their nondrinking siblings on cognitive tests.

The researchers believed this may have occurred because of the benefit that moderate alcohol intake confers upon the cardiovascular system.

I believe it's also quite possible that moderate alcohol intake over the course of many years allowed the test subjects to better achieve regular relaxation, and to produce less cortisol.

I do not recommend alcohol consumption, however. There are many better ways than drinking alcohol to help the cardiovascular system, and to relax.

The side effects of many common pharmaceutical drugs can mimic the symptoms of Alzheimer's. Elderly people are especially vulnerable to drug side effects, because of their frequent use of medications and because the aging process generally leaves their livers less able to break down and eliminate various drugs. And because older people usually have fewer remaining neurons, each of these neurons is subjected to a relatively greater amount of each drug.

Sedatives—including such drugs as Valium, and sleep-inducing barbiturates—often cause cognitive problems. Just as excitement and stimulation biologically aid consolidation of new memories, sedation impairs the laying down of new memories. Even a mild beta blocker, which blocks the effects of adrenaline, interferes with the creation of memories. If a person takes sedatives over a long period, memories of that time can be scattered and dulled.

Cognitive and behavioral symptoms also commonly arise when sedative dosages are decreased or eliminated. Withdrawal symptoms include anxiety, agitation, and possibly delirium and even seizures.

Another negative effect of some sedatives, and also narcotics (including morphine, codeine, Darvon, and Percodan), is that they decrease normal biological drives such as appetite and the desire for movement. When this happens, the patient can become malnourished, or extremely sedentary. As mentioned previously, a very sedentary lifestyle can contribute significantly to depression and cognitive decline, and malnourishment can cause a variety of cognitive problems.

Other drugs that sometimes have a deleterious effect on cognition are antidepressants (such as Elavil, which interferes with acetylcholine production). The brain can be harmed by drugs taken to lower blood pressure, and by drugs used for Parkinson's disease. Steroidal hormones can also cause serious mental side effects.

If you are taking any of the aforementioned drugs, you should find out about any possible cognitive side effects. Then, if you begin to suffer from any of those side effects, you should speak to your physician about altering the course of your medication.

Recreational drugs can also take a heavy toll upon the brain. Thus far, use of recreational drugs among the aging has not been a significant problem; this is gradually changing, though, as the baby-boom generation reaches midlife.

The recreational drugs with the most obvious cognitive side effects are stimulants (such as cocaine and amphetamines), and marijuana.

All powerful stimulants, including cocaine, are notably harmful to the brain, and also to the endocrine system. These drugs cause an immediate oversecretion of all the stimulating catecholamine neurotransmitters, followed by a sharp drop in the availability of these neurotransmitters. When these neurotransmitters have been depleted, consolidation of new memories becomes almost impossible. That's why some cocaine abusers experience a "blackout" of memories during their binges. Cocaine also has a depleting effect upon the "feel good" neurotransmitter dopamine.

Marijuana has less severe effects, but is still markedly harmful to the creation of short-term memories, because of its interference with the production and utilization of acetylcholine. Acetylcholine disturbance can be compensated for by ingestion of choline, the nutritional precursor of acetylcholine, which is found in lecithin. Still, marijuana use can make it difficult to return acetylcholine levels to normal.

I've had a number of patients who were chronic abusers of marijuana. One patient in his mid-thirties had used marijuana almost every day for many years, and suffered from a considerable deficit of short-term memory. Fortunately, though, when he began a brain longevity program, not only did his memory problem clear up, but he also felt much less desire to smoke marijuana. He told me that the brain longevity program had helped him to feel "less tense," and that he simply no longer needed marijuana to calm his nerves.

Another very common cause of memory loss and cognitive impairment is simple malnourishment. Often this malnourishment is caused by lack of specific vitamins, rather than by a lack of calories. Therefore the malnourished person may look deceptively well nourished, or even overweight.

Even a moderate deficiency of some vitamins—including C, B_{12}, riboflavin, and thiamine—can disrupt cognitive function.

Several of the B vitamins are *vitally* important to brain function. Thiamine and B_{12} are both needed to produce acetylcholine. B_{12} also helps build the myelin sheath that protects nerve fibers, and, in addition, prevents pernicious anemia, which can rob the brain of oxygen. Thiamine prevents nerve damage from beriberi, and prevents brain damage in alcoholics. (As noted earlier, a deficiency of thiamine causes Korsakoff's psychosis). Niacin prevents pellagra, which has symptoms that resemble psychosis, and helps many people to feel relaxed, because it promotes formation of the tranquilizing neurotransmitter GABA. One patient of mine who had chronic insomnia for many years was able to relax at bedtime and sleep well whenever he took a dosage of 400–500 mg of niacin. He sometimes takes a smaller dosage, of approximately 100–200 mg, to feel relaxed during the day. If you take niacin, please remember that it usually causes the skin to redden in a "flushing effect."

Several minerals are necessary for optimal function of the brain, including iron, iodine, zinc, and copper.

Another nutritional factor that can cause mental lassitude is weight-loss dieting. Caloric restriction may result in hypoglycemia, which can create an array of negative mental symptoms, including inability to concentrate, fatigue, difficulty in consolidating memory, and mood swings. Severe caloric restriction, to the point of malnutrition, can even cause death of neurons. We'll examine nutrition in much more detail in Part Three.

Another factor that contributes to cognitive dysfunction is a chronic lack of oxygen to the brain. This problem may be relatively subtle, and the person suffering from it may not be aware of it. Nevertheless, a consistent shortage of oxygen in the brain will slow cognitive processing, reduce energy, and impair memory consolidation and retrieval. If this is a long-term problem, it will contribute to the death of millions of neurons.

There are two common causes of restricted oxygen to the brain: cigarette smoking and lack of exercise. Smoking not only destroys the lungs, but causes constriction of the blood vessels that supply oxygen to the brain. Exercise, which we'll discuss at length in chapter 16, is absolutely vital to proper circulation of blood to the brain.

Cognitive function can also be hurt by excessive exposure to a number of environmental pollutants, including ingredients in some chemical-laden consumer products, as well as "heavy metals," such as lead or mercury.

Lead poisoning, which is most common in children, but also occurs in adults, causes severe swelling of the brain, and results in marked mental impairment.

Exposure to mercury can produce very harmful mental effects. In fact, in the nineteenth century, it was exposure to mercury used in the manufacture of felt hats that created the phrase "mad as a hatter." Currently, some physicians believe that mercury in the silver composite material used to fill cavities in teeth contributes to the onset of Alzheimer's.

The brain can also be damaged by exposure to small amounts of arsenic and other substances, found in insecticides and industrial waste, that enter our water supply and food chain.

The presence in the body of virtually all toxins can be detected through medical testing. If you think you may have been exposed to an environmental toxin, consult a physician.

A final factor that may contribute to cognitive dysfunction is allergy—especially food allergies. As a rule, older people are less susceptible than younger people to allergies. Even elderly people, however, occasionally react to foods with either an allergic response or a less severe "sensitivity." This response can include various cognitive symptoms such as depression, forgetfulness, migraine headaches, anxiety, and hyperactivity. Occasionally these symptoms can be so severe that they mimic symptoms of Alzheimer's. Even muscular coordination can be impaired by a severe allergic response.

As you'll soon see, all food allergies can be detected and avoided. Sometimes, when a patient eliminates offending foodstuffs from his or her diet, no other mental or psychological treatment is necessary.

*   *   *

Obviously, a multitude of problems can beset the aging brain. Now we'll find out how to solve those problems.

Part Three will tell you how to start your own brain longevity program. It covers the four basic elements of the program: (1) nutritional therapy (including dietary change, intake of specific food supplements, and use of natural medicinal tonics); (2) stress management (including stress reduction and meditation); (3) exercise therapy (including cardiovascular exercise, mental exercise, and mind/body exercises); and (4) administration of pharmaceutical medications.

You've seen what the ravages of time can do to your brain.

Now let's see what you can do for *yourself.*

A Case in Point

Small Improvements Can Bring Great Joy

M.P., seventy-eight years of age, was a patient whom many people had given up on. But her husband was not one of them.

M.P.'s husband loved her deeply, even though he was already losing her, in slow and painful stages. M.P. had Alzheimer's disease, and it was so advanced that her doctor, she said, had offered her no hope. She also stated that her physician had essentially given up on her therapy program and planned no pharmacologic treatment.

M.P.'s husband, however, refused to give up on his wife. He was a very bright and aggressive man of seventy-eight, who looked about fifty-five. After a long and successful career in business, he had become a writer. He had been married to M.P., a former fashion model and ballerina, for more than forty years, and was determined to keep her with him, alive and healthy, for as long as he possibly could.

When I first consulted with M.P., I determined that she was hovering between stage 4 and stage 5 on the Global Deterioration Scale. Stage 4 patients have a decreased ability to function independently; they cannot manage their finances, travel by themselves, or perform complex tasks. Their primary memory deficits, though, tend to be related to short-term memory.

Stage 5 patients manifest a somewhat greater inability to access long-term memory. Stage 5 patients often forget the names of their family members, and sometimes forget major events in their lives.

For many people, the loss of long-term memory is much more emotionally painful than the loss of short-term memory—because, to some extent, we *are* our long-term memories.

Similarly, loss of long-term memory is especially painful for family members, because remembrance of shared events gives family life much of its richness, depth, and cohesion. Loss of short-term memory can be terribly annoying, but loss of long-term memory is, in a sense, a form of death.

At first, M.P.'s brain longevity program was very challenging for her, because she was in the habit of smoking cigarettes and having a drink or two every evening. I strongly recommended that she curtail both of these habits as much as she possibly could. For someone like her, teetering on the brink of acute brain degeneration, these habits were critically harmful.

Her husband was very supportive, and helped her in every way he could. For example, each evening, when he made her cocktails, he put less and less alcohol in them. After a few weeks, she was consuming almost no alcohol.

Also, because of chronic back pain, M.P. had some difficulty doing the mind/body exercises. She could do the kirtan kriya, though, and was conscientious about doing it every day. When she forgot to do it, her husband reminded her.

Along with the other elements of her program, she took relatively high dosages of deprenyl, phosphatidyl serine, and *Ginkgo biloba*.

Slowly she began to improve. Then, once her recovery gained momentum, she began to exhibit more pronounced signs of cognitive regeneration. She began to be considerably more articulate, and no longer struggled to find the proper word. She had much more mental energy, and became significantly more involved with the daily routine of her life. Her concentration increased in strength and duration.

Partly because of these improvements in her cognitive abilities, her general mood improved. She began to act more buoyant and confident.

The last time I consulted with M.P. she was much more clearly in stage 4, instead of hovering between stage 4 and stage 5.

To M.P., her improvement was a great victory. She had achieved what is generally considered a medical "impossibility."

M.P.'s husband was thrilled by her improvement. He felt as if he had gotten his wife back.

If you were to see them today, holding hands and chatting, you might think to yourself, "What an attractive and happy couple. I hope that's how I end up."

PART THREE

Designing Your Own Brain Longevity Program

11

The Brain Longevity
Diet

It's now time to take an exciting step: your first therapeutic step on the road to your own brain regeneration.

Years from now, you may remember this day as the day when you began to change the direction of your life. Until now, your life's direction may have been inadvertently characterized by the steady, implacable degeneration of your brain and body. You may have felt that this steady decline was inescapable—even normal. You may have believed that "aging" and "deteriorating" were synonymous. *They are not.*

"Aging" merely refers to the passage of time. And time can be used for regeneration—not just degeneration.

The power to regenerate lies within you. If you want to, you can tap into it.

The choice is yours.

The Regenerative Power of Nutritional Therapy

Nutritional therapy—which includes dietary change, the use of natural medicinal tonics, and supplementation with specific, concentrated nutrients—will be one of the four pillars of your brain regeneration program. The other three are stress management, exercise (including cardiovascular exercise, mental exercise, and mind/body exercises), and use of pharmaceutical medications.

None of these four pillars is more important than the others. All four are synergistic, and all four may be necessary for the successful regeneration of your brain.

The only element that I exclude from the programs of some patients is administration of pharmaceutical medications. Patients who have only mild age-associated memory impairment— or who have no pathology and simply wish to optimize their cognitive function—may not require pharmaceutical drugs. Also, some patients need pharmaceutical medications only in the early stages of their programs.

Engaging in nutritional therapy is the best way for you to begin your brain longevity program, and you can start as soon as your next meal. The results can be quick and dramatic; patients often respond to nutritional therapy virtually overnight. For example, one of my patients—a forty-eight-year-old man with mild age-associated memory impairment—purchased a few supplements immediately after he first consulted with me, just to "get the ball rolling." The next morning he took a couple of capsules of phosphatidyl choline, a *Ginkgo biloba* tablet, and a 100-mg multiple-B capsule. When he arrived for his follow-up consultation around noon, he was beaming. He said he felt as if he'd "been lifted out of a fog." His cognitive function was sharper, and his mind was already working with greater clarity.

Of course, he had probably just allowed his body to produce somewhat more of the neurotransmitter acetylcholine than it had been producing, and this had, in all likelihood, accounted for his subjective sense of increased cognitive clarity. To this patient, though, his response felt almost miraculous, and it encouraged him to pursue his brain longevity program with tremendous enthusiasm.

Not incidentally, this patient's first burst of improvement was followed by several others, as he added the other elements of his program. In a matter of months he reported that he "felt like a kid again." But nothing ever had as dramatic an impact as that first boost to a new plateau of function. Nutritional therapy is really that powerful.

One of the primary benefits of nutritional therapy is that it helps to repair the damage that has been done by cortisol. It also prevents further such damage. As you'll recall, cortisol has three primary negative effects: It disrupts the supply of the brain's only source of fuel, glucose; it interferes with the function of neurotransmitters; and it causes the eventual death of neurons, by creating free-radical molecules. As you'll see in this chapter, proper nutritional therapy counters all of these devastating effects. It restores and stabilizes the brain's supply of glucose; it nourishes neurotransmitters; and it protects neurons from free radicals.

Nutritional therapy also helps to repair damage done by another terrible destroyer of the brain: impaired blood circulation. Impaired circulation, as you may remember, is directly responsible for approximately 20 percent of all cases of severe cognitive dysfunction in the elderly, and I am certain that it is a powerful contributor to mild age-associated memory impairment. Also, although there is no irrefutable evidence that impaired circulation contributes to Alzheimer's disease, I believe that it often exacerbates Alzheimer's symptoms.

The other great benefit of nutritional therapy is that it directly supplies neurons with the "building materials" they require for proper function. Because your brain is "flesh and blood," it needs the same nutritional "building blocks" that other organs in your body need. With proper nutrition, your brain can create new dendrites, and forge new synaptic connections—even until the final day of your life.

It's possible that you are already ingesting all of the nutrients that your brain needs for regeneration. But it's not likely. If you're eating a diet that approximates the average American diet, you are almost certainly failing to consume the nutrients you need to achieve brain longevity. In fact, you may be slowly poisoning yourself. Approximately one out of every three Americans is committing slow suicide, every day, at the dinner table.

How the Average American Diet Contributes to Degenerative Disease

It may sound like hyperbole to you when I say that approximately one-third of all Americans are gradually poisoning themselves. But, strong as this statement is, the facts back it up.

It is a fact that eight out of every ten Americans gets cardiovascular disease or cancer. It is also a fact, according to the National Institutes of Health, that 35 percent of all cancer deaths and 30 percent of all cardiovascular disease deaths are *directly* related to diet. A substandard diet is the number-two preventable cause of death in America today, right after smoking. Smoking kills about 425,000 people a year, and dietary mistakes kill at least 350,000.

Of course, some people say, "Everybody dies of *something*, sooner or later, so you might as well die from something that makes you feel good." But if these people had witnessed firsthand the awful, endless suffering that comes from cancer, from a crippling stroke, or from Alzheimer's, they might rethink their philosophy. Take my word for it, it's better to die later than sooner, and in peace, not in pain. And it is better to die as your *self*, rather than as a poor, brain-destroyed victim of Alzheimer's.

People simply do not *have* to die from their diets.

In historic terms, our epidemic level of diet-related degenerative disease is a relatively recent phenomenon. Virtually all public health studies show that diet-related degenerative disease was relatively uncommon approximately one hundred years ago, when the typical diet was much different. This holds true even when the shorter lifespans of one hundred years ago are taken into consideration.

Diet-related degenerative disease, even now, is not a worldwide phenomenon. It's relatively rare in many countries—particularly in vegetarian-oriented countries. Death from diet is, essentially, a "disease of affluence." One of the most tragic ironies in the world today is that about one-third of the people on the planet are undernourished, while another one-third are eating themselves to death.

The American diet changed radically starting about one hundred years ago, as our nation increasingly enjoyed the economic benefits of industrialization. From 1910 to 1980, consumption of fat increased from an average of 125 mg per day to 156 mg. In addition, the ratio of dietary unsaturated-to-saturated fat rose precipitously during this time, to a current ratio of about five to one, instead of a healthy ratio of one to one. Over that same period, consumption of complex carbohydrates dropped from 37 percent of the diet to 21 percent. Also, from 1910 to 1980, consumption of simple sugar increased from 12 percent to 25 percent of the total diet.

One reason dietary patterns have changed is that so many people now dine outside the home. About one-fifth of all meals are now eaten in restaurants. Also, even when we do dine at home, we tend to eat foods that have already been processed, with fat and sugar added to them.

The biggest societal change that affected diet was simply an increase in standard of living. Once, "a chicken in every pot" was a utopian dream. Now, for most people, it's reality—for better *and* for worse.

As a result of these changes, the average American diet is now 33 percent fat. When this fat consumption is added to the 25 percent of our diet that is sugar, we see that a whopping 58 percent of our diet is nothing but fat and sugar.

Because of this gross imbalance, we are eating more calories than ever before. Caloric consumption is rising so quickly that people are rapidly becoming much heavier. In the last one hundred years, the weight of the average American has increased by about twenty-five pounds (even when adjusted for increases in height). Most disturbing, about half that weight gain has occurred just since 1976. In 1976, 22 percent of all Americans were significantly overweight, but in 1996, 30 percent were.

As the intake of fat and sugar has risen, the consumption of healthy foods has declined. Currently, only about 9 percent of all Americans eat the five or more servings of fruits and vegetables that most health experts recommend. More than half of all Americans consume *no* fruits, vegetables, or fruit juices at all on an average day. Only 16 percent of all Americans eat a serving of a high-fiber bread or cereal during an average day.

Furthermore, even when we do eat healthy foods, these foods tend to be relatively depleted in nutrients, compared to the foods that people consumed one hundred years ago. Modern food has been devitalized and robbed of nutrients by the conversion to monoculture (the growing of only one crop on an area of farmland). This practice severely depletes the nutrients in soil, and is possible only through the use of chemical fertilizers.

In addition, our food supply has been degraded by the heavy use of pesticides and herbicides, by increased hybridization, and by the chemical growth stimulation of animals. These factors have produced food that looks glossy, healthy, and rich, but is really just a step above junk food.

The modern food processing industry has also despoiled our food supply. For example, a carrot may start out as a *relatively* healthy foodstuff when it's pulled out of the ground, even though it may have been grown in depleted soil. But then it is trucked to a processing factory, where some nutrients are removed so that the carrot will resist spoilage and look attractive, while other nutrients are added. Then the carrot is packed in a fluid, and shipped to a storage warehouse, where it is freeze-dried. It spends weeks or months there, in a state of suspended animation. Then it's thawed, washed, cooked, colored orange with dye, and crammed into a can. Then it spends another month on a warehouse shelf before it's shipped to a grocery store. At the store, it spends *another* month on the shelf. Then it's transported to a restaurant or a home, where it is microwaved, salted, and buttered.

Finally, it ends up on your plate. You look down at it. It still *looks* like a carrot. But it's not. Now it's a carrot cadaver.

Ironically, in underdeveloped countries, where people do not have the "luxury" of eating cadaverous, depleted, high-fat foods, death rates for diet-related diseases are extremely low. For example, the death rate for breast cancer—which is closely linked to excessive consumption of fat—is exceedingly low in most underdeveloped nations. In El Salvador and Thailand, breast cancer rates are more than *twenty times* lower than in the United States. In Japan, which is economically developed but is still characterized by a mostly vegetarian diet, breast cancer rates are about six times lower than America's.

Cardiovascular diseases show similar patterns of occurrence.

Obviously, dietary mistakes are taking a terrible toll on Americans. And they are taking an even greater toll on *stressed-out* Americans.

Stress Increases Nutritional Needs

If you are under stress—as are most people with memory loss—your nutritional needs are magnified. Stress "burns" extra nutrients, just as physical activity does. Therefore, people under stress need additional nutrients, just as athletes do.

In one revealing study by the U.S. Department of Agriculture, researchers discovered that subjects who were given significantly more work than normal, with strict deadlines, experienced a 33-percent drop in the mineral content of their blood.

One of the minerals that was most depleted was magnesium, which is excreted in excessive amounts when cortisol levels rise. Because magnesium is a "calming mineral," its loss increases vulnerability to stress. Thus, loss of magnesium is not only *caused by* stress, but also *causes* stress—leading to a degenerative spiral.

Furthermore, magnesium is usually abnormally low in the neurons of Alzheimer's patients. Some researchers believe that this deficit is partly responsible for one of the most common signs of Alzheimer's—a buildup of calcium in neurons. Magnesium is calcium's "counterpart," and the two minerals normally keep each other in balance.

Other nutrients depleted by stress are the antioxidant vitamins C and E, which help protect your brain from free radicals. Vitamin C, in particular, is "burned up" by stress, in part because large amounts of the vitamin are stored in the adrenal glands.

Stress also increases the body's needs for proteins and carbohydrates. Stress speeds up the metabolic rate, which increases the demand not just for food "fuel," but also for the partial proteins, called amino acids, that are used in a host of neurological activities.

Stress, via cortisol, also increases the physical craving for carbohydrates. Cortisol production triggers the release of a brain chemical called *neuropeptide Y*, which causes the desire for carbohydrate consumption. This biochemical mechanism is the reason that many people overeat sweets and starchy foods when they are under stress.

As you can see, there is much that is wrong with the average American diet. Americans pay a terrible price for this dietary indiscretion—and they pay for it with the slow degeneration of their brains and bodies.

Now let's look at a much smarter way of eating: a diet that will create *regeneration*.

The Brain Longevity Diet

There is absolutely nothing complex, unappetizing, or difficult about the Brain Longevity Diet. In fact, it is not even a diet in the usual sense of the word. I do not advise patients on the Brain Longevity Diet to eat specific foods, in specific amounts, at specific times. I have always been very skeptical of that kind of diet, which I consider extremely contrived. For one thing, hardly anyone ever stays on that kind of denial-oriented diet for more than a few months. It's just too much trouble, and it's not emotionally or physically satisfying. Also, a rigid, denial-based diet cedes all power and control to whoever *created* the diet. I don't believe in that at all. I don't want to control my patients. I want them to learn *self*-control, the only kind of control that ever really works, and the only kind that lasts.

Therefore, the Brain Longevity Diet is not a set of menu plans, but a group of *principles*. And these dietary principles, like the other principles of the brain longevity program, are simple, clear, and doable. Like the rest of the program, they revolve around good science and good sense.

Here are the basic principles:

Eat a low-fat diet. What's good for the heart is good for the head. The brain is flesh and blood, and blood doesn't circulate well when it's full of fat. Besides, fat literally "rots your brain," as I'll soon show.

Eat a nutrient-dense diet. Your brain needs an immense assortment of nutrients, and you can't get them in empty calories. Don't stress your organs of digestion, assimilation, and elimination with "non-food." Make every bite count.

Avoid hypoglycemia. Your brain's only fuel is glucose. When your blood sugar is low, your brain functions poorly. When it gets extremely low, neurons die. When you go on a starvation diet, you starve your brain. If your diet is extremely severe, you can starve parts of your brain to *death*.

Eat a relatively low-calorie diet. Don't go hungry, but go light. Caloric restriction is one of the few proven methods of achieving longevity. However, if you eat low-fat and nutrient-dense foods, you'll *naturally* tend to eat "low-cal."

Eat a balanced diet. I *don't* mean you should eat equal amounts of the "four basic food groups." That's the unbalanced, high-fat style that's caused so many health problems. Eat a diet that's a balance of whole grains, vegetables, fruits, and non-animal-based protein, along with some low-fat dairy and some low-fat meat (if you feel you must have meat).

Take supplements. I know some "experts" say you can get enough nutrients in a good diet. But enough for *what*? In my opinion, following a good diet does not necessarily provide enough nutrients to regenerate your brain.

Eat real food. Not processed food. Not pesticide-poisoned food. Not embalmed food. Real food for real people—despite the ads you see—is mostly found in your grocery's produce section.

Feed your neurotransmitters. They need special nutrients, and they probably aren't getting enough of them. When you consciously "feed your head," you'll get a huge "brain boost."

That's it. End of lecture. It's really that simple.

Of course, this diet may be simple to describe, but it may not be so simple for you to follow—not if you're now eating the typical American diet.

Now I'll be somewhat more specific about the general type of diet you should be eating.

I recommend to my patients that they be especially careful about their diets in the *early* stages of their programs, when the most dramatic "brain healing" occurs. During this pivotal phase, which lasts a couple of months, I advise them to eat about 50 percent of their calories as whole grains. These grains can be cereals, breads, and other baked goods. They can also be eaten in soups, stews, pastas, and casseroles. Almost any whole grain is acceptable, and a wide variety of them should be eaten, to keep the diet interesting and satisfying.

Another 25 percent of total caloric intake should be made up of fruits and vegetables. Beans, especially, are exceptionally nutritious and high in protein, and can be prepared in a multitude of pleasing dishes. Because they're a high-protein, hearty food, they're a good substitute for meat.

Whenever possible, the fruits and vegetables should be fresh. It's also wise to find produce that was organically grown. Herbicides and pesticides can have a gravely deleterious effect upon cerebral function.

To meet your brain's demand for protein, soy products are especially valuable because they're low in fat and high in the amino acids that make up neurotransmitters. Soy protein is also an effective free-radical scavenger, because of its high content of *genisten,* a potent antioxidant. Soy tends to boost "good" high-density lipoprotein cholesterol, and it reduces triglycerides. It is also rich in two amino acids, glycine and arginine, that control insulin output and help stabilize blood sugar.

Soy products may also be of benefit for females experiencing menopause, because soy products contain compounds called *phytoestrogens*—natural substances that exert mild estrogenic activities. Studies of women in China and Japan indicate that those who consume high amounts of phytoestrogens from soy products suffer relatively fewer menopausal side effects. If you are allergic to soy or have difficulty digesting it, other high-protein, nonmeat foods include yogurt, cottage cheese, almonds, mung beans, lentils, chickpeas, and grains like millet and basmati rice.

Ingestion of moderate amounts of low-fat or nonfat dairy products can be helpful, but people in most developed countries tend to overemphasize their value. Yogurt is probably the best dairy product, primarily because of its probiotic actions in the intestines, where it provides the helpful bacteria that aid digestion.

Meat is an acceptable part of a brain longevity program, but it's by no means necessary. Adequate protein can be consumed without eating meat, and virtually all meat is high in fat. Even the leanest types of white chicken are much higher in fat than almost any of the other high-protein foods I recommend. Many people, however, feel attached to the idea of eating meat, and I find it counterproductive to make a major issue out of it.

If you think, though, that you can chow down on bacon for breakfast, a Big Mac for lunch, and a sirloin steak for dinner— and still be on a brain longevity program—forget it. Those days are over. You've got a choice to make: your burger or your brain.

If you do eat meat, you should try to confine consumption to three times weekly. When you eat meat, you should eat only about three ounces. That's about the size of a deck of cards. If you eat fish, you can have a larger portion. This may not sound like as much meat as you want, but it's as much as your *body* wants. Until approximately World War II, this amount of meat was the average that was consumed. Until that time, most people just weren't "lucky" enough to afford large quantities of meat.

If you do eat a diet that is composed mostly of grains, vegetables, and fruits, you'll be helping more than just your brain.

You'll also cut your cancer risk by *at least* half, according to the National Institutes of Health, and you'll cut your risk of cardiovascular disease by approximately 70 percent. You'll also greatly reduce your risk of diabetes, and reduce by 80 percent your risk of the most common form of adult-onset blindness (macular degeneration). Also, you'll have more energy, your sex drive will probably increase, and you'll very likely lose weight.

Furthermore, a primarily vegetarian diet will probably boost your immunity to common diseases. This will happen not only because your immune system will be better nourished, but also because you'll be ingesting a rich supply of a group of newly discovered nutrients called *phytochemicals.* Especially abundant in green, cruciferous vegetables (cabbage, broccoli, brussels sprouts, etc.), phytochemicals have powerful pharmacologic, antidisease properties. They not only help prevent disease, but also support the immune system's reaction to disease.

There's much more to nutritional therapy than simple common sense, though. There are specific dietary methods you can use to take firm control of your cognitive function, moods, and memory.

How to "Feed" Your Neurotransmitters

By now you know that there are several key neurotransmitters that are of absolute importance in memory, focus, learning, energy, and happiness. The materials that compose four of the most important neurotransmitters—acetylcholine, norepinephrine, serotonin, and dopamine—*come directly from your diet.*

So let's look at how you can nutritionally build high levels of these important neurotransmitters.

MANUFACTURING ACETYLCHOLINE:
YOUR "MEMORY NEUROTRANSMITTER"

As you know, acetylcholine is the primary carrier of thought and memory. If you don't have enough acetylcholine in your brain, you will definitely suffer from memory loss and cognitive dysfunction. In fact, *a deficit of acetylcholine is probably the single most common cause of age-related cognitive impairment.* The brains of virtually all Alzheimer's patients are notably low in acetylcholine, and it is my belief that the brains of almost every person with age-associated memory impairment are also low in acetylcholine.

Restoring acetylcholine to a proper level is extremely easy; you may be able to do it in literally a matter of hours. All you have to do is ingest the specific nutrients that acetylcholine is made from. The most important of those nutrients is choline, which is present in high amounts in lecithin.

Choline can be purchased as a supplement in any health food store. Most people, however, prefer to ingest it by taking lecithin, which is also available in every health food store, and in most grocery stores. Lecithin tends to be cheaper than choline, and it won't give your breath a "fishy" odor, as choline sometimes does.

Lecithin is also very useful in helping your body to digest and transport fat. It keeps cholesterol soluble, and also helps produce the bile acids that are made from cholesterol.

The type of choline that your brain needs most is called *phosphatidyl choline.* This type of choline is a major component of each of your brain cells. If your brain does not get enough phosphatidyl choline nutritionally, it will literally "cannibalize" brain cells to obtain this crucial nutrient.

Choline, ingested as lecithin, is often prescribed by doctors as part of their treatment for Alzheimer's. However, by the time Alzheimer's is clinically apparent, it's often too late for choline to have a significant impact. By this time the brain has suffered severe structural damage, and a deficit of acetylcholine is only a secondary problem. Even so, some minor benefit may be derived.

Clinical evidence strongly indicates, however, that lecithin can be of great value in *preventing* deterioration of the brain, if it is used therapeutically in the early stages of memory impairment. People with mild age-associated memory impairment typically respond very well when lecithin is administered. In my own practice I have seen patients with mild to moderate memory disorder respond positively to lecithin. It's practically a "wonder drug" for some mildly impaired brains.

You probably already ingest about 1,000 mg of lecithin each day, because it is very commonly found in foods, and is also frequently added to foods. Foods that are highest in lecithin are soybeans and soybean oil, egg yolks, wheat germ, peanuts and peanut butter, liver, ham, and whole wheat products.

To ingest lecithin in *therapeutic dosages*, however, you need to take lecithin supplements. You just can't eat enough lecithin-rich foods to get the effects you need for brain regeneration. Lecithin supplements are inexpensive, absolutely nontoxic, and easy to digest, and are available in capsule, granule, liquid, tablet, and powder form. I recommend the capsule form, since patients seem to prefer it. You should take approximately 2,500 to 3,000 mg four times daily, for a total daily dosage of approximately 10,000 to 12,000 mg. A chlorophyll-based "green drink" is one abundant source, supplying about 2,000 mg of lecithin per serving.

It's very important that you also take vitamin C, and vitamin B_5 (pantothenic acid) with your lecithin, because these vitamins are needed to transform lecithin into acetylcholine.

To potentiate acetylcholine production, you should take approximately 1,000 mg of vitamin C, three times a day (for a daily dosage of 3,000 mg). Some physicians consider this a high dosage, but I consider it very prudent, and recommend even higher dosages for many patients. In some people, however, this much vitamin C can cause mild, temporary stomach and intestinal upset. If this occurs, lower the dosage until you are free of any gastrointestinal symptoms.

No less than 100 mg per day of B_5 should be taken. Again, this is considered by some doctors to be a "megadose" of the vitamin. But a great many nutritional experts believe that B_5 can be beneficial in dosages as high as 500 mg. B_5 has no toxicity level, and causes no side effects whatsoever.

In addition to vitamins C and B_5, it's also wise to take B_6 and zinc, which also aid the synthesis of acetylcholine. Usually, a good multivitamin will supply enough of these cofactors.

This one simple nutritional formula—lecithin + B_5 + C—is an *absolute must* for anyone on a brain longevity program.

Another way to help build acetylcholine levels is to take the nutrient DMAE (dimethylaminoethanol). DMAE is present in small quantities in the brain, and is concentrated in some seafoods, including sardines. It aids in the production of acetylcholine, particularly when it's taken with B_5 and calcium pantothenate. Studies have shown that DMAE can elevate learning and memory, and also help learning disorders that are linked to hyperactivity.

DMAE is somewhat stimulating to the central nervous system, so you should initially try it in low dosages—about 40 mg twice daily. You can build up to about 200 mg daily, if you do not feel overstimulated. Even when stimulation does occur, though, there is rarely a "rebound effect" of lethargy, as there often is with other stimulants, such as caffeine.

In general, the effects of DMAE will increase gradually. You may not notice any improvement in your mental abilities for the first two weeks.

Do not underestimate the critical importance of nutritionally fortifying your brain's supply of acetylcholine. It is the foundation of nutritional therapy for memory.

MANUFACTURING NOREPINEPHRINE AND DOPAMINE, YOUR "ENERGY NEUROTRANSMITTERS"

Remember how important norepinephrine is in creating long-term memories? This stimulating neurotransmitter—the "first cousin" of adrenaline (or epinephrine)—is the substance that makes us remember exciting or traumatic events. If it weren't for norepinephrine, people would not have vivid, enduring memories of emotional events.

Besides transporting and "locking in" long-term memories, norepinephrine is one of your brain's primary "happiness" chemicals. It elevates your mood, and gives you energy and optimism.

Without enough norepinephrine, you will have a depressed mood, and an inability to concentrate, to cope with stress, and to move memories to long-term storage.

...ine is not quite as important to cognitive function as ...phrine, but it's still a powerfully stimulating brain chem-... Dopamine, as you may recall, is the primary neurotransmitter that controls bodily movement. It commonly declines as people age, and this accounts for the loss of coordination and muscular control that elderly people almost always experience. A gross deficit of dopamine causes the extreme loss of muscular control that is identified as Parkinson's disease.

Dopamine helps to improve mood, burn fat, increase sex drive, enhance immunity, and promote longevity. An extreme shortage of dopamine can cause severe cognitive dysfunction.

Dopamine and norepinephrine are manufactured in much the same way. The primary nutritional building blocks of both neurotransmitters are the amino acids *tyrosine* and *phenylalanine*. To potentiate the action of these amino acids, folic acid, magnesium, and vitamins C and B_{12} can be taken.

Both phenylalanine and tyrosine can be purchased at health food stores or—more economically—from manufacturers through the mail. (See the "Resources and Referrals" appendix.)

A typical daily dosage of each amino acid—for persons with no frank cognitive pathology—would be in the 500-to-1,000-mg range. For my patients who show signs of moderate clinical depression, I may recommend dosages of up to 1,500 mg daily of each amino acid.

Tyrosine and phenylalanine can also be ingested in most high-protein foods, including poultry, seafood, and soy and dairy products.

When you take tyrosine, it's important to take it *before* you eat anything with a high content of carbohydrates. If you eat carbohydrates prior to taking tyrosine, it will interfere with tyrosine's ability to enter the brain.

To enter the brain, tyrosine must "compete" with other amino acids, including the amino acid *tryptophan*. When you eat high-carbohydrate foods, they cause tryptophan to enter the brain instead of tyrosine.

If you are not taking tyrosine supplements—and are depending for mental stimulation solely upon tyrosine in foods—

the same "no carbohydrate" rule applies: *You must eat high-protein foods first.* Then, after about an hour, you can eat carbohydrates. By then the tyrosine will be in your brain, and will help stimulate your mind for several hours.

When you eat carbohydrates first—and favor the uptake of tryptophan—you will get a calming effect, because tryptophan produces the calming neurotransmitter serotonin.

In short: For stimulation, eat protein. For relaxation, eat carbohydrates.

If you want to be alert during your workday, you should eat a high-protein breakfast. However, it's quite possible that you will feel a natural desire to eat a high-carbohydrate breakfast, because your blood sugar falls as you sleep. Most people do, in fact, prefer carbohydrates in the morning: bread, cereal, sugar, fruit. But if you resist the urge, by midmorning you'll probably be glad you did.

At lunchtime, a high-protein meal is likely to keep you more alert than a high-carbohydrate meal.

In the evening, when you want to relax, feel free to eat carbohydrates. They'll increase your tryptophan uptake, and you'll soon be manufacturing the calming serotonin.

MANUFACTURING SEROTONIN, YOUR "FEEL GOOD" NEUROTRANSMITTER

Serotonin is your brain's major "contentment chemical." If you don't have enough of it, you're almost certain to feel a nagging sense of emotional malaise. If you are saddled with this feeling, you may gravitate toward medications like Prozac, which increase serotonin.

Serotonin also controls your sensitivity to pain, and helps you sleep. It is manufactured by ingestion of the amino acid tryptophan. Without tryptophan, there can be no serotonin.

Until several years ago, millions of people took tryptophan tablets, mostly as an aid to sleep. However, the Food and Drug Administration removed tryptophan tablets from the over-the-counter marketplace after a single contaminated batch—manufactured by one overseas company—caused some tragic health problems, including several deaths. Needless to say, exercising greater control over the manufacturing process of tryptophan would have been a prudent course for the FDA to have taken. But in this situation, some critics charged that the FDA overreacted. Now the only way to ingest tryptophan is from dietary sources, or to purchase it with a doctor's prescription through a compounding pharmacy.

Tryptophan, as mentioned above, competes with tyrosine and other amino acids to enter the brain. To enter the brain, tryptophan requires ingestion of carbohydrates. This causes the body to release insulin, which in turn causes almost all the amino acids *except* tryptophan to be absorbed quickly by cells. Tryptophan gets "left behind," because it's a larger molecule than the others. When tryptophan gets left behind, and is the only amino acid remaining in the bloodstream in high concentrations, it soon gets a "free ride" to the brain. Therefore, to assimilate tryptophan, you should eat the *opposite* way from the way you eat to assimilate tyrosine. You should eat high-carbohydrate, low-protein foods, and make sure you eat the carbohydrates before the protein.

Because carbohydrate consumption stimulates the uptake of tryptophan—and the manufacture of serotonin—I believe that carbohydrate craving, in many cases, is really a craving for serotonin, and the emotional contentment it triggers.

Some of my patients who were chronic overeaters of carbohydrates were not overeating for the classic psychological reasons, such as reward, pleasure, or indulgence. Instead, they had been trying to self-medicate their serotonin deficit.

For example, one thirty-eight-year-old female patient of mine had long been a chronic overeater of carbohydrates. Because of this, she was overweight, and because she was overweight, she hated to exercise. Thus she was locked into a degenerative spiral. However, when she simply changed the timing of her carbohydrate consumption—to optimize serotonin manufacture—her entire eating pattern changed. She lost her cravings, lost weight, began exercising, and felt better than she had in many years.

It's interesting to note that the latest purported wonder drug for obesity, dexfenfluramine (Redux), is a compound that simply increases serotonin assimilation by the brain. This drug may soon prove to be very valuable for many people, but I prefer that people try to solve their problems without using pharmaceutical medications. I am not antagonistic to the use of pharmaceutical drugs, but I have found that changes that occur without drugs are usually more lasting.

I have also noticed that patients with seasonal affective disorder often crave carbohydrates. This is because seasonal affective disorder, or "winter blues," often results in a serotonin deficiency. As a rule, when the seasonal affective disorder is cured—through the use of exercise, melatonin replacement therapy, meditation, and "bright light therapy"—the carbo-craving abates.

Feeding your neurotransmitters is a vitally important way to control your cognitive function and moods. But it's just as important to do one other simple thing that will help you feel sharp all day, every day: Keep enough "fuel" in your brain.

How Low Blood Sugar Can Damage the Brain

One of the ways that cortisol robs you of your optimal cognitive function—day in and day out—is by disrupting the level of your brain's blood sugar. The brain, as I've mentioned, runs on only one "fuel"—glucose, or simple sugar—and it requires a full 25 percent of all blood being pumped by the heart to supply this fuel. *Any* disruption of your glucose levels has a powerful and immediate impact upon your brain. When you miss a meal, you may feel lightheaded and irritable, and have poor long-term and short-term recall. This occurs because your brain isn't getting enough fuel. The "power plants" in your neurons (the mitochondria) are struggling to help build memory traces, but they just don't have the power they need.

If this "power outage" to neurons lasts more than just a few minutes, neurons can be badly damaged, and can even die. Most of us have probably lost millions of neurons just from blood sugar disruptions.

As noted previously, cortisol disrupts blood sugar by stimulating overproduction of insulin. When this happens, sugar stored in your liver as glycogen rushes out of your liver and into your bloodstream, where it's converted to glucose. Then this glucose enters your cells. For a few minutes you surge with energy, and your cognitive function hits peak levels. But then, because your blood has been "robbed" of its supply of sugar, you quickly begin to lose energy. Your brain, which is extremely sensitive to glucose deprivation, is hit hard—and fast.

Most people who experience this type of hypoglycemic episode are tempted to react to it by reaching for a candy bar or a cup of coffee, to stimulate more adrenalin\insulin\glucose. Of course, this offers only a quick fix, and ultimately exacerbates the problem.

In fact, as you probably know, hypoglycemia is often caused not by stress, but by simply eating too much sugar. Ingestion of excess sugar causes the same surge of insulin that stress does.

Unfortunately, it's often difficult for people to ascertain how much sugar is too much. I believe that as many as one out of four of my patients has at least a mild inability to process dietary sugar without oversecreting insulin. For those people, even a small sugary snack can cause mild hypoglycemia, if the snack is eaten at the wrong time, or is not accompanied by a more "lasting" fuel.

This "blood glucose intolerance," or "carbohydrate sensitivity," is sometimes the result of a lack of dietary chromium. Chromium (or chromium picolinate) is the mineral that increases insulin efficiency, and helps maintain stable blood sugar levels. Chromium also plays an important role in helping to control cholesterol and triglycerides.

I generally advise patients to be sure that their multivitamin supplement contains about 200 mcg of chromium. It is almost impossible to achieve ingestion of this level of chromium just from dietary sources; to do this, you would have to eat more than 10,000 calories per day.

Some of my patients also use chromium as part of a weight-loss regime, because it helps naturally curb the appetite by stabilizing blood sugar.

Chromium also helps my patients to maintain high levels of

the "anti-aging" hormone DHEA. DHEA levels can become depleted if the body produces too much insulin, because insulin interferes with an enzyme that helps produce DHEA. In one study, patients' levels of DHEA dropped by an average of 10 percent after they discontinued taking 200 mcg of chromium daily.

You should be aware that one report in 1996 noted that chromium picolinate caused chromosome damage to cells grown in a laboratory. Theoretically, chromosome damage can lead to cancer. However, I do not believe this one negative report merits discontinuation of chromium.

Another way to help stabilize blood sugar levels is to eat a diet rich in soy products. Soy is abundant in two amino acids, glycine and arginine, that help to control insulin fluctuations. Therefore, soy helps maintain an even level of blood sugar.

Another important way to stabilize blood sugar levels is to maintain proper function of the liver. The liver stores part of your "emergency supply" of glucose, and anything that makes liver function sluggish will compromise the delivery of that emergency supply. Alcoholics, for example, are often hypoglycemic, partly because of damage to their livers.

If you wish to maintain stable blood sugar levels, one thing you should definitely avoid is "crash" dieting, which wreaks havoc upon blood sugar stability. Unfortunately, many people still engage in this type of dieting, even though it's been proven ineffective for weight loss. It doesn't work because it lowers the body's metabolic "set point," and "magnifies" every calorie that's consumed—often for *weeks* after the diet ends. This, of course, often causes a weight gain that is greater than the amount of weight that was lost during the diet. People who do engage in this folly, however, should realize that it doesn't damage just their bodies. It also damages their brains. Depriving the brain of its only energy source damages and kills neurons.

By far the best way to avoid hypoglycemia is simply to eat a prudent diet, rich in complex carbohydrates and protein. It may help to eat a number of small meals and snacks throughout the day. Also, your diet should be relatively low in foods that convert very quickly to blood sugar. When foods "break down" into glucose very quickly, they cause a "rollercoaster" of blood sugar. Foods that break down slowly help to stabilize blood sugar.

Conventional wisdom says that foods rich in complex carbohydrates—such as carrots or whole wheat bread—are always the best defense against a blood-sugar "rollercoaster ride." But that's not always true. Take a look at the following index of foods, which are ranked in order of how quickly they're converted into sugar. You'll note that many sweet foods, such as orange juice or table sugar (sucrose), are actually converted to glucose *more slowly* than many foods that are high in complex carbohydrates. Potatoes, for example, are converted to glucose much more quickly than table sugar.

As you can see, all foods high in fruit sugar, or fructose, are relatively slow to convert to glucose. Therefore, fructose can be of value to you as a sweetener.

GLYCEMIC INDEX

Glucose	100	Spaghetti	50
Potato	98	Orange juice	46
Carrot	92	Grape	45
Honey	87	Apple	39
White rice	72	Yogurt	36
Wheat bread	72	Tofu	35
White bread	69	Milk	34
Rice	66	Grapefruit	26
Banana	62	Fructose	20
Sucrose (table sugar)	59		

As you can see, the fundamental elements of the Brain Longevity Diet are nothing more than good science and good sense. This is *not* a difficult, unpleasant diet that you'll only be able to follow for a few months. It's a lifetime dietary program of moderation and sensible eating, which revolves around simply eating wholesome, nutritious foods, instead of junk foods.

It is, in short, the same basic dietary advice your mother gave you long ago: Eat your vegetables, take your vitamins, don't skip breakfast, don't live on sweets, and don't eat like a pig. That was good advice then, and it's still good advice.

To optimize your cognitive function, though, and achieve brain longevity, you will doubtless want to "fine-tune" your nutritional therapy. There are a number of ways to do that.

That's what we'll look at next—fine-tuning your nutritional program for a lifetime of optimal mental function.

A Case in Point

Brain Longevity Programs Can Help Correct Other Health Problems

S.C., forty-seven years old, was a science writer who heard about my work from a professional associate. He decided to begin a brain longevity program in order to optimize his cognitive function.

At our first consultation, S.C. showed no objective evidence of any significant neurological problems; he performed adequately on various memory and cognitive function tests.

Subjectively, however, S.C. believed that his cognitive function had declined in recent years. In his twenties and thirties, he told me, he had worked extremely hard, but had rarely experienced mental fatigue. In his forties, though, he had begun to become more mentally fatigued during the normal course of his workday. This fatigue had caused him to drink more coffee while he was working, and to take more breaks during the day. Even so, he was generally unable to do as much work as he had in his twenties and thirties.

He said that his recall of vocabulary words, which was an important component of his professional ability, had diminished noticeably, and that he had begun to rely much more heavily upon his thesaurus. Also, he said, he had more trouble focusing intently for long periods.

In addition, S.C. frequently felt a sense of mild emotional malaise, which he described as "a blah feeling." He said that he had come to feel that his life consisted mostly of work and family responsibilities, and that he had little time or energy left for the recreational activities that had once given him a great deal of pleasure.

Physically, his health was relatively good, though he was experiencing mild to moderate arthritis in both hands, and especially in his right hand. The joints in his fingers were swollen, and his range of motion was limited. The condition, he said, had existed for about two years.

I was anxious to work with S.C., because I am generally able to elicit the highest levels of cognitive function in patients who have experienced only mild declines in cognition. In these people, I am consistently able not just to halt decline, but to restore cognitive function to peak performance levels.

S.C. began his program enthusiastically. It was not a difficult regimen for him to follow, because he already had a healthy and active lifestyle.

Aspects of his brain longevity program that already were a part of his lifestyle included regular cardiovascular exercise, regular mental exercise, supplementation with vitamins and minerals, and meditation. The primary changes he instituted included ingestion of lecithin, DMAE, *Ginkgo biloba*, a chlorophyll-based "green drink," ginseng, and additional antioxidants. He also began doing the mind/body exercises, and eating much less red meat.

Within about one month, S.C. received a powerful boost from his brain longevity program. He gained notably better access to his remote memory for language, and he was able to work for longer periods without becoming mentally fatigued. He remarked to me that he felt as if there were "more hours in the day." His productivity gradually began to increase.

After about three months on his program, an extremely interesting thing happened. He told me that his arthritic symptoms—swelling of the joints, pain, and stiffness—had begun to subside. The improvements, he said, were most noticeable in his right hand, where the condition had been more pronounced.

About two months later he called back and said that both of his hands were completely free of any signs of arthritis. I scheduled him for an appointment, to examine him myself. His hands, just as he had said, were free of any apparent arthritic condition. He had full range of motion, no soreness, and no swelling.

Because his brain longevity program consisted of a wide, synergistic range of lifestyle and nutritional modifications, there was no practical way to determine what particular aspects of his program had caused the improvement. I did, however, have a couple of theories.

It was possible that his increased nutritional supplementation was providing him with the nutrients that his body needed to remain resistant to arthritic symptoms. Arthritis can sometimes be exacerbated by a deficiency in minerals, including phosphorous, magnesium, calcium, and manganese, and also by a lack of vitamins E and C. His brain longevity program was providing him with more of these nutrients than he had previously been receiving. Perhaps this had helped relieve his arthritis.

It was also possible that his arthritic symptoms had been relieved by the detoxifying elements of his program. The inflammatory symptoms of arthritis can be significantly aggravated by toxins in the bloodstream. By eating less red meat, he was subjecting his body to fewer of the toxic byproducts that are released during the metabolic processing of high-fat foods. In addition, the chlorophyll-based product that he was drinking every morning helped to detoxify his blood and his cells. Some of the nutrients in his "green drink," including magnesium and chlorophyll, act as natural "cleansing" agents.

S.C.'s arthritic symptoms have yet to return. I believe it's quite possible that they never will return. He also became able to function at an extremely high cognitive level. He told me that he had fully regained the mental vigor that he'd had in his twenties and thirties. In conjunction with the rejuvenation of his fluid intelligence, he experienced a significant improvement in his general mood. He no longer was plagued by his "blah" feeling, and began to be more involved with some of his favorite recreational activities.

S.C. was extremely pleased with the improvement in his cognitive function. But he was even more excited about the relief of his arthritic symptoms, because he had not expected that to happen.

In truth, I hadn't been expecting it, either. But it did not take me completely by surprise, because many of my brain longevity patients have gained relief from a wide variety of physical ailments (including migraine headaches, asthma, chronic pain, gastrointestinal distress, impotence, chronic fatigue syndrome, high blood pressure, and cardiac irregularity).

Brain longevity programs are "powerful medicine." They help the brain, and they help the body.

12

Fine-Tuning
Your Nutritional Therapy

One evening I had the honor of dining with the legendary neu-robiologist Dr. Candace Pert, who discovered the beta endorphin receptor. I was telling her about my work with nutritional therapy and cognitive function, and she concurred with my emphasis on improving blood circulation to the brain. She told me, "What's good for the heart is good for the head." I thought, at the time, that it was a brilliant statement—clear, concise, and correct. In the years since, the clinical responses of my patients to enhanced cerebral circulation have validated her pronouncement.

To state the obvious, if there's one thing the brain needs, it's blood. Shut off that supply, and the brain begins to die in a matter of moments. Everyone knows this. And yet, many people are blithely unconcerned about gradual decreases in their brain's supply of blood. It's as if they think, "As long as I have enough blood in my brain to maintain consciousness, every-thing's fine."

Not so! When cerebral circulation declines, so does cognitive power.

The second-most-common cause of severe cognitive decline in the elderly is multiple minor strokes. This problem, multi-infarct dementia, accounts for 20 percent of all dementias. Often this problem is as disabling as Alzheimer's. Sometimes it happens at the same time as Alzheimer's, and magnifies mental decline.

Further, it's been proved that just having high blood pressure significantly impairs cognitive function. In one study, cognitive decline in older patients with high blood pressure was so apparent that this decline in brain power could be used to predict the likelihood of strokes.

I am also convinced that some patients suffering from age-associated memory impairment are experiencing a decline in cerebral circulation. One reason I believe this is that many of my patients with mild memory impairment respond positively to substances that enhance their cerebral circulation. These substances, such as *Ginkgo biloba*, often achieve dramatic results quickly.

Improving cerebral circulation creates a number of benefits for the brain: it supplies the brain with more oxygen and glucose; it provides the *micronutrients* that neurons need to thrive; it aids neuronal cellular metabolism by carrying away the intracellular debris that can damage and eventually kill brain cells; and it helps protect neurons from free-radical damage.

It's often difficult, however, for patients in midlife, or later, to maintain optimal cerebral circulation. One major problem is that blood pressure typically rises as we age. On average, the blood pressure of Americans rises by fifteen points between the ages of twenty-five and fifty-five, but this increase is certainly not inescapable; a similar rise does not occur in all other countries. In countries where a vegetarian diet is the norm, there is generally little elevation of blood pressure in older people.

There are a host of methods that help keep blood pressure low, and help maintain optimal circulation. These include exercise, stress management, and nutritional therapy.

In this chapter we'll consider just the nutritional factors that help circulation; in subsequent chapters we'll discuss exercise and stress management.

A circulation-boosting diet should be low in fat and sodium, and high in antioxidants. Vitamin C, in particular, is helpful in keeping blood pressure down. Studies indicate that low blood levels of vitamin C tend to raise blood pressure by an average of approximately 16 percent (systolic) and 9 percent (diastolic).

High-fiber diets also help circulation, by helping to reduce cholesterol.

Of course, being significantly overweight is also very deleterious to circulation. So is smoking. The single *worst* thing you can do for circulation, though, is simply to *eat too much fat.*

The Toll That Fat Takes on the Brain

Excess dietary fat has two devastating effects upon the brain: it impairs cerebral circulation, and it creates millions of free radicals.

Excessive consumption of fat impairs cerebral circulation by clogging arteries with "bad" low-density lipoprotein (or LDL). LDL decreases the elasticity of the brain's blood vessels.

High fat intake also creates huge numbers of free radicals, because fat oxidizes extremely quickly—often almost instantaneously. In fact, it oxidizes so quickly that if you pour oil into an open container, it will become infused with air in just a few seconds. This infusion of air (or oxidation) will quickly turn the oil rancid, and rancid oil contains some of the most destructive free radicals that exist.

When the free radicals from fat meet your neurons, they quickly damage the neurons, and begin to kill them. One reason your neurons are especially vulnerable to free-radical damage is that the brain itself is composed largely of fat. Each of your neurons is approximately 60 percent fat. In a sense, parts of your brain can become "rancid"—from oxidation—over the course of your life. As you age, portions of your brain can literally "rot."

Some forms of fat, though, are much worse for your brain and body than others. There are three basic types of fat: *saturated* (which is the most harmful), *polyunsaturated* (which is the next most harmful), and *monounsaturated* (which is the least harmful).

When fat is "saturated," it means that it is saturated with hydrogen atoms, which make fat molecules pack together tightly. This results in a thick consistency, like lard. Unfortunately, saturated fat doesn't dissolve at all well in the body; it retains its lard-like consistency, and builds up on the walls of your blood vessels. Eventually it can close some of your vessels entirely, and cause a disruption of blood flow to your heart (a heart attack), or a disruption of blood flow to your brain (a stroke).

Saturated fat buildup can also damage the walls of your blood vessels, and actually cause blood to leak out. Frequently this happens in the brain, and contributes significantly to cognitive dysfunction. If cerebral hemorrhage is sufficiently severe, it can even cause death.

Saturated fat also enters every cell in your body, including your brain cells. When too much fat enters a cell, it causes the cell wall to thicken, harden, and lose its ability to allow nutrients to come into the cell. It also prevents waste from leaving the cell. This badly damages the function of the cell, and can eventually kill it.

Polyunsaturated fat is not as deadly as saturated fat, but it is still one of the most damaging things you can eat. When fat is polyunsaturated, that means it is less saturated with hydrogen atoms, and isn't so "lardy." Many oils, for example, are polyunsaturated.

The problem with fats that aren't lardy, though, is that they oxidize even *faster* than saturated fats, and are quickly turned into free radicals. As you've probably noticed, if you leave polyunsaturated cooking oil out of your refrigerator for even a few hours, it becomes rancid.

Examples of polyunsaturated fats are safflower oil, sunflower oil, corn oil, and soybean oil.

The least harmful fats are those that are mostly monounsaturated. Because monounsaturated fats have fewer "hydrogen bonds" than polyunsaturated fats, they're more chemically stable. Therefore, they don't become free radicals nearly as easily as polyunsaturated fats.

Monounsaturated fats have several other very positive qualities. They help "bad" LDL cholesterol to keep from oxidizing.

They also increase the efficiency of "good" cholesterol (high-density lipoprotein). In addition, monounsaturated fats bolster the ability of vitamin E to protect against free radicals.

Examples of monounsaturated fats include olive, canola, flaxseed, fish, and macadamia nut oil. Of these, olive oil and canola oil are the most palatable and affordable, and easiest to find.

Below is a list of unsaturated fats, ranked from best to worst. Also noted is the percentage of polyunsaturated fat in each.

1. Macadamia nut oil (3%)
2. Extra virgin olive oil (8%)
3. Flaxseed oil (16%)
4. Canola oil (22%)
5. Peanut oil (33%)
6. Sesame seed oil (41%)
7. Walnut oil (51%)
8. Soybean oil (54%)
9. Corn oil (61%)
10. Sunflower oil (69%)
11. Safflower oil (77%)

The absolute *worst* form of fat, though, is fat or oil that has been changed to a solid or semisolid form, such as margarine or shortening. This type of fat—called *hydrogenated* or partially hydrogenated—has been transformed into a particularly destructive form of fat called "trans-fatty acid." Trans-fatty acids glob together in your cells—including your brain cells—and wreak havoc on normal cellular function.

Margarine is *the highest dietary source of fat for Americans.* For most people, it's an even greater source of fat than meat.

One study showed that women who ate four or more teaspoons of margarine per day had a 66-percent higher chance of contracting cardiovascular disease than women who ate about one teaspoon per month. Also, women who eat relatively high levels of the trans-fatty acids found in margarine and shortening have a much higher chance of contracting breast cancer, the number-one cancer killer in women. When men eat this form of fat, they greatly increase their risk of prostate cancer. Therefore I agree with Andrew Weil, M.D., who recommends we not use margarine at all.

Mediterranean countries, where olive oil is the primary form of fat that is ingested, have much lower rates of cardiovascular disease than does the United States.

Currently, many nutritional experts advise people to eat no more than 30 percent of their calories as fat. More-cautious nutritionists and physicians recommend keeping fat to about 20 percent of the diet. I advise patients to try to keep their fat consumption down to about 15 to 20 percent of their diets. In the diets of most people, a 20-percent level of fat consumption would still allow about 50 to 60 grams of fat per day.

It's important that a patient in the first stage of his or her brain longevity program try especially hard to control fat intake. After the momentum of brain regeneration has begun to take hold, you can be somewhat less careful about fat consumption. In the early days of your program, though, it's good to "clean your blood" in order to "clear your head."

If you do restrict much of the fat from your diet, you will almost certainly lose weight. Fat is fattening—there are more than *twice* as many calories in an ounce of fat as in an ounce of protein or carbohydrate. Fat also doesn't "rev up" your metabolism, as does the ingestion of complex carbohydrates. If you eat complex carbohydrates, they require *23 percent of the calories* in the food to convert the complex carbohydrates into body fat. But when you eat fat, it only requires 3 percent of the calories in the food to convert it into body fat.

If you begin a brain longevity program, you will probably lose weight, for several reasons. You will probably eat less fat, and therefore consume fewer calories. Your endocrine system will begin to function more efficiently, producing the hormones that help "burn" fat, such as human growth hormone. You will probably do less "stress eating," as the stress-management techniques in the program calm your nerves. And you will probably exercise more, because you'll feel more energetic.

If you do lose weight, you will almost certainly increase your longevity—including your brain longevity—for reasons I'll explain in the following section.

As the pounds drop off, a regenerative spiral is created.

How Caloric Restriction Increases Brain Longevity

Laboratory research indicates that longevity in test animals can be increased dramatically merely by decreasing caloric intake. Caloric-restriction experiments on rats and other animals have extended lifespan by up to 50 percent. If this same longevity increase were to extend to humans, it could theoretically allow us to live to approximately 120 years of age, without a severe decline in quality of life.

Although this may sound overly optimistic, it does have important implications.

Most important to me, as a brain longevity practitioner, is evidence that caloric restriction helps keep the brain from deteriorating during the aging process. Experiments conducted by the "guru" of caloric restriction, UCLA's Roy Walford, M.D., indicate that caloric restriction prevented the decline of dopamine receptors in the brain cells of animals. If this can be carried over to humans—and I believe it can—it would mean that the action of one of the most important neurotransmitters could be enhanced. Because dopamine typically declines in the elderly—causing serious restrictions in bodily movement (as well as Parkinson's disease)—the protection provided by dopamine during the aging process would be a major achievement.

Another of Dr. Walford's experiments indicated that function of brain cells' dendrites was also improved by caloric restriction. Again, if this applied to humans, it would be a major breakthrough in brain longevity. As I've mentioned, the ability to grow new dendrites is one of the most important aspects of brain plasticity. In recent years, researchers have found that new dendritic connections can be forged up until literally the last moment of life. This helps our brains to keep regenerating for as long as we live. Anything that might stimulate this regeneration is obviously quite valuable.

The caloric restriction that Dr. Walford recommends is not terribly severe. Dr. Walford himself eats approximately 1,500 to 2,000 calories per day. Although this is about 500 to 1,000 calories per day less than most men eat, it is still not a painfully ascetic dietary regime.

"Underfeeding" promotes longevity by providing a number of physiological advantages: It places less strain on the organs of digestion and assimilation; it produces fewer free radicals; it boosts levels of antioxidant enzymes by as much as 400 percent; it increases immune strength by up to 300 percent; it lowers blood insulin levels and cholesterol; it increases glucose tolerance; and it lowers blood pressure.

Many of my patients are very resistant to the concept of caloric restriction, for an obvious reason—it *sounds* difficult—but most people are already relatively cautious about overeating. I simply advise patients to be aware that eating less will probably be very good for their brains and their bodies.

The most important aspect of caloric restriction is simply to avoid being significantly overweight. It's a well-established fact that overweight people do not enjoy the same length of life, or quality of health, as people who are not overweight. If you are relatively thin—about 20 percent under the average weight for your height—you will live, according to national averages, about 40 percent longer than the heaviest 20 percent of people who are your height.

If you *do* try to lose weight, do it *slowly*. Any quick weight loss is a form of metabolic Russian roulette. You will have only about one chance in ten of keeping off weight that was lost during a crash diet.

If you follow my Brain Longevity Diet guideline of eating about 50 percent of your diet as whole grains, and about 25 percent as fruits and vegetables, you will probably reach your ideal weight relatively quickly. This happens for a simple reason: grains, vegetables, and fruits are less fattening than filling. You should be able to eat an abundant amount of them and still maintain your ideal weight.

Now you've gotten most of the fundamental information on what you should be *eating* for your Brain Longevity Diet. But before we move on to supplements and natural medicinal tonics, let's take a look at three special nutritional issues: sexual nutrition, nutrition for insomnia, and cerebral allergies.

How to Achieve "Sexual Longevity"

One of the most disquieting aspects of aging is the decline of sexual function. Loss of libido, and of sexual vitality, can destroy relationships and harm self-image.

Men, in particular, are often troubled by a decline in their sexuality during midlife, because many men directly equate their sexuality with their masculinity. Unfortunately, in most men, sexual decline during the aging process is a biological fact of life. The good news is that this sexual decline can generally be corrected.

About half of all men over forty experience at least occasional impotence. As men approach age fifty, this problem often becomes exacerbated. In one British study of 802 men over age fifty, half of those who were sexually active reported that they had experienced poor erections since turning fifty. *More than one-third* of the men in the study reported that *they no longer engaged in sexual intercourse.*

Females, too, commonly report a decrease in sexuality in their postmenopausal years. Some women who undergo hysterectomies note an especially sharp drop in libido following the surgery, particularly if no hormonal replacement therapy is prescribed for them.

The most obvious reason for age-associated sexual decline is the decline in testosterone in both males and females. This hormone is primarily responsible for triggering the libido in *both* sexes. Testosterone often drops sharply at approximately age fifty, in both males and females, and a drop-off can result in a marked decrease in sexual desire.

Other neurological factors also figure in age-associated sexual decline. Three neurotransmitters—dopamine, acetylcholine, and norepinephrine—play important roles in sexuality, and all often decline in midlife. When this happens, it can contribute significantly to a lessening of the sexual urge, and to diminished sexual ability in males.

Dopamine is a key element in sexual desire. When dopamine is increased in Parkinson's patients, through administration of the drug L-dopa, they commonly report an increase in sex drive.

Acetylcholine is vitally necessary for the sense of relaxation that males must feel in order to achieve erections and orgasms. It also helps control blood flow to the genitals in both sexes.

Norepinephrine, the excitatory neurotransmitter, must be present in adequate amounts for both sexes to feel sexual arousal. Often, when people complain that they are "too tired" to desire sex, they are experiencing a lack of physical excitation due to a norepinephrine deficit.

Of course, production of each of these three neurotransmitters can be stimulated nutritionally, as indicated in the preceding chapter.

In recent years, researchers have also discovered that the gas nitric oxide, which is present in the body in small amounts, is needed for penile erections, and for enhanced blood flow to the female genitalia. Nitric oxide is manufactured in the body by the amino acid *arginine*. If arginine levels are low, there can be a deficit of nitric oxide. This can decrease sexual performance in males, and sexual sensitivity in females.

A number of other nutrients are also important for establishing and maintaining sexuality in midlife. Vitamin B_1 and vitamin A are important in nerve transmission. Vitamin E and vitamin C help maintain proper levels of sex hormones. Vitamin B_5 helps the adrenal glands to make steroid hormones. And vitamin B_3, or niacin, helps dilate the blood vessels and capillaries, which is necessary for sexual arousal.

Of course, maintaining optimal blood circulation is also an

important element in ensuring sexual vitality. *Anything* that interferes with circulation, such as a high cholesterol level, can dampen sexual ardor.

One possibly promising substance for ameliorating age-associated sexual decline is the homeopathic formulation called *Avena sativa,* which is prescribed for impotence and for sexual debility. *Avena sativa,* though discounted by some researchers, has shown sexual restorative qualities in several studies. In one double-blind crossover endocrinological study, 90 percent of male patients given the controversial substance showed some evidence of enhanced libido and improved sexual performance.

Ginseng, described in detail in the following chapter, is also widely used to enhance sexual vigor. In one interesting recent experiment at Southern Illinois University, male rats given a diet that included ginseng took an average of just fourteen seconds to initiate sexual contact with female rats, while male rats given no ginseng took an average of one hundred seconds.

Two of the pharmaceutical medications that I often prescribe also often increase sex drive and improve sexual function. One is deprenyl, which markedly increases levels of dopamine, the neurotransmitter that is closely associated with sex drive. The other is DHEA, the hormone that can be converted by the body into sex hormones.

The only medication approved by the FDA for sexual dysfunction is yohimbine, which is derived from the bark of the yohimbe tree. Many health-food stores sell capsules of unrefined yohimbe bark, but there is no evidence that it is effective. Yohimbine, which must be prescribed by a physician, should be used cautiously, because overuse may cause kidney damage, particularly in diabetics.

Nutritional Therapy for Insomnia

Too often, even the "naturalistic" nutritional therapies for insomnia consist of just using nutrients or herbs to "drug" an insomniac's imbalanced neurochemistry. I recommend a much more enduring approach that consists of restoring metabolic balance to the brain biochemistry, so that it doesn't need to be drugged with "nutritional downers."

One of the primary metabolic imbalances that leads to chronic biochemical insomnia is a deficit of melatonin. Melatonin, a hormone secreted by the pineal gland, governs the "circadian rhythms" that determine our sleep cycles. In the evening, melatonin production generally increases, causing drowsiness, and heightening the ability to fall asleep and stay asleep. In the morning, melatonin production declines, creating a daytime period of arousal.

It's widely believed that seasonal affective disorder (SAD)— the form of clinical depression that strikes some people during the short daylight hours of winter—is linked to excessive production of melatonin. During the darkest months of the winter, melatonin production increases. Why? Because melatonin production is halted when light strikes the eye. Light causes photoreceptors in the eye to "tell" the pineal gland to stop producing melatonin. Theoretically, this reaction evolved as a simple survival mechanism; when the sun came up, it biochemically stimulated people to stop producing calming melatonin, and to be active. Then, when the sun went down, it increased melatonin production, and biochemically created a desire for sleep.

Seasonal affective disorder is especially common in northern latitudes, where winter daylight is much shorter. There, SAD strikes about one in every thousand people. In the southern latitudes, where there is more sunlight, incidence is only about one in sixteen thousand. Some researchers think SAD causes the higher rates of suicide and alcoholism in places such as the Scandinavian countries.

To reverse SAD, clinicians expose their patients to bright, full-spectrum lights for a length of time each day that mimics summertime daylight hours. The positive response rate to this therapy is extremely high.

Experimenting with this form of therapy on your own is easy and safe. Just buy four to six fluorescent bulbs, six feet long, and turn them on when you awaken in the morning. Stay near these lights for about an hour in the morning, or longer if it's convenient. It's important, though, to use *full-spectrum* lights (or "grow lights"), because they contain the various wavelengths that most effectively stimulate the pineal gland to halt melatonin production.

Many people naturally feel more energetic in the summer, as a response to decreased melatonin production. In some cases, people become excessively energetic during the long days of summer, experiencing "summertime hypermania."

Frequently, people with insomnia are merely experiencing a mild form of "summertime hypermania." They simply aren't producing enough melatonin to be able to sleep well at night.

This is especially common in midlife and beyond. Aging people have a deficit of melatonin, because of atrophy of their pineal glands. The pineal grows less vital every year, and in many elderly people it becomes calcified and nonfunctional. For many years, anatomy experts believed that *everyone's* pineal gland became nonfunctional in their elderly years. More recently, though, some researchers have come to believe that the pineal does not always cease to function in aging people, and that it can even be "revived," and function as well as it did in youth.

To substitute for the decline of melatonin production during the aging process, you can take melatonin orally. Available in health-food stores, it is inexpensive and nontoxic. Many of my patients with insomnia take 1 to 3 mg of melatonin each evening around bedtime. One of the leading melatonin researchers, however, takes only 0.1 mg nightly.

Some of the mind/body exercises that I recommend increase melatonin production by stimulating the pineal gland. In my practice, I've found that patients who regularly perform the mind/body exercises require much smaller dosages of melatonin. In fact, they frequently cannot tolerate the relatively high dosages required by people who don't do the exercises. Often, when they take a full 3-mg tablet, it makes them feel groggy.

Maintaining adequate levels of melatonin does more than just help sleep. Melatonin plays an important role in immune function, and animal studies indicate that melatonin also increases longevity. In one study, the lifespan of mice was increased by 50 percent, merely with application of melatonin.

The common decrease in melatonin during aging probably accounts for the fact that older people often get less sleep than younger people. Often, of course, older people say that they "need" less sleep than they did when they were young. Actually, they probably "need" just as much sleep, but have learned to live without it, simply because they don't get it.

Melatonin is not the only nutritional aid to sleep. In fact, all of the nutrients that help produce acetylcholine will promote better sleep. Acetylcholine controls the brain's calming, or *cholinergic*, system of chemicals. The cholinergic system is essentially the opposite of the stimulating adrenergic system, which is governed primarily by adrenaline.

As you may recall, the primary nutrient that produces acetylcholine is phosphatidyl choline, derived from lecithin. Ingestion of lecithin should be accompanied by ingestion of the nutrients that lecithin needs for synthesis into acetylcholine; these nutrients are vitamin B_5 and vitamin C, and (to a lesser extent) zinc and B_6. The nutrient DMAE also helps synthesize acetylcholine from lecithin, but DMAE can stimulate the central nervous system, so it should always be taken in the morning instead of the evening.

Taking large amounts of lecithin at night will not "drug" you to sleep. Maintaining high acetylcholine levels *all day long*, however, will optimize function of your cholinergic nervous system, and help you to sleep in the evening.

Another powerful aid to sleep is the amino acid tryptophan. Millions of people once used tryptophan as a safe and healthy alternative to sleeping pills. Now the only way to purchase tryptophan is with a doctor's prescription at a compounding pharmacy. (See "Resources and Referrals.") The best way to obtain it, however, is to ingest it in foodstuffs. As mentioned earlier, to metabolize tryptophan, you should eat a meal or snack high in carbohydrates.

Another "sleep aid" amino acid is GABA. GABA is a very calming nutrient that is especially helpful at controlling the "racing thoughts" of an overactive mind. A nontoxic, natural, and non-habit-forming "cousin" to the benzodiazepine sedative drugs, such as Valium and Xanax, GABA causes relaxation, as Valium or Xanax does, but doesn't have the disturbing side effects of the benzodiazepines.

Also, some herbs, such as valerian and chamomile, are mildly sedating.

Vitamin B_3, or niacin, attaches to the same receptors in brain cells as the benzodiazepines and GABA. Therefore it has a mild calming effect on many people. It is especially effective when taken *with* GABA, shortly before bedtime. Niacin usually causes the skin to flush, or redden, for about twenty minutes, because it dilates capillaries. Some people find this mild tingling and warmth pleasurable; others find it annoying. If you don't enjoy the skin flush, you can substitute for niacin with niacinamide, which exerts approximately the same actions, but causes no flushing.

Other B vitamins also have a strong calming effect on many people, and so do calcium and magnesium.

A deficiency of any of the above mentioned nutrients can create agitation and restlessness. These nutrients will not narcotize you, as a sleeping pill does. Instead they will help balance your brain biochemistry, and naturally allow you to get as much sleep as you need.

Another obvious aspect of insomnia that many people ignore is caffeine consumption. The stimulation from caffeine can take two to four hours to peak, and stimulation can persist for up to twenty hours. Therefore, if you have an insomnia problem, you should try to limit caffeine intake to just the morning hours, and to avoid caffeine entirely after about 3:00 P.M. You should also be aware that chocolate contains small amounts of caffeine, and that many over-the-counter pain remedies contain large amounts of caffeine. Patients on brain longevity programs tend to avoid caffeine, because they usually have abundant energy without it.

Cerebral Allergies and Brain Dysfunction

One of the more controversial elements of cognitive dysfunction is the possible impact of "cerebral allergies," or allergies that affect the brain. On one side of this controversy are the physicians and researchers who believe that a wide segment of the population—up to 60 to 80 percent of all people—have at least a minor physical reaction to various foods, and to certain environmental substances, such as chlorine and formaldehyde. On the other side of the controversy are physicians who believe that allergic reaction to foods and chemicals is relatively rare, and usually involves only a few common foods, such as wheat or milk. This view is often held by conventional allergists.

My belief is that many people *do* suffer mild responses to a wide variety of foods and chemical substances. I do not, however, agree with the doctors who believe that this occurs in 60 to 80 percent of all people.

Many allergic reactions do seem to cause at least minor cognitive dysfunction, ranging from mild depression to a vague feeling of malaise. In severe cases, intellectual reasoning declines significantly, and patients may feel markedly agitated or profoundly depressed.

Allergic reactions occur when the immune system mistakenly identifies a substance as a dangerous "foreign invader" (such as a virus or bacteria). When this happens, one of the reactions is an attempt by the body to "wash away" the invader, by releasing fluids. This is the reaction that causes your eyes to water, your nose to run, and your tissues to swell. In the brain, this swelling can cause cognitive disturbance, or a headache. Other immune-based biochemical changes can occur, such as a release of adrenaline.

The best defense against allergic response is to eat sensibly, and to balance your body's biochemistry, so that your immune system will be less likely to mistake normal foods for allergens.

If you do feel you may have a food or chemical allergy, eliminate the suspected food or chemical from your diet or environment. Then reintroduce it, and monitor yourself for allergic response. If, in your opinion, you do have a reaction—or perhaps a less severe "sensitivity"—seek treatment from an allergist or a naturopathic physician.

In the next chapter we'll examine the nutritional substances that have the most dramatic, immediate effects upon cerebral function. These concentrated nutrients and *natural* medicinal tonics will help you to achieve your peak mental abilities.

These nutrients, I believe, will prove to be the "mental wonder drugs" of the twenty-first century.

A Case in Point

Even Some Late-Stage Alzheimer's Patients Can Improve

When W.N., eighty-five years of age, first consulted with me, I feared that he might never get any better. He was a stage-6 Alzheimer's patient, rapidly approaching the final, most devastating stage of Alzheimer's, stage 7.

Sometimes, when patients advance to early stage 6, I can help them slow progression of the disease, but am unable to help them return to higher levels of cognitive function.

W.N., a very successful Russian immigrant, had many of the classic characteristics of stage 6, and virtually all of the characteristics of stage 5. He could not remember his children or his ex-wife, he couldn't understand much of what he read, he couldn't tell me what month or day it was, he couldn't remember his date of birth, and he couldn't remember who was the current president. He was frequently disoriented, was obsessive about hanging up his clothing, and didn't respond to humorous remarks. He couldn't remember the name of his sister-in-law, even though he saw her frequently, and he kept forgetting that he and his wife were having a new home built.

His wife, who was also of European origin, was terribly worried about him, and felt, quite understandably, that she was quickly losing him.

His problems had begun about five years earlier. Until that time he had remained very active in his career, running a manufacturing company. He had also been very physically active, jogging almost every day. However, when he was about eighty, he'd experienced a traumatic death in his family. Shortly after that, he'd experienced a great deal of stress with his business. From that point on, he had begun to decline mentally and physically.

He had developed a bleeding ulcer that was so severe that he'd needed a transfusion. His cognitive function had plummeted.

Around this time, while he'd been climbing a hill, he had passed out from lack of oxygen. Shortly after this experience, his mental decline had accelerated.

He had gone to a well-known medical center, where he'd been given a battery of cognitive function tests. Doctors there had diagnosed him with senile dementia. They'd placed him on a course of tacrine, which increases acetylcholine function. But according to his wife, the medication had had no discernible positive effect, and his decline had continued.

When he began his brain longevity program, I advised him to keep taking the tacrine, because there was no evidence that it was causing him to suffer from liver damage, as it does in some patients. Also, I hoped that if the tacrine was combined with ingestion of phosphatidyl choline, derived from lecithin, it would be more effective. The latest research indicates that the value of tacrine, which stimulates the cholinergic system, can be amplified by ingestion of choline, which provides the cholinergic system with its nutritional "building blocks."

I also placed him on 300 mg daily of phosphatidyl serine, 1,500 mg daily of acetyl-L-carnitine, and large dosages of *Ginkgo biloba* and the vitamin-B complex. In addition, I prescribed 800 international units daily of vitamin E; daily ingestion of a chlorophyll-based "green drink"; and pregnenolone hormonal replacement therapy.

As part of his mental exercise program, I recommended that he sing to his wife, because both of them enjoyed that. Interestingly, song lyrics often persist in the memories of Alzheimer's patients, because the lyrics are stored not only in the language centers of the brain, but also in the areas that process music. Having this doubled association increased his recall success, and this success encouraged him to continue the mental exercise.

About six weeks after his program had begun, I called his wife, to see how he was doing. Because his progression had been so advanced, the most I was hoping for was that he would not have deteriorated further.

But when I asked how he was, his wife said, "He's better!" She began to rattle off a list of improvements. She was very excited and extremely pleased, and so was I.

In just his first six weeks, W.N. had begun to participate much more in his daily routine. He no longer followed his wife around the house all day long, as he previously had. He was reading again, and taking much more interest in current affairs. One evening, she said, they had gone to the opera, and he had read along with the translation of the lyrics, and had laughed in the appropriate places. He now remembered the name of his sister-in-law, and had much better access to his vocabulary.

After his initial surge of progress, W.N.'s improvements began to plateau. But then he had another spurt of improvement.

I am hoping that he will continue to improve.

But even if he doesn't, his condition now is far superior to what it was when he began treatment. For an early-stage-6 Alzheimer's patient, this is a medical miracle.

13

Key Nutrients and Natural Tonics for Peak Mental Performance

Now I'll tell you about some very special nutrients that are so powerful they often have a pharmacologic effect upon the brain, producing dramatic results quickly. Some of these nutrients can be ingested as nutritional supplements. Others come in the form of natural medicinal tonics.

Let's start by looking at particular nutritional supplements, and the roles they can play in cognition. After that, I'll describe natural medicinal tonics that will boost your brain power.

Every day, you should take several key nutrients. Some of these nutrients are in standard multiple vitamins. They may not, however, be present in sufficient quantities in a multiple vitamin to reverse cognitive dysfunction, or to stimulate optimal cognitive function. Often, nutrients in multiple vitamins are present only in sufficient quantities to prevent frank pathology from vitamin deficiency. Obviously this falls far short of promoting optimal function of your body and brain.

It's also important to take enough of these nutrients to make your brain strong enough to withstand the ravages of time. Remember, you're trying to achieve not just *current* optimal cognitive function, but also brain longevity. You want your brain to work perfectly for the rest of your life. To achieve this ambitious goal, you will have to undertake a nutritional regimen that is high in both quantity and quality of nutrients.

One quick word about the so-called Recommended Daily Allowances: *Nonsense!* I believe they're just too low. These daily allowances, until recently, were called "Minimum Daily Requirements." But then someone with a good sense of public relations realized that most people want more than just the "minimum." So they changed "Minimum" to "Recommended"—but still left the amounts at approximately the same low levels.

The same government agency that assigns the RDAs also assigns the nutrient levels for research animals in government labs. Ironically, for its research monkeys, the agency assigns nutritional needs according to "*optimum* intake." As a result, the agency recommends that monkeys be given an amount of vitamin C that's *higher* than the *human* RDA.

I'm sure you've heard nutrition "experts" tell you that you can get all of the nutrients you need in a normal diet. They then generally describe the foods that provide these nutrients, and they're things like rutabagas, caviar, mutton, and persimmons— as if we all *ate* that kind of stuff.

The next time you hear that line of logic, you might remind the expert that it would take twenty oranges a day to get a single gram of vitamin C, or twenty pounds of liver to get 50 mg of B_6.

From a normal diet, you *can* get enough nutrients to keep from contracting beriberi or rickets. But I'm sure you have higher goals than that.

Another criticism of high amounts of vitamins is that they might cause an overdose.

It is true that a few vitamins, taken in gross excess, can cause health problems. Extremely high amounts of vitamin A can be toxic (although I have never spoken to a physician who has actually seen this occur).

When you compare the safety of vitamins to the safety of pharmaceutical drugs, however, it's easy to see that drugs are *far* more dangerous. In one typical seven-year period, from 1983 to 1990, the federal Poison Control Centers reported that there were 2,556 fatalities directly caused by medically prescribed drugs—but no deaths from vitamins.

I am not claiming that no harm can ever come from vitamins, if they are taken in *grossly excessive* amounts. Vitamin B$_6$ can cause some problems if it is taken in extremely high dosages, and the mineral iron can promote free-radical damage if ingested in large quantities. Pregnant women who take more than 10,000 units daily of vitamin A increase the risk of serious birth defects by 240 percent and should always consult their obstetrician before taking any vitamin supplements or other concentrated nutrients.

All in all, though, there are very few risk factors associated with intake of high dosages of vitamins. Most of the risk factors that exist are theoretical rather than practical. For example, if taken in *extremely* high dosages, in the absence of other B vitamins, B$_6$ can cause temporary, mild nerve damage; to cause this damage, though, a person must take 1,000 to 6,000 mg per day. However, even "megadose" B-vitamin tablets contain only 50 to 100 mg.

While you don't have to be overly worried about taking large doses of some nutrients, you should be *sensible* and always consult your physician first.

Here are the nutrients you need to stock your "cognitive arsenal." They are in alphabetical order—for a particular reason. I did not rate them from "most important" to "least important," because they're *all* important. They all work synergistically, and none of them, if used alone, will give you the results you want.

Vitamins

VITAMIN A

A powerful antioxidant, it protects the membranes of brain cells, which are easily damaged by free radicals. It also helps the circulatory system; in one study, it reduced risk of heart attack and stroke significantly. It's especially good at neutralizing the harmful "singlet oxygen" that's found in air pollution and cigarette smoke.

Take it with beta carotene, another form of vitamin A. If you're pregnant, take small dosages only, to prevent possible birth defects. For most people (but not pregnant women), a reasonable daily dosage would be at least 10,000 units. Many people, though, take multiple vitamins that contain 25,000 units of vitamin A, and 15 mg of beta carotene.

B VITAMINS

Absolutely vital for neuronal growth and vitality. The four B vitamins that are most important for your brain are B_{12}, B_6, B_1, and folic acid.

B_{12}. Almost 25 percent of all people age sixty to sixty-nine are deficient in B_{12}, and up to 40 percent of all people over eighty, according to a major study. One primary reason for this is that the substance that breaks down B_{12} in your stomach—hydrochloric acid—declines as you age. A B_{12} shortage can mimic the classic signs of age-associated cognitive decline: poor memory, a reduction in reasoning skills, and mood disorders. A deficiency of B_{12} is 300 percent more common among people who don't take vitamin supplements. An appropriate daily dosage of B_{12} can be anywhere from 100 to even 1,000 mcg. Some doctors prescribe sublingual administration of B_{12}. Others administer it with intramuscular injections, which often provide a boost of energy.

B_6. This vitamin helps convert stored blood sugar into glucose, the brain's only fuel. It helps protect blood vessels, and appears to protect significantly against heart attacks. People in midlife and beyond need about 20 percent more B_6 than younger people for optimal cognitive function, but they usually don't get it, because the metabolism of B_6 declines after age forty. Most Americans ingest only about *half* of even the low RDA of B_6.

Because of its beneficial effects upon circulation, B_6 has been shown in studies to successfully improve memory. It's also an immune stimulant, and can be very helpful in mediating against premenstrual symptoms. An appropriate daily dosage is in the range of 100 mg.

B_1 (thiamin). Thiamin, B_1, is involved in innumerable metabolic processes in the brain and peripheral nervous system. It is also a powerful antioxidant, and increases the abilities of B_6 and vitamin E to destroy free radicals. If you drink alcohol, it's especially important to ingest enough B_1, because excessive alcohol consumption can cause a deficiency of B_1, resulting in the severe psychiatric condition called Korsakoff's psychosis. A prudent daily dosage is 50 to 100 mg.

Folic Acid. According to some studies, folic acid has been helpful in relieving depression, even when used in dosages as low as 400 mcg. It can also enhance cerebral circulation. One study showed that people with low levels of folic acid were twice as likely as people with adequate levels to have narrowed arteries in their necks. Psychiatric symptoms also appear to be much higher in people, particularly elderly people, who have low folic acid levels.

In one study, low folic acid levels increased likelihood of dementia by 300 percent. Folic acid is especially effective at breaking down the common chemical *homocysteine*, which is a neurotoxin. An appropriate daily dosage would be 400 mcg, the amount found in many multiple vitamins.

Vitamin B_3 (niacin). Niacin helps to manufacture neurotransmitters, convert carbohydrates to glucose, and lower cholesterol. It can also have a calming effect, because it potentiates the power of the calming neurotransmitter GABA. Niacin causes a mild flushing of the skin, but another form of B_3, niacinamide, does not. An appropriate daily dosage is 100 mg to 200 mg.

Vitamin B_5. Absolutely vital to the synthesis of the brain's primary memory neurotransmitter, acetylcholine, B_5, also called pantothenic acid, also helps form a protective sheath around the spinal cord. A gross deficiency of B_5 can lead to paralysis. B_5 is also helpful for arteries. A reasonable daily dosage is about 100 to 200 mg.

VITAMIN C

So vital for brain function that its levels in the brain are almost *fifteen times higher* than they are outside the brain, vitamin C is probably the strongest antioxidant in existence. It increases the antioxidative potential of other nutrients. For example, vitamin C has the remarkable ability to "revive" vitamin E as an antioxidant, even after E has been oxidized itself.

Vitamin C is one of the best nutrients at promoting longevity. In a large study at UCLA, people who ingested at least 300 mg daily of vitamin C lived more than six years longer than those who ingested less than 300 mg. Furthermore, vitamin C cut deaths from cardiovascular disease by 40 percent.

A full 25 percent of all Americans, though, don't get even 60 mg of vitamin C per day. As we age, this deficiency begins to take a physical toll. In a study of hospitalized elderly patients, more than two-thirds had a deficiency of vitamin C in their white blood cells.

Vitamin C is an important ingredient in the creation of several neurotransmitters, including acetylcholine, dopamine, and norepinephrine. Therefore, intake of this vitamin can improve cognitive function. In one interesting study, administration of vitamin C raised students' scores on IQ tests by an average of five points.

Vitamin C boosts immunity, improves arterial function, reduces cholesterol, and is at least partly helpful in preventing a host of diseases (everything from asthma to periodontal disease to some forms of cancer).

To get the maximum efficiency from vitamin C supplementation, stagger your intake throughout the day. Your body can fully metabolize about 500 mg at a time, but is able to metabolize only about half of the *next* 500 mg you take (in the same dosage). If you take 1,500 mg, your body metabolizes only about one-fourth of the "last" 500 mg. Thus you quickly reach a point of diminishing returns. To get the most "bang for your buck," you should take vitamin C in dosages of no more than 1,000 mg., several times daily.

A reasonable daily dosage for optimal physical and mental function is about 3,000 mg. However, the "godfather" of vitamin C research, Dr. Linus Pauling, recommended dosages of 7,000 to 10,000 mg daily. In my opinion, this is overkill, unless you are using the vitamin medicinally (to speed recovery from a minor illness, for example).

If you take more C than your body can tolerate, you'll notice a buildup of intestinal gas, and may experience diarrhea. If you do reach this "bowel tolerance" level, back off your intake until the symptoms go away. These symptoms arise partly because vitamin C helps to kill the "good" bacteria in your intestine, so you should replenish this digestive bacteria by eating yogurt with lactobacillus.

Vitamin C is one of the compounds being considered for testing as a preventive agent for Alzheimer's, in high-risk patients, by the national Alzheimer's Research Centers. (The other compounds under consideration include vitamin E, coenzyme Q-10, and deprenyl.)

Vitamin E

Not only does vitamin E protect neurons from damage by free radicals, but it even *restores* damaged neurotransmitter receptor sites on neurons. Therefore it can not only prevent deterioration of the brain, but also actually *reverse* an important element of deterioration.

Some Alzheimer's researchers believe that vitamin E can help prevent Alzheimer's, and even slow the progression of the disease, once it already exists. Recently, in the *Proceedings of the National Academy of Sciences*, a geriatric researcher noted that a daily dosage of 400 IU of vitamin E may "help protect the brain and its memories from the ravages of time."

Studies have shown that vitamin E, when taken with selenium, can improve mood and cognitive function in the elderly.

Vitamin E is one of the most potent antioxidants, and is unquestionably of great value to the circulatory system. One study showed that vitamin E decreased oxidation of "bad" cholesterol by 40 percent. Numerous studies strongly indicate that vitamin E decreases risk of heart attack and stroke. In one large study, heart disease was reduced by more than 40 percent in people who took at least 100 units of vitamin E daily.

Vitamin E increases immune function, helps the body fight cancer, retards the onset of cataracts, helps relieve arthritic symptoms, and significantly slows "brain aging."

Leading brain researchers recommend a daily dosage of 800 international units of vitamin E, but because my patients are on full-spectrum, synergistic programs, they often do not require this high a dosage. I generally recommend 400 IU daily, only rarely going as high as 800.

If taken in extreme megadoses, such as 3,000 units daily, vitamin E can cause headaches and raise blood pressure. Because vitamin E has a mild ability to prevent clotting of blood, patients on anticoagulants should use vitamin E only under the strict supervision of a physician. Because vitamin E is fat-soluble, any regular daily dosage higher than 800 IU might accumulate to toxic levels.

Minerals

MAGNESIUM

An important nutrient that may in the future prove to be of *absolute* importance. It's been proven that the brains of Alzheimer's patients have a deficit of magnesium, and a toxically high level of its counterpart, calcium. It's been theorized that, in healthy brains, which have a normal ratio of magnesium to calcium, magnesium helps to avert the deadly consequences of calcium toxicity.

Magnesium helps to maintain the metabolic viability of neurons, and helps to minimize brain damage resulting from lack of blood flow (ischemia).

Magnesium is also a powerful free-radical scavenger, helps increase the antioxidative power of vitamin E, and promotes circulation by deterring blood clotting and decreasing blood pressure. A study in Europe indicated that low intake of magnesium increased risk of sudden death from heart attack by about 50 percent.

An appropriate daily dosage to achieve brain longevity is 200 to 300 mg. If magnesium is taken in very high dosages (600 to 700 mg), it sometimes causes diarrhea.

Selenium

This may well be the most effective mineral antioxidant. It is particularly effective at preventing oxidation of fat, which is especially beneficial to the brain, since about 60 percent of the brain is composed of a form of fat.

Selenium levels in the blood typically decline as we age. After age sixty, they can drop by almost 10 percent, and beyond seventy-five, they can drop by more than 20 percent.

Selenium significantly boosts immunity, and appears to improve circulation. If taken in relatively high dosages, selenium sometimes creates an anti-anxiety effect. An optimum dosage is about 50 to 100 mcg daily.

Zinc

Another nutrient that has powerful anti-aging properties. However, a zinc deficiency is quite common in people age fifty and older. It's been estimated that up to 33 percent of all people over fifty have at least a minor deficiency in zinc. This generally occurs because of inadequate *intake* of zinc. Almost 90 percent of all people fail to meet even the so-called RDA for zinc on most days. One reason for this is that you would have to eat almost 2,500 calories per day to get enough zinc, unless you were carefully targeting ingestion of foods rich in zinc. This, again, belies the theory that people can get all the nutrients they need from a normal diet.

Zinc plays an important role in brain metabolism. It's part of an antioxidant "chain reaction" that *destroys* many of the free-radical molecules in the brain. It also bolsters the strength of neuronal cell membranes, which protects neurons from damage.

Zinc helps rid the brain of lead, which enters the brain from sources like auto exhaust, and which can be profoundly damaging to cognitive function. It boosts immunity, promotes sexual function, and potentiates the actions of vitamin A.

A recommended dosage of zinc for brain longevity patients is approximately 30 to 50 mg daily.

Amino Acids

In addition to the above listed vitamins and minerals, some amino acids (or partial proteins) are also of special value.

Phenylalanine. The major nutritional precursor of the energizing neurotransmitter norepinephrine, phenylalanine helps brighten mood, stimulate energy, and improve memory. To feel energetic and to have a good long-term memory, it's absolutely vital that you have sufficient intake of phenylalanine. Some people take phenylalanine supplements, although this is not always necessary.

Glutamine. The major nutritional precursor of GABA, the calming neurotransmitter, glutamine can also improve clarity of thought, and can increase alertness—probably because it helps produce glutamic acid, which neutralizes metabolic wastes in the brain. Some people ingest glutamine prior to events that require increased alertness.

Methionine. Another amino acid that helps to "clean" the brain of toxins, methionine acts as a powerful antioxidant, and helps prevent the accumulation of heavy metals in the brain, such as mercury or cadmium.

Arginine. This amino acid is partly converted in the body to a chemical called spermine, which helps the brain to process memories. Low levels of spermine are sometimes a biological indicator of age-associated memory impairment. Arginine is also an effective stimulator of the metabolism, and is used by some people as part of a weight-loss formula.

Tryptophan. As mentioned previously, tryptophan is easily available in supplement form, but can be ingested in foodstuffs (especially by eating high-carbohydrate foods). It is the major nutritional precursor of serotonin, the primary "feel good" neurotransmitter. If you frequently feel agitated, or have insomnia, this may be caused by a deficit of serotonin.

For your convenience, here is a list of the most important nutritional supplements for brain longevity, and a general range of dosages I recommend to many patients, depending on their needs:

NUTRITIONAL SUPPLEMENTS

Daily Dosage

Vitamin A	10,000–25,000 IU
Vitamin B$_{12}$	100–1,000 mcg
Vitamin B$_6$	50–200 mg
Vitamin B$_1$	50–100 mg
Folic Acid	400 mcg
Niacin	100–200 mg
Vitamin B$_5$	100–200 mg
Vitamin C	3,000 mg
Vitamin E	400–800 mg
Magnesium	200–300 mg
Selenium	50–100 mcg
Zinc	30–50 mg
Multi vitamin/mineral	1–2 tablets (may contain all of the above)
Amino acids	one serving, protein powder

The vast majority of the above listed nutrients are appropriate for all patients, even when taken in high dosages. Further, all of these nutrients at moderate levels are absolutely vital for all people. Your brain has always needed each one of them, and always will.

Now let's look at an especially powerful form of nutritional therapy—use of natural medicinal tonics. Once you begin using some of these natural brain tonics you'll wonder how you ever lived without them.

Natural Medicinal Tonics

In modern Western medicine, you don't often hear the word *tonic.* A tonic is a substance that is used to tonify, or strengthen, the function of an organ, gland, or system. Often this organ, gland, or system is already working at a normal or near normal level, but is *improved* by the tonic.

Modern Western medicine, however, pays little attention to improving normal function. Western modalities focus mostly on relieving pathologies instead of optimizing function. The problem with waiting for something to break is that it usually does. If, on the other hand, it is tonified regularly, it might never "break."

In Eastern medicine, however, tonics play a major role.

They also play a major role in my brain longevity programs.

Even if you feel that your cognitive function is normal, you should try some of these tonics. They might lift you to a new level.

GINKGO BILOBA

One of the most important natural medicinal tonics, *Ginkgo biloba* powerfully enhances cerebral circulation, and has wondrous effects upon the brain. An extract from the leaf of the common ginkgo tree, it has been subjected to more than two hundred controlled, double-blind experiments, and many have indicated that ginkgo increases cognitive ability. It has even been used with some success in cases of Alzheimer's.

In a 1995 study, reported in the journal *Human Psychopharmacology*, forty Alzheimer's patients received either 80 mg of ginkgo or a placebo, three times daily for three months. Patients were assessed with a battery of cognitive function tests, and with EEG examinations. Among the patients taking ginkgo, significant improvement was noted in psychopathology, psychomotor performance, neurophysiology, and cognitive function. Memory and attention span began to increase in the first month of treatment. The substance was well tolerated, and no side effects were noted. The group on the placebo showed no objective improvement.

Please note, though, that the daily dosage of 240 mg used in this study is substantially higher than the dosage taken by most people who use ginkgo only as a tonic.

Studies have indicated a similar positive response to ginkgo among patients with other forms of impaired cognition. In one study, 79 percent of patients with cerebrovascular insufficiency showed significant improvement after taking ginkgo.

In another study of patients with degenerative dementia (or progressive cognitive decline), patients using ginkgo scored higher on cognitive assessment tests, and experienced higher levels of alertness, than patients on a placebo.

Ginkgo often elicits a very fast response. In one double-blind crossover study, a single 600-mg dosage of ginkgo caused patients with memory loss to experience a significant improvement in short-term memory within *one hour*. No immediate response was shown, however, in patients receiving dosages of 120 mg and 240 mg.

Like virtually all medicinal substances used for impaired cognitive function, ginkgo is better at preventing cognitive problems, and improving minor cognitive problems, than at reversing profound cognitive dysfunction. Therefore it may prove to be of most value in *delaying progression* of cognitive decline, and thus effectively preventing debilitating, late-stage symptoms.

As mentioned earlier, the primary mechanism of action of ginkgo is to improve cerebral circulation, so it is of special value for patients with dementia caused by multiple minor strokes. This type of dementia accounts for approximately 20 percent of all cases of Alzheimer's-like symptoms.

Ginkgo improves circulation, in part, by quelling the action of a substance called *platelet-activating factor*, which interferes significantly with cerebral circulation.

Because it is so beneficial for cerebral blood flow, ginkgo is used by many people who suffer from migraine headaches, which are closely associated with disturbed cerebral circulation. In one study, 80 percent of migraine sufferers experienced cessation of headaches after using ginkgo.

It has also shown promise in the treatment of impotence caused by circulation disorders, and in the treatment of various other circulatory disorders. Studies have shown that ginkgo lowers blood pressure, and expands peripheral blood vessels.

Ginkgo has demonstrated an ability to increase the brain's tolerance for oxygen deficiency. It is effective at slowing the progression of macular degeneration, an eye disease that develops gradually, usually in older people, and is one of the leading causes of blindness. It is believed that impaired circulation to the eyes is a major contributing factor to macular degeneration.

I strongly recommend ginkgo to virtually all of my patients. For people in midlife, who have no apparent cognitive dysfunction, a daily dosage of 90 mg is often sufficient. If cognitive decline has begun, this dosage level may be increased to between 120 and 160 mg. If frank pathology exists, patients may be advised to take 200 to 320 mg daily. For most people, however, 120 mg is sufficient. Dosages should be spread evenly throughout the day, in three administrations.

Some supplement companies have begun to add other antioxidants to their ginkgo products, and this may improve the products' effectiveness.

Even if you engage in only a partial program of brain longevity, you should use ginkgo.

LECITHIN

Along with ginkgo, phosphatidyl serine, and ginseng, lecithin is extremely important.

You probably now ingest about 1,000 mg of lecithin daily as part of your normal diet, but this is not a high enough quantity to promote brain longevity. As noted, lecithin's active ingredient, phosphatidyl choline, is the nutritional building material for acetylcholine, the primary neurotransmitter of thought and memory.

Many studies and experiments have shown that ingestion of lecithin, or phosphatidyl choline, can improve cognitive function. I have already recounted several of these studies. Like ginkgo, though, lecithin is much more effective as a *preventive* agent than a curative agent. Most of the studies in which lecithin was given to Alzheimer's patients indicate that, even though most patients have a shortage of acetylcholine, lecithin is not effective at reversing Alzheimer's.

In early-stage memory disorders, lecithin can be of significant benefit. Innumerable studies have also indicated that, in cognitively healthy people, it can *heighten* mental abilities.

Besides being the "main ingredient" of acetylcholine, phosphatidyl choline is used to repair and maintain neurons. In addition, it is used outside the brain in the metabolism of fats, in the regulation of cholesterol, and in the production of the myelin sheaths that surround nerves. For maximum effectiveness, lecithin may be taken with vitamin B_5, and also with the nutrient DMAE.

DMAE, however, may be somewhat stimulating for many people, and it should not be taken by people with bipolar, or "manic," depression, because it can exacerbate the depressive phase of the cycle.

Phosphatidyl choline can be ingested not only by taking lecithin, but also by taking *choline bitartrate* or *choline chloride.* Both of these nutrients, though, can create a slightly "fishy" odor, and occasionally cause diarrhea.

Lecithin can be purchased in health-food stores and supermarkets. It is often about 30 to 55 percent pure phosphatidyl choline. Check the label of your lecithin to determine how much of the active ingredient is present.

Lecithin is nontoxic, and can be taken in very high dosages without side effects. A reasonable dosage would be about 1,500 mg daily, for a person with no significant cognitive impairment. If early-stage memory impairment is present, this dosage can be doubled or tripled. Patients with severe memory disorders may take up to 10,000 mg daily. Patients with profound memory disorder, however, should not expect this substance to dramatically impact their condition.

PHOSPHATIDYL SERINE

An extremely beneficial brain tonic, phosphatidyl serine (or PS) is chemically similar to the phosphatidyl choline found in lecithin. It is less abundant in lecithin than phosphatidyl choline is, however, and it is not easily found in other common foods. Therefore it should be taken in capsule form.

Shown in a number of studies to improve cognitive function significantly, PS is a naturally occurring form of fat, or *phospholipid,* that is found in every cell in the body, but it is far more abundant in the brain than in other organs. It is especially abundant in the cell membranes of neurons, and is important for keeping those membranes easily permeable, so that nutrients can enter and wastes can exit.

It also helps brain cells to conduct nerve impulses, and to release adequate amounts of neurotransmitters. Both of these actions enable neurons to communicate better with one another.

Many studies indicate that PS is helpful for people with age-associated memory impairment. It also helps to optimize cognition in people who have no cognitive impairment.

In one study, a group of memory-impaired patients with an average age of sixty-four showed significant cognitive improvements after taking PS. They improved on a number of memory tests, including tests for recall of phone numbers, of misplaced objects, and of written material. In addition, they had an improved ability to concentrate while reading, conversing, and performing tasks. Researchers said that PS had enabled these patients to "roll back the clock" twelve years—by helping them to achieve an average "cognitive age" of fifty-two.

In a study of healthy subjects, it was discovered that PS significantly lowered production of stress hormones, and another study showed that PS increased the presence of calming alpha brain waves by 15 to 20 percent, apparently by enhancing the brain's acetylcholine-based cholinergic system. It has also been shown to relieve depressive symptoms in a significant percentage of patients with clinical depression.

PS can be purchased in most health-food stores. A reasonable dosage for a brain longevity patient would be 100 to 300 mg daily, depending upon the patient's degree of cognitive decline. Anything less than 100 mg is ineffectual.

In the past, PS was generally derived from the brains of animals. Now, because of technological advances, PS is derived from soy lecithin.

Many of my patients report to me that PS has had a dramatic, positive impact upon their cognitive function.

ACETYL L-CARNITINE

A naturally occurring substance that aids cognition, ALC improves the energy metabolism in the brain's "power plants" (the mitochondria) by boosting energy transfer across the mitochondrial membrane. It also reduces intracellular generation of the free radicals that are caused by oxidation of fatty acids.

ALC also has the fascinating ability to improve communication between the two hemispheres of the brain. The only other substance known to do this is the pharmaceutical drug Piracetam. When this improvement in communication occurs, it spurs creativity and helps patients achieve a more "balanced" cognitive ability.

In one study of ALC, 279 patients with mild to moderate cognitive decline consumed either a placebo or 1,500 mg daily of ALC. Those taking ALC significantly improved their scores on objective mental function tests. Those on the placebo showed no improvement.

In another study, subjects were tested for their ability to exit a maze. After they were given ALC, the time it took them to exit the maze was reduced by 43 percent.

In an interesting study of the ability of ALC to improve communication between the brain's two hemispheres, right-handed subjects were tested for their ability to exit a printed maze. First they used their right hands, then their left hands. At first they did better with their right hands, which is the usual response among right-handed subjects. After they took ALC, however, they did almost as well using their left hands. This suggests improved hemispheric coordination.

ALC is also effective for patients with early age-associated memory impairment. In one large study, patients with this disorder who ingested ALC improved their scores on cognitive tests, and also reported improvements in mood.

ALC is so promising that a major drug company, Sigma Tau, is investing considerable funding in the final stages of efficacy testing, at Stanford University, in hopes of patenting the compound for use in Europe.

The only problem with ALC is its expense. A one-month supply—a bottle of one hundred capsules (with 500 mg each)—costs about seventy-five dollars, even if purchased through a discount buyer's club. Thus, it's by far the most expensive natural medicinal tonic for the brain.

For many of my patients, I prescribe 250 mg of ALC daily. If a patient suffers from substantial cognitive decline, however, I recommend up to 500 mg three times daily. I strongly recommend that patients take ALC *with* phosphatidyl serine, because the two substances potentiate each other.

GINSENG

This herb has astonishing neurological effects, and is particularly adroit at stopping the overproduction of cortisol.

Ginseng, as you may know, is generally regarded as the "Cadillac" of Asian medicinal tonics. It is used very widely in America, Europe, and the Far East, and has been employed medicinally for thousands of years.

High-quality ginseng is very prized among practitioners of traditional Chinese medicine. A Chinese emperor once paid the equivalent of thirty thousand dollars for one particularly well-developed root. In recent years, roots have sold for up to ten thousand dollars in America. Though it's ridiculous to pay this much for ginseng, these high prices illustrate the herb's allure.

Ginseng became a major commodity in Europe in the late 1600s, after the King of Siam gave a gift of ginseng to Louis XIV. In America, ginseng was a popular medicinal tonic as early as the mid-1700s. In fact, it was the primary crop harvested and traded by Daniel Boone, who sometimes brought up to fifteen tons of ginseng from the frontiers of Kentucky, where it grew wild, to the eastern United States. In Kentucky, ginseng is still an $11-million-per-year crop.

According to the Eastern perspective, ginseng is a vitalizing and harmonizing agent that repairs "yang energy." It is not used by traditional Chinese medicine (TCM) practitioners as a specific curative agent, but is used to strengthen various organs, glands, and energy systems, so that *they* can cure disease. In traditional Chinese medicine, it is considered effective for relieving fatigue, impotence, and the general effects of aging.

Ginseng is an *adaptogen*—a compound that helps the body to adapt to physical and psychological stressors. It does this, according to the Western interpretation, by heightening the productivity of the adrenal glands.

It is considered by Western practitioners to be a "balanced stimulant," because it achieves arousal without provoking a nervous or jittery response. It does this by simultaneously stimulating both the adrenergic (or adrenal) nervous system, and the cholinergic (or "calming") nervous system. It arouses the adrenergic system via the adrenals, and it activates the cholinergic system via the brain's "reticular formation."

To my brain longevity patients, however, the most valuable attribute of ginseng is its unique biochemical ability to curtail release of cortisol.

As mentioned previously, adrenaline and cortisol are both excitatory hormones, but cortisol has a longer-lasting effect. Because cortisol stays in the system longer than adrenaline, it is more disruptive than adrenaline.

Ginseng stops excessive cortisol release by decreasing the demand for cortisol. It does this by stimulating the production of adrenaline (but not necessarily the release of adrenaline). When the supply of adrenaline is increased, the body does not need to release as much cortisol in response to stressful situations.

Many studies have shown that when ginseng is regularly ingested, the adrenal response to a stressful situation is faster—and that more adrenaline is released. As a reaction to this abundant secretion of adrenaline, the hypothalamus and the pituitary—which control the output of both adrenaline and cortisol—"decide" not to produce high amounts of cortisol. Further, ginseng biochemically enables the adrenals to "shut off" more quickly, once the stressful situation has passed. It therefore has the superb ability to make the stress response more efficient. In medical jargon, ginseng "tightens" that response.

Numerous studies have shown that ginseng heightens cognitive function, apparently because of its ability to evoke a stable state of arousal.

In one of the early controlled experiments on ginseng, telegraph operators who are given ginseng were able to do their work considerably faster, while making 10 percent fewer mistakes.

In another experiment, 80 percent of subjects taking ginseng increased the speed of their reactions to a cue.

Yet another experiment showed that students using ginseng improved their scores on cognitive function tests by an average of more than 50 percent. These tests stressed quick reaction time and reasoning skills.

Other studies have shown that ginseng increases mental and physical stamina and helps people resist stress-related diseases.

Many brands and varieties of ginseng are available. Among the most popular is the original variety of ginseng, called *Panax ginseng*, which once commonly grew wild but is now mostly commercially grown in China, Japan, Russia, and South Korea. Another high-quality variety of ginseng is the North American type, *Panax quinquefolium*, which grows in the wild in the northern United States and in the Appalachian mountains. This type of ginseng is also sometimes grown commercially, primarily in Wisconsin. In Russia, a potent variety known as *Siberian ginseng* grows wild. Siberian ginseng is also grown commercially in Russia, China, Korea, and Japan. This variety is the one most frequently found in formulations designed to boost cognitive function.

There is disagreement about which type of ginseng is best. Some experts believe North American ginseng has the highest amounts of active ingredients, while others believe Siberian ginseng is a more potent adaptogen.

Furthermore, among the three major types of ginseng, there are various grades of quality. For example, wild ginseng is generally considered more potent than commercially grown ginseng. The potency of ginseng is also related to the quality of the soil in which it was grown, the duration of its growth, the weather in which it was grown, and the methods by which it was processed.

Thus, because the quality can vary widely, it's wise to buy ginseng from a trusted retailer or buyer's club. For its cognitive effects, as mentioned, I prefer Siberian ginseng.

A reasonable daily dosage of ginseng may range from 750 mg to 1,500 mg, depending upon your medical condition and the quality of the ginseng.

One of the ginseng products that I recommend to my patients is a Chinese patent medicine called *Ching Chun Bao*. It contains Royal Manchurian, perhaps the most potent form of ginseng, and several other Chinese herbal medicines.

Ching Chun Bao was first formulated during the reign of the third emperor of the Ming dynasty; thus it has a long and rich history of use. Ancient Chinese physicians claimed that Ching Chun Bao "prolonged life and maintained youth." In recent years, practitioners at the Hangzhou Traditional Chinese Medical Institute performed double-blind studies with the compound on animals and on people. In all those studies, the researchers noted either objective or subjective improvement after use of the formulation. Patients given Ching Chun Bao reported increased energy, enhanced resistance to fatigue, and improvements in memory and cognitive function. Some of the postmenopausal females who used it reported resumption of menstruation. Animals given the product grew faster than nontreated animals, and had increased resistance to disease.

I recommend ingestion of four to eight Ching Chun Bao tablets daily to my brain longevity patients.

DMAE

A relatively recent addition to the family of cognitive tonics, DMAE, or dimethylamine ethanol, has already proven to be of considerable benefit. It helps the body to create acetylcholine, the primary neurotransmitter of memory and thought.

DMAE produces acetylcholine when it is combined with phosphatidyl choline (derived from lecithin), and vitamin B_5. In some patients, it has generated effects that were almost as striking as those elicited by potent pharmaceutical drugs such as tacrine.

DMAE definitely increases memory—particularly short-term memory, which is very dependent upon adequate levels of acetylcholine. It also elevates concentration and learning ability.

In some of my patients, DMAE—which stimulates the central nervous system—has improved mood and subjective perceptions of well-being.

Occasionally, patients will feel overstimulated by DMAE.

When this happens, I reduce their dosages. Even in those cases, though, DMAE generally does not cause a "rebound effect" of lethargy, as do most stimulants. Instead, it provides a stable plateau of stimulation. However, it can sometimes cause insomnia.

Patients with epilepsy, or with bipolar depression, are generally advised not to use DMAE, because it can exacerbate both of those conditions.

A prudent daily dosage of DMAE is in the 50-to-100-mg range.

GREEN JUICE PRODUCTS

These products can include a relatively wide variety of substances, many of which appear to enhance the function of the brain. The most common substances found in these products are blue-green algae, wheatgrass, barley grass, oat grass, spirulina, chlorella, and dulse. In addition, many of these products are fortified with a number of other natural brain tonics, including astragalus, lecithin, beet juice powder, bee pollen, ginkgo, and green tea extracts.

Because of this broad range of ingredients, these products offer the patient a veritable smorgasbord of micronutrients. Often these micronutrients are obscure chemical compounds that are not present in most common foodstuffs.

Of particular value to brain longevity patients are the combinations of amino acids (or partial proteins) that are abundant in green juice products. These are called *peptides*, and they can be transformed by the body into *neuropeptides*. As you may recall, neuropeptides, such as beta endorphins, are one of the primary links between mind and body.

Besides supplying peptides, the green juice products are also rich in the nine essential amino acids that cannot be manufactured by the body, and must therefore be ingested as nutrients. These nine important amino acids are *tryptophan, lysine, leucine, methionine, phenylalanine, valine, threonine,* and *isoleucine*. As I'm sure you recall, two of these amino acids—tryptophan and phenylalanine—are the primary "building blocks" for the important neurotransmitters serotonin and norepinephrine.

The green juice products are also among the few common nutritional sources of chlorophyll, which activates the enzymes that produce vitamins E, A, and K. Interestingly, chlorophyll has almost the same molecular structure as hemoglobin, which carries oxygen throughout the body.

These products are also extraordinarily rich in trace minerals, in which many people with cognitive decline are deficient. These minerals are the catalysts that enable vitamins and enzymes to perform their various functions.

I advise patients to take their green juice product first thing in the morning, as part of their wake-up routine. For most people, these products create a pleasant feeling of stimulation. This stimulation is not like the rollercoaster ride of caffeine stimulation, but is instead an influx of *stable* energy. Occasionally, patients report that their green juice product is too stimulating. When this occurs, I reduce the dosage.

There are many brands of green juice products, but my personal favorite contains a broad array of nutrient sources. Many of my patients who use a green juice product report a noticeable increase in their cognitive abilities, as well as an increase in their general levels of energy and well-being.

GREEN TEA

Green tea can be helpful in three ways: It is a powerful antioxidant; it is a rich source of "flavonoids," which reduce risk of stroke; and it contains caffeine, which can be an effective cognitive enhancement agent, when used cautiously.

Green tea contains antioxidant *polyphenols*, including *catechins* and *quercetin*, which can increase antioxidant activity in the blood by as much as 50 percent. This increased activity occurs about half an hour after drinking the tea.

Green tea also improves the efficiency of the liver's enzyme detoxification system. Therefore it is able to help rid the body of toxins before they are able to damage cells.

It's interesting to note that although green tea has recently been heralded in the media for its health-promoting properties, black tea may be almost as beneficial. Black tea, the common form of tea consumed in most Western countries, does not contain catechins. But it does have other antioxidants that green tea lacks.

Black tea and green tea are both rich in flavonoids, which are vitaminlike compounds that naturally occur in tea, and also in fruits and vegetables. Flavonoids tend to make blood cells less prone to clotting. Therefore they can help reduce risk of stroke, including the "mini-strokes" that can cause symptoms similar to Alzheimer's. In one recent study, men with a high flavonoid intake had a 73-percent lower risk of stroke than a control group, over a fifteen-year period. The men in the study got about 60 percent of their flavonoids from tea.

The caffeine in tea can also benefit cognition, if it is ingested in prudent amounts. Other drinks that contain caffeine, such as coffee and colas, can also aid thought and memory, if used properly.

Caffeine, in fact, is the most widely used cognitive-enhancement product in our society. Numerous tests have proved that, when used in moderate amounts, caffeine boosts concentration and alertness. Because it is a stimulant, it increases output of adrenaline, and can temporarily improve memory and mood.

Coffee also contains several substances that are biochemically similar to opiates. Therefore it can cause simultaneous stimulation and relaxation.

Far too many people overconsume caffeine, however. This occurs, I think, because people simply do not have enough natural energy. Instead of getting enough sleep, nutrients, and exercise to provide the energy they need, people depend upon caffeine to push them through the day. The short-term price for this dependency is nervousness, irritability, insomnia, and a "rebound effect" of lethargy and mental lassitude. The long-term price is burnout of the adrenal glands, and a body that has been exhausted by artificial stimulation.

Further, it's now clear that caffeine, if used in excess, can increase levels of artery-damaging LDL cholesterol. Caffeine has also been linked to breast cysts in females.

Research indicates that up to 200 mg of caffeine can be consumed every day with no apparent health risk. I take a more cautious approach, and recommend no more than 100 mg daily.

Following are the amounts of caffeine found in a single serving of various beverages.

CAFFEINE CONTENT
(in milligrams)

Coffee		Tea	
"drip" style	110–150	1 minute brew	9–33
espresso	100–150	3 minute brew	20–46
percolated	64–124	5 minute brew	20–50
instant	40–108		
decaffeinated	2–5		

Soft Drinks

Dr. Pepper	61
Colas	30–60
Mountain Dew	52
Mellow Yellow	51
Tab	44

COENZYME Q-10

Useful for many brain longevity patients, primarily because it increases the energy-generating potential in each of the body's cells, including the neurons, coenzyme Q-10 or CoQ, is found in virtually every cell in the body and helps the cells' "power plants" (the mitochondria) to produce energy.

CoQ is synthesized from the amino acids phenylalanine and tyrosine, so anyone who does not get enough of these nutrients may have a deficit of CoQ. Symptoms of this deficit might include fatigue, mental lethargy, or depression.

Besides supplying energy, CoQ has been shown to be effective as a nutritional adjunctive therapy for congestive heart failure, angina pectoris, high blood pressure, and atherosclerosis. In animals, it has been shown to increase lifespan. Studies at Harvard Medical School have shown it to be a powerful antioxidant in the brain.

CoQ has been thoroughly tested for safety, and has no side effects.

Based on recent research, the optimal daily dosage for most people is 100 mg.

Another relatively similar coenzyme that some researchers believe can be helpful for cognitive function is *NADH.* NADH is present in all of your body's cells, and plays a central role in producing energy. Recent exciting research indicates that the combination of coenzyme Q-10 and NADH potentiates the neuroprotective effects of both substances.

Following is a list of the most appropriate natural medicinal tonics for brain longevity, with general dosages. These dosages, however, may not be appropriate for all patients, because people have widely varying needs. Patients often take more than one tonic.

NATURAL MEDICINAL TONICS

Daily Dosage

Gingko biloba	60–320 mg
Phosphatidyl choline (from lecithin)	1,500–10,000 mg
Phosphatidyl serine	100–300 mg
Acetyl L-carnitine	250–1,500 mg
Ginseng	750–1,500 mg
Ching Chun Bao	4–8 tablets
DMAE	50–100 mg
"Green juice" products	one serving
Green tea	1–2 servings
Coenzyme Q-10	100 mg

As the preceding three chapters have shown, brain function can be powerfully affected by nutritional therapy.

These chapters have demonstrated that much of the benefit

derived from nutritional therapy comes from its ability to compensate for the harmful effects of stress.

Now it's time to deal *directly* with stress.

In the next chapter we'll examine ways to *reduce and eliminate stress.*

A Case in Point

Nootropic Medications Can Have a Wide Range of Effects

T.G., forty-two years old, was a patient who had a strong desire to have a steel-trap memory. T.G. was a cattle trader, based in the western United States, who conducted all of his transactions by computer. Every month, millions of dollars passed through his trading network, and it was imperative that he hold dozens of details in his mind at all times. If just a couple of details slipped his mind, it could cost him or his clients many thousands of dollars.

Several years before I met him, T.G. had been hiking high in the Colorado Rockies, when he had exercised too strenuously at too high an altitude, and it had caused high-altitude pulmonary edema, which had robbed his brain of oxygen. The result had been a swelling of his brain, and loss of brain cells.

Since that injury, T.G. had suffered from intermittent lapses of memory, and from cognitive dysfunction. Much of the time his ability to think and to remember was quite adequate. But often, he said, his memory would become "fuzzy," and he would forget important information. He would also sometimes experience a slowing of his cognitive processing skills, and an inability to focus intently. These cognitive lapses most frequently occurred when he was tired, stressed, or mildly ill. His job was almost always stressful, and it started at four-thirty every morning.

T.G. had tried to keep his mental lapses from affecting his work, but it had been difficult. His job required a high level of cognitive function at all times.

When he began his brain longevity program, I placed him on a high dosage of *Ginkgo biloba*, to increase the circulation to his brain. I also recommended that he begin a conscientious exercise program, to potentiate his cerebral circulation.

In addition, I prescribed piracetam for him. I believed it would help not only to spur his recovery from oxygen deprivation (hypoxia), but would also have a positive impact upon his impaired memory.

At that time, piracetam was not considered by most researchers to be a memory-enhancing medication, but I believed that I knew even more about piracetam than many researchers did.

My knowledge had come to me quite by accident. In the year before I began treating T.G., I had gone to Brussels to meet with a number of European doctors who were working with nootropic medications. One afternoon, one of the physicians I had contacted showed up unexpectedly at the apartment where my wife and I were staying. It was an elegant apartment— owned by my wife's father, who was then a diplomat stationed in Brussels—and it featured a closed-circuit television system, so that we could see guests as they entered the lobby downstairs. The gentleman who was on his way up looked very distinguished.

When I greeted him, I missed his name.

He told me he was from Romania.

"Romania!" I said. "Then you must have known Dr. Ana Aslan." She was the late creator of the rejuvenation drug Gerovital.

"Yes, I did know Ana," he said. "Sometimes I used the medication she developed, and sometimes she used mine."

His medication? I was confused. "I'm sorry," I said, "but I didn't catch your name when you came in."

"Giurgea," he said, "Cornelius Giurgea."

"Dr. Giurgea!" I exclaimed. It was like meeting some fantastic guitar player in a dark club, and he says, "Hi, I'm Eric Clapton." Dr. Cornelius Giurgea was the famous inventor of piracetam, the nootropic medication that does more than $1 billion in sales every year.

I'd been hoping to meet Dr. Giurgea, but had been expecting to meet someone who looked much older. Dr. Giurgea looked about twenty-five years younger than his age.

I got Dr. Giurgea to tell me the story of piracetam's development. He told me that he had developed it expressly for a single patient, one of his country's greatest wartime heroes, who had incurred a brain injury that had caused severe vertigo. The compound that Dr. Giurgea had developed—an early version of piracetam—had cured the war hero's vertigo. In fact, the war hero had recovered so fully that he had begun to ride motorcycles—until the day he crashed his motorcycle, and suffered another head injury, which caused significant memory impairment.

Lacking a new drug to apply to the memory disorder, Dr. Giurgea put his patient back on high dosages of piracetam. The patient experienced another astounding recovery.

"So you see," Dr. Giurgea told me, "some of these medications that we develop for the brain, they can help the brain to thrive in many ways."

From that meeting, I gained the knowledge—before most other researchers—that piracetam could mitigate memory impairment in some patients with head injuries.

About a year later, I applied this bit of knowledge to T.G.

After he began taking piracetam, T.G. experienced a wonderful turnaround. He was careful to take his piracetam regularly, and he also adhered to the other elements of a complete program.

His memory became as sharp as the blade of a knife, and he became able to focus his mind with laserlike intensity.

These days, T.G. no longer requires regular administration of piracetam. He uses it only upon occasion. Often, if he is tired or feeling stressed, he will use a small amount of piracetam to help restore his mental vigor.

His memory problems have been gone for well over four years, and I am hopeful that they will never recur. They probably won't. Unless, of course, he starts riding motorcycles.

14

Stress Management and Optimum Brain Power

I recall with crystal clarity the most recent conversation I had with one of the great men of modern medicine, Herbert Benson, M.D., the pioneer of stress management.

However, almost *any* conversation with Dr. Benson can be memorable, because of the force of his personality, which is that of "a saint-soldier," as the Eastern philosophers say. He combines the compassionate, wise demeanor of a saint with the fierce dedication of a soldier. Therefore, when he makes a point, it sticks with you, because of the personal power with which he presents it.

The point he made the last time we spoke was that to most modern people, having a relaxed state of mind feels extraordinary—even though this should be the mind's ordinary condition. "The normal state of the mind," he said, "is *not* uptight. It's relaxed, creative, intuitive, vibrant, and intelligent. It's almost magical. I call the fully relaxed mind the 'magical mind.'"

I'll never forget that phrase, "the magical mind." Helping my patients to achieve "magical minds" has become one of my constant goals.

To achieve this, I help my patients to manage their stress, because a "magical mind" is possible only when stress is held firmly in check. Make no mistake: *Optimal cognitive function requires a relaxed mental state.*

Most of my patients, when I first consult with them, have no idea how important stress management is to optimal cognitive function, and to brain longevity. Many of them don't even know what stress actually is. They think the word refers to an outside force that causes them to feel tension. That's not stress, though—that's a "stressor."

Stress is the feeling that can result from a stressor. This may seem like a trivial distinction, but it's vitally important. It means that if you don't *perceive* a stressor to be stressful, then it's not one.

This chapter is about learning how to stay stress-free, even when your life is full of stressors. It's easier than you may think.

In the chapters on nutritional therapy, you learned how to guard against stress nutritionally, and how to compensate nutritionally for stress when it occurs. In effect, you learned strategies for putting *matter over mind.* In this chapter I'll tell you how to stop the physical effects of stress with mental techniques. You'll learn how to put *mind over matter.*

When you learn how to do this, you'll achieve a great victory. You will be able to drastically reduce the number of times when stressors overwhelm you, making you feel like a "leaf in the wind," buffeted by forces beyond your control. And as your vulnerability to stressors begins to diminish, several critically important physical changes will occur in you: Your cortisol levels will decrease; your blood pressure will drop; you will more easily make new synaptic connections in your neocortex; your brain waves will shift more frequently to the relaxed, high-focus alpha and theta frequencies; and your neurotransmitters will function far more efficiently.

Each of these changes may significantly improve the *current power* of your brain. Your memory may become sharper. Your thought processes may operate more quickly and easily. You may become happier. Your brain may regenerate.

And your life may get better.

You will also be better able to achieve *brain longevity*, and to enjoy your current high level of cognitive function for the rest of your life.

Before I tell you how to rid yourself of stress, though, let's look at some of the most common *causes* of chronic, long-term stress.

In the past, you've probably seen various stress indexes—such as the well-known Holmes-Rahe index—which rank stressors on a scale of one to one hundred. I think the existing stress indexes can be helpful, but I believe they all share a common failing, in that they don't factor in the individual's *perception* of the stressor; they seem to presume that all people respond to particular stressors uniformly, and that's simply not true. People respond *differently* to stressors. As I've mentioned, the critical element in stress is not what *happens* to you, but how you *respond* to it.

For example, in most stress indexes, being fired from a job is rated as a mid-range stressor. But being fired from a job can affect two people quite differently. One person may love the job, and badly need the money it provides. Another person might hate the job, and not need the money. Obviously those two people will respond differently to the job loss.

In my stress index, I have assigned the usual "stressor ratings" to various stressors. But I have also added a "multiplier" that reflects your own *perception* of the stressor. The multiplier is on a one-to-ten scale, based on how much stress you felt from the stressor.

For example, if being fired from your job didn't bother you very much, you should multiply the "stressor rating" by just two or three. But if being fired *devastated* you, you should multiply by nine or ten.

This index applies only to stressors that occurred within the past twenty-four months.

THE BRAIN LONGEVITY STRESS IMPACT INDEX

Event	Stressor Rating	Personal Perception Multiplier (1–10)	Score
Death of your child	100	_____	_____
Death of your spouse	99	_____	_____
Life-threatening illness	95	_____	_____
Prison term	80	_____	_____
Divorce	78	_____	_____
Marital separation	68	_____	_____
Death of a parent or sibling	68	_____	_____
Fired from your job	65	_____	_____
Pregnancy	60	_____	_____
Hospitalization for serious illness	58	_____	_____
Marriage	57	_____	_____
Foreclosure on a mortgage	57	_____	_____
Serious illness in the family	55	_____	_____
Birth of a child	50	_____	_____
Demotion at work	50	_____	_____
Lawsuit against you	50	_____	_____
Retirement	49	_____	_____
Sexual problems	45	_____	_____
Laid off from work	43	_____	_____
Problems with boss	40	_____	_____
Major business change	40	_____	_____
Major change in finances	39	_____	_____
Move to new town	38	_____	_____
Death of a close friend	38	_____	_____
Change careers	38	_____	_____
Change in frequency of arguments with spouse	35	_____	_____
Change in sleep habits	31	_____	_____
Problems with co-workers	30	_____	_____
Assuming a mortgage of over 25% of net earnings	29	_____	_____

Event	Stressor Rating	Personal Perception Multiplier (1–10)	Score
Birth of first grandchild	28	_____	_____
Children leaving home	27	_____	_____
Problems with extended family	25	_____	_____
Significant lifestyle change	24	_____	_____
Illness of more than one week	23	_____	_____
Promotion at work	23	_____	_____
Change in political or religious beliefs	20	_____	_____
Assuming a mortgage of over 20% of net earnings	18	_____	_____
Change in social life	17	_____	_____
Change in diet	15	_____	_____
Vacation	10	_____	_____
Minor legal problem	10	_____	_____
		Total Score	_____

If the sum of your multiplied scores (your total score) is less than 500, you are leading a relatively *stress-free* life. If it is 500 to 1,000, you have a *low-stress* life. If it is 1,000 to 2,000, you have a life of *moderate stress*, and should work hard to minimize your response to your stressors. If your score is 2,000 to 3,000, you have a *high-stress* life, one that is almost certainly creating short-term cognitive dysfunction, and that may eventually contribute to age-associated cognitive decline. If your score is higher than 3,000, you are in the *danger zone*; your stress levels are far too high, and are a serious threat to your physical health, emotional well-being, cognitive function, and brain longevity.

If you had a high total score on the Stress Impact Index, it means that you are habitually experiencing the "stress response." It is the *stress response* that physically endangers you.

I covered the stress response in chapter 6, but let's review it again very briefly.

The Destruction Caused by the Stress Response

The human stress response is badly outdated. For most of us, it's no longer necessary for survival on a day-to-day basis, and yet we're still stuck with it. If the human body could be engineered like a machine, the stress response would have been modified several generations ago.

The stress response was created tens of thousands of years ago, by the process of evolution. It was created at a time when virtually all threats were physical, and could be overcome only with physical action. Currently, however, most threats are not physical but psychological. Today's stressors usually consist of factors like demanding bosses, impending deadlines, honking horns, broken machines, and empty bank accounts. To deal with these stressors, we don't need the physical reactions that the stress response causes. But we *experience* these physical reactions, whether we need them or not.

In brief, here's what happens when you activate your stress response:

1. You release adrenaline, causing your blood sugar to rise, your blood pressure to increase, your heartbeat to accelerate, your arteries to constrict, and your digestion to slow. For a limited time, your mind and muscles work very efficiently.

2. If the stressor is severe, or persists for more than just a couple of minutes, you also secrete cortisol. This "locks in" a long-lasting stress response.

A small amount of stress, over a very short period, is healthy. It causes a mild degree of excitation, and helps people to become involved in productive activity. This healthy level of stress, sometimes called *eustress*, actually helps prevent *unhealthy* levels of stress. When you have absolutely *no* stress, you soon become bored, and then boredom itself causes unhealthy stress levels.

Further, a very mild degree of stress, at intermittent moments, is good for your brain. It causes you to release norepinephrine, the excitatory neurotransmitter. You need norepinephrine to move your short-term memories to long-term storage. You also need it to help give you a positive mood.

Therefore, your key to successful stress management is to keep just a mild, healthy degree of stress in your life. Your stressors will then feel like challenges, not problems. Then, when you meet those challenges, your brain will engage in creative thinking, grow new dendrites, and make new synaptic connections.

Unhealthy levels of stress occur primarily when you feel as if your ability to deal with your stressors is inadequate. That creates the nerve-racking, depressing, annoyed feeling that we all identify as stress.

If you experience unhealthy levels of stress only very occasionally, it will do little damage. But if you experience prolonged, high-level stress on a daily basis, it will profoundly disturb your physical, intellectual, and emotional health. If you do experience this type of chronic, uncontrolled stress, you will soon become a victim of one of life's most damaging phenomena, the "general adaptation syndrome."

Watch out for this syndrome! It can "cook your brain."

How the General Adaptation Syndrome "Burns Up" Your Brain

In 1956, the endocrinologist Hans Selye became one of the preeminent pioneers of stress research, when he wrote the first major book on the damage that stress does to the body. In that book, *The Stress of Life*, Selye described how stress gradually assaults the body, through a mechanism that he called the "general adaptation syndrome," which is the broad set of changes your body goes through when it is chronically subjected to the stress response.

There are three stages to this set of changes. The first is the "alarm reaction," when you secrete adrenaline and cortisol, causing your entire body and mind to spring into action against the stressor. The second stage is the "stage of resistance," in which your mind and body try to pinpoint the threat, and activate only the most *appropriate* resistance mechanisms. During this phase, the secretion of adrenaline and cortisol decreases, while the "battle" against the stressor is fought only by the most appropriate organs or systems. Then, however, comes the most insidious phase: the "phase of exhaustion."

During the phase of exhaustion, the specific, appropriate organs or systems that are "fighting" the stressor wear out, and become depleted. Your mind and body then "draft" other organs and systems to "join the battle." When this happens, there is again a surge in the secretion of adrenaline and cortisol.

During the exhaustion phase, *most* of the organs and systems in your body are affected, and some are badly harmed. Often there is substantial enlargement of the cortex of your adrenal glands. There is also often a shrinkage of your thymus, spleen, and lymph nodes. There is generally a decrease in the number of your immune system's white blood cells. Excess stomach acid is secreted. As a rule, your blood pressure increases. Your sex hormones almost always decline.

Of course, when these changes occur, illness often follows. It's common for people who suffer from the general adaptation syndrome to have chronic high blood pressure. It's also common for them to develop minor illnesses. Sometimes, high levels of chronic stress can even contribute to catastrophic illnesses, including heart disease and cancer.

Mortality and illness among the chronically stressed rises sharply. For example, an older person who has lost a spouse is ten times more likely to die within one year of this loss than an older person whose spouse is still alive. Similarly, when a person gets divorced, his or her probability of significant illness over the next year increases by 1,200 percent.

Even recovery from injury is hampered by chronic stress. In one recent study, skin wounds among highly stressed subjects took an average of forty-nine days to heal completely, while skin wounds among nonstressed subjects took only thirty-nine days to heal.

Research even indicates that stress can significantly increase levels of "bad" LDL cholesterol.

It's not only the body that suffers from stress, though. The brain does, too. When the exhaustion phase of chronic stress hits, learning ability and concentration nosedive, partly because of the effects of cortisol. In one revealing study, students with high levels of chronic stress scored 13 percent lower on IQ tests than students with low stress.

High blood pressure caused by chronic stress also reduces cognitive function. As I've already shown, "what's good for the heart is good for the head." And few things are worse for the heart (and the head) than high blood pressure.

In addition, the exhaustion phase of the general adaption syndrome causes a deficit of the important neurotransmitter norepinephrine—particularly in the frontal lobe of your neocortex, where much of your abstract thinking takes place.

Chronic stress causes norepinephrine to be shunted away from your limbic system. As you'll recall, your limbic system controls your emotions. Because of this lack of norepinephrine in the emotional center of your brain, chronic stress can cause you to experience biological depression, anxiety, and malaise. If your chronic stress lasts long enough, it can even biochemically create anhedonia—the inability to feel any emotional pleasure.

Another unwanted mental effect of chronic stress is its influence on brain waves. A person experiencing stress has a predominance of "uptight" beta waves, rather than "calm" alpha and theta waves. Beta waves are also less conducive to learning and concentration than alpha or theta waves.

Finally—and most harmful of all—chronic stress creates chronic oversecretion of cortisol. And cortisol, as mentioned previously, wages a "three-stroke attack" on your brain: It starves the brain of its only energy source, glucose; it interferes with neurotransmitter function; and it leads to the eventual death of brain cells.

Another tragic consequence of unrelenting stress is its assault on the mechanism that naturally shuts off your cortisol production. This cortisol shut-off usually occurs when the threats against you have passed. As you'll recall from chapter 8, when your limbic system's hippocampus is healthy, it has the ability to give your endocrine system "feedback," and tell it when to quit producing cortisol. But when your hippocampus becomes damaged by chronic stress, this feedback mechanism turns into the destructive "feedforward mechanism." The feedforward mechanism keeps demanding that you secrete more and more cortisol, even when you no longer need it. This unfortunate phenomenon is especially common in older people, whose hippocampi have been compromised by many years of stress.

When the feedforward mechanism occurs, a degenerative cycle is created. This degenerative cycle, I believe, sometimes turns mild age-associated memory impairment into full-blown dementia.

As you can see, chronic stress is a killer. It kills the body, the intellect, and the emotions. Now let's see how we can *protect* ourselves against the physical and mental ravages of stressors.

There are two basic psychological methods for keeping stressors from becoming stress. If you employ both of these psychological methods, you will be able to avoid most of the damage that stress can do. Thus you'll be able to put mind over matter.

The first method consists of learning *coping skills.* There are a great many such skills that a person can use, but psychiatrists and stress researchers have discovered that there are three primary coping skills that provide the greatest protection from stress: taking control of the stressor; developing a social support system; and learning how to release stress.

Besides these important coping skills, there is one other important psychological method of defeating stress. This is remarkably effective—even though it's very simple. It consists of engaging in a mental exercise that evokes the *opposite physical condition* of the stress response. This opposite condition, discovered by Dr. Herbert Benson, is the "relaxation response."

There are several mental exercises that can evoke the relaxation response. Most of them are just basic forms of meditation. For stress management, meditation is as powerful as a "wonder drug."

I will discuss meditation in the next chapter. The remainder of this chapter will be about the three coping skills that can save your brain.

Why "Control Freak" Should Not Be an Insult

Taking control is probably the most critical element in defeating stress. If you can control a stressor, you will probably perceive it as a *challenge*, and will approach it with confidence and a relaxed mental state. If you can't control a stressor, you'll probably see it as a *threat*, and it will cause you to feel stress.

Some stress researchers, in fact, define stress as *any difficult situation that you can't control.*

If you can control a difficult situation, it will probably be *good* for your brain. It will coax you to make new synaptic connections between neurons, as you attempt to resolve the situation. To meet your challenge, you'll use your "associative brain"—the parts of your neocortex (mostly in the temporal and frontal lobes) that are most active in creative problem-solving. The neurons that perform your associative functions are among your most plastic, adaptive neurons. They thrive on challenge.

But if you perceive your situation as out of your control, you will be much less likely to engage these neurons in creative problem solving, and much more apt to secrete the hormones that will "cook" your brain.

A number of studies have shown that *loss of control* drastically increases stress. One important element of control is predictability. If a person knows when a stressor will occur, it vastly reduces his or her stress response. For example, during World War II, peptic ulcers increased by 300 percent in the outskirts of London, where aerial bombing was sporadic and unpredictable. In the center of the city, however, where bombing occurred regularly, there was only one-sixth as much of an increase in ulcers, because although the city-center residents were bombed much more often, they were able to predict when the bombing would occur.

In experiments on rats, those that were subjected to painful shocks without warning showed many more signs of stress than did rats that were *warned* before they were shocked.

Having control is tremendously important in cutting down on job stress. The primary factor in determining job stress, most experts agree, is a person's degree of *control* over the work situation. If people are free to make their own decisions, they feel much less stress on the job than people who must constantly defer to others. Therefore, jobs that have high demands, but also high degrees of authority, are actually less stressful than jobs with fewer demands but less authority. Thus, being a nurse is often more stressful than being a doctor.

Another situation that illustrates the importance of having control is that of the medication of pain patients in hospitals. Experiments have shown that when doctors allow pain patients to administer their own pain medication, as often as they like, those patients use less medication than do patients who have no control over their medication.

People who have the least sense of control—and the highest levels of stress—are often those who have a personality trait called "learned helplessness." These are people who have *tried* to take control of various situations in their lives, but who have frequently failed. In general, people with this trait have elevated levels of cortisol, and have difficulty functioning at high cognitive levels.

This trait can wax and wane in people, depending upon the situations in which they find themselves. The trait has even been provoked in short-term experiments. In one experiment, some subjects were given a task to perform that was impossible, and others were given a similar task, but one that *was* possible. Most of those who had been given the impossible task soon showed signs of poor motivation and high levels of stress. The group with the *possible* task stayed motivated, and had low levels of stress. Then both groups were given another, identical task, which was possible to perform. On this task, most of the group that had first been given the impossible task performed much worse than the people in the other group. They had quickly developed the trait of learned helplessness.

Not all of the group given the impossible task adopted the trait of learned helplessness, however. Some of them remained motivated and stress-free, even after they had failed at the impossible task.

This same *resistance* to learned helplessness has also been exhibited in animal experiments. About one-third of a group of dogs in an experiment on learned helplessness were able to remain free of the trait. Interestingly, most of the dogs who stayed free of the trait were dogs that had been obtained from the dog pound, rather than dogs born and reared in laboratories. This suggests that the "school of hard knocks" is a good place to learn resilience against stressors.

Now let's look at the best, most widely accepted ways to *gain control* over stress.

How to Take Control

One of the most important ways to keep the feeling of control in your life is simply to know when you've *really* lost control, and when you haven't. Far too often, people feel out of control when they're really not.

The great stress researcher Robert Sapolsky, Ph.D., noted this failure to recognize loss of control when he did some experiments with monkeys. He wrote about these experiments in his excellent book about stress, *Why Zebras Don't Get Ulcers*. Dr. Sapolsky found that certain monkeys, after winning skirmishes with other monkeys, showed various signs of victory, such as engaging in grooming behaviors. Apparently, after winning their fights, these monkeys felt in control. Other monkeys, however, would win a fight, but then act exactly the same as they had before the fight. They gained no apparent sense of being in control. For some reason they couldn't differentiate between victory and defeat. These monkeys had much higher cortisol levels than the monkeys who realized they were in control.

Many people suffer from this same inability to realize that they really are "in the driver's seat." Even when they are in control, they feel out of control. In humans, just as in animals, this activates the stress response. If this feeling persists chronically, as it frequently does, it generally elicits the destructive general adaptation syndrome.

Feeling that you're out of control when you're really not is a form of learned helplessness. Often this attitude is "locked in" by several self-defeating styles of thinking.

One of these faulty "thought styles" consists of jumping to negative conclusions. Many people just *assume* they have problems, when they really don't. They might think, "I'm sure the boss doesn't like me, because he's so demanding." Never assume the worst. It may appeal to the pessimist in you, but pessimism feeds chronic stress.

A similarly distorted style of thinking is *overgeneralizing*. If you draw broad negative conclusions from limited information, you're asking for trouble. Often, people think things like, "I *never* know what's going on around here, because *everybody* leaves me out of things." Or: "I haven't found a girlfriend yet, so I don't think I ever will." Try to just *know what you know*, and resist sweeping, negative generalizations.

Another self-defeating style of thinking is always to feel as if you must relinquish control in order to get along with other people. Many people always try to "go along" with others, just to be liked. There's nothing wrong with being nice to people, but if you habitually defer your own desires, just to fit in, you'll probably end up feeling like a victim, and a "leaf in the wind." Don't be afraid to say what you need. If you're being unreasonable, people will tell you.

Another destructive "thought style" is thinking that to be in control, you have to be in *total* control. This just isn't true. You don't have to control every detail to stay in control of the "big picture." Learn to appreciate the control you *do* have, and not to fixate on the "fine print." After all, a life of absolute control would be a life with no surprises, and no challenges.

People who suffer from the out-of-control feeling of learned helplessness almost always have far *more* control than they realize. Often, learned helplessness results from getting "stuck" in the past. People get "stuck" when they constantly relive the traumas that occurred when they really didn't have much control over their lives. Specifically, many people can't "get over" their childhoods, mostly because they suffered painful events then that they really couldn't control. As adults, they are haunted by these painful events, and subconsciously create similar events, so that they can rectify the situation and "set the record straight." For example, a woman who had an emotionally cold father might repeatedly fall in love with distant, remote men, thinking that if she changes them, she will rectify the past.

But this just doesn't work, because no amount of replaying the tragedies of your youth can make those tragedies go away. To move beyond your childhood traumas, you've got to grapple with them directly—instead of "acting them out" in your current daily life. The most widely accepted way to do this is to work with a therapist, and *confront* your traumas. Another way is to engage in advanced meditative techniques. Directly confronting your childhood traumas is difficult, but it frequently enables you to let the past *stay* in the past. When you're able to do this, you can live your adult life with a feeling of control, and shed the out-of-control attitude that haunted your childhood.

There is still another very effective method that will help you to feel a sense of control over your life. This method is to realize that you can't always control what happens to you, but that you can usually control how you react to it. That probably just sounds like common sense—because it is—but it's critically important, because it can enable you to keep stressors from becoming stress.

My coauthor, Cameron Stauth, once used this method to overcome a phobia of flying. During one particularly uncomfortable flight, in a thunderstorm, Cameron realized that he couldn't control the flight, but that he *could* control his physical reactions to it. So he began doing some deep breathing and other stress-control exercises, and soon experienced a strong sense of relief. When he focused on controlling his *reactions* to the flight, he regained much of his sense of overall control. After that, flying didn't really bother him, because he always knew he had an "ace in the hole": *self*-control.

Another powerful technique that can help you control your reaction to a stressor is *denial.* It isn't an effective long-term strategy for stress control, because it can keep you from eventually solving your problem. In the short term, though, it can be an excellent way to keep from becoming overly stressed. For example, in one study of heart-attack patients, it was found that patients benefited greatly if they used the coping strategy of denial during the first twenty-four hours after their heart attack. Those who denied the seriousness of their problem had less anxiety, less of a problem with cardiac arrhythmia, and a lower rate of mortality.

Using denial is often a good way to keep from panicking in a crisis. If you pretend your problem isn't serious, you can often solve it with a clear head and steady hands, but if you face it head-on right away, it may overwhelm you.

In a study of parents with seriously ill children, those who used denial had the lowest cortisol levels. If their children did not recover, however, the parents who had used denial ultimately fared worse than those who hadn't used it. When reality finally crashed down on the parents in denial, their cortisol levels spiked up much higher than the cortisol levels of the more realistic parents. Thus, denial is an effective temporary tool, but not a long-term panacea. You have to know when to let go of it and face reality.

Keeping a healthy and strong *perception* of your control is extremely important—but it's also vitally important to maintain and exert *actual* control, in the "real world."

If you want to stay free of chronic stress, you have to be in essential control of your own life, on a day-to-day basis. If you're not really the "captain" of your own ship, you'll be an easy target for every stressor that comes along.

These days it's in vogue to criticize people who like to feel in control. It shouldn't be. Control isn't a vice. It's a powerful psychological need, just as important as the need for freedom or love.

The key to successfully staying in control of your life—*without* aggravating other people—is to try to just control your *own* life, and not other people's lives. People are resented as "control freaks" not when they control their own lives, but when they meddle in the lives of others. I believe many people who do try to control others do it precisely because they feel out of control of their own lives. They're "acting out" their own lack of control.

When you feel that, for the most part, you *are* able to control your own life, you'll be better able to occasionally *give away control*, without feeling resentment or fear. When you achieve this psychological condition, you'll be more resilient; you'll be better able to "bend without breaking." This resilience will be of great value to your brain and body. In a recent Harvard study of people one hundred years of age and older, researchers found that the primary trait shared by most centenarians was *resilience*—the ability to bend without breaking.

I believe that you can achieve the highest degree of control by simply letting go, and realizing that a higher power is the *real* controller. If you can reach this feeling, you'll have a powerful sense of control over your life.

If you do try to control your own life, you'll be forced to confront an "addiction" that almost all of us have, to some extent: *addiction to stress*. It's quite true that *moderate* stress feels so good that it can become addicting. Most of us enjoy the nice jolt of adrenaline that moderate stress causes. This jolt peps us up, stimulates our mood chemistry, and quickens our thought processes. A quick zap of stress enlivens us just as much as a strong cup of coffee does. Often, of course, the stress soon becomes unmanageable, and destabilizes our biochemistries. But for those first few minutes it feels exciting, and we often try to create *more* moderate stress. In a way, we're like the lab rats that keep activating the electrodes that stimulate their brains.

In our modern, hyper-stress society, it's hard not to be an "adrenaline junkie." Every day, it seems, you get your first "shot" of adrenaline "for free"—whether you want it or not. When it wears off, it's hard not to go back for another.

Therefore, your first step in taking *real* control of your life, in the real world, is to realize that you've got to *stop indulging in stress.* You've got to "just say no" to adrenaline.

There are dozens of other ways to take practical control of your daily life.

One of the best is to make lists of your goals. For maximum benefit, make three different lists: one to cover your goals for the entire year, one to cover your goals for the next month, and one to cover your goals for the next day or two.

Prioritize these goals. Force yourself to be very clear about exactly what you want *most.* But be realistic. An unreachable goal will just set you up for stress.

Then, after you're sure what you want, make up *action* lists— "to do" lists. Again, it helps to have three such lists: long-term, medium-term, and short-term. But put your maximum focus on your *short-term* action plan. That's the one that will guide you through today.

Each item on each of your to-do lists should be prioritized. You'll probably find that only the top of your list really *needs* to get done. Don't jump into an easy job at the bottom of the list just to "warm up." Dive into the tough stuff. Do what matters, and don't sweat the details.

Keep your expectations high, but realistic. If you aren't moving toward your goals fast enough, adjust your list—not your life. Push yourself as hard as you comfortably can, but remember that if you make your tasks too hard, you'll perceive them as stressors instead of challenges.

Don't be afraid to fail. The best way to avoid this fear is to keep your *ego* detached from your goals. If you believe that failing to reach a goal will mean you're worthless, you *will* be afraid to fail; there'll be too much riding on the outcome. Remember that you're a human *being,* not a human *doing,* and that your achievements do not define you. Strive for excellence, but realize that perfection is impossible.

As much as you can, make your goals internal, rather than

external. For example, don't make it your goal to *be* rich. Make it your goal to *feel* rich. There are millions of rich people who feel desperate for more money, and millions of middle-class people who feel prosperous and satisfied. More than two hundred years ago, Benjamin Franklin wrote, "Wealth is not his that has it, but his that enjoys it."

One of the best ways to *feel prosperous* is to work at a job you love. If you love what you do for money, the money you make will feel like enough. If you *hate* what you have to do for money, no amount of it will feel satisfying.

If you do dislike your job, don't try to buy happiness by spending every penny you make. You'll just lock yourself into your job with debt.

There is one goal that should always be at the top of your list. That goal is to *be happy*. There are many paths to happiness; some are easy to follow, and some are hard. Only *you* know the path that's right for you. But if you give up on happiness, you give up on life. Happiness—or joy, or hope, or contentment—is the well-spring of all energy, and the primary vitalizing force of life. It is our birthright as human beings to be happy.

As you are devising your goals and your action plans, you should ask the members of your immediate family what *they* expect you to accomplish. Maybe they expect less than you thought. If so, you'll probably feel relieved. If they expect *more* of you than you expect of *yourself,* find out why, and try to reconcile the difference. You don't *need* to be a slave to the expectations of your spouse, or children, or parents. Don't be afraid to stand up to people. If you do, they'll respect you more than if you "jump through their hoops."

Learn to say no. Don't be lazy, and don't be contrary. But *be yourself.* If your *true self* is not good enough for your boss or your spouse or anyone else, it's *their* problem. As Shakespeare said, "This above all: To thine own self be true." I know this is dangerous advice, because you might be tempted to use it to indulge in selfish, petty, narcissistic behavior. But that kind of behavior would not reflect the *real* "you." It would reflect the "you" that is living in the past, acting out old hurts and grievances. The *real* "you" wants to take care of others, but knows you can't take care of others unless you also take care of yourself.

It's also very important to stay as free as possible from technology-induced exhaustion. Much of your stress probably comes from invasive technological sources, such as ringing telephones, or having the stereo and TV on at the same time. This may feel normal to you, but it can definitely frazzle your nerves. Stay in control of technology, before it takes control of you. If you can, *simplify* your life.

If you take control of your life, you will probably love your life. Even when your life is filled with stressors, you will *experience* it as mostly stress-free.

Once, Mohandas Gandhi was asked, "You have been working at least fifteen hours a day, every day, for almost fifty years. Don't you think it's time you took a vacation?"

Gandhi replied, "I am always on vacation."

Clearly, the Mahatma often had little control over his stressors. But he had tremendous control over his *stress*.

How Support Vanquishes Stress

Support is the second critical element in your psychological triumvirate against stress. Along with *control* and *release*, it is invaluable in enabling you to put mind over matter.

If you have a strong support network of friends, family, and trusted colleagues, you can endure powerful stressors without internalizing them as stress. Also, if your stressors do overwhelm you, and become stress in your life, your support network can help you to minimize the stress before it wreaks havoc on your brain and endocrine system.

One study of people with no support networks vividly depicts how vulnerable to stress people are when they bear it alone. In this five-year study of 1,350 patients with severe coronary disease, the patients with no support system (no spouse or intimate friends) were three times more likely to die than those who had spouses or close friends. In the group without a support system, the mortality rate was 50 percent. In the group that had support, it was just 17 percent.

A person's support system, though, does not always have to consist of an extremely close confidant, such as a spouse or an intimate friend. It appears as if just good friends, or a strong sense of community, can also help a great deal. This concept was supported by the "Roseta study," a well-known examination of a small town in New Jersey. Roseta was a close-knit town mostly populated by Italian-Americans who adhered to Old Country traditions and customs. Within this supportive network of camaraderie and community, the people of Roseta enjoyed remarkably good health. The Rosetans did not lead conventionally healthy lifestyles; they ate high amounts of red meat, had normal rates of obesity and high blood pressure, and were typical in their drinking and smoking habits. Nonetheless, they had extraordinarily low rates of stress-related diseases, including cardiovascular disease and peptic ulcers. For example, their heart disease rates were about 350 percent better than the national average. When Rosetans moved away from their nurturing hometown, however, they quickly succumbed to stress-related illnesses at the national rate.

This same phenomenon has been mirrored by many other American ethnic communities. Small, insular communities of Greeks, Italians, Japanese, and Yugoslavians all have enjoyed relative immunity to stress-related diseases. But when residents left their close-knit communities, they lost this immunity.

Another study backs up the idea that an adequate support network can consist of just good friends. This study—of seven thousand residents of Alameda County, California—showed that people with good friends and associates were just as healthy as married people.

The stress researcher Robert Sapolsky showed that just *talking* to a relative stranger can help. Dr. Sapolsky measured the cortisol levels of patients who were undergoing a painful cardiac catheterization. He found that those who did not speak to their doctors about their fears had significantly higher cortisol levels than those who did reach out and voice their fears.

Dolores Krieger, Ph.D., has shown that offering patients emotional support by just *touching* them can profoundly improve their physical well-being. Dr. Krieger, a professor of nursing, developed a healing modality that she calls "therapeutic touch." It consists of touching patients in a caring way, and trying to focus "healing energy" upon them. In one fascinating experiment, Dr. Krieger showed that nurses who used therapeutic touch were able to increase at least one statistically measurable index of their patients' health (hemoglobin values).

Many studies and experiments corroborate the healing value of touch. Some of the most dramatic studies involve infants. Infants who are *not* frequently held tend to have mortality rates that are about 35 percent higher than those of infants who are physically nurtured. Additional studies have shown that infants who are massaged have lower stress hormones as well.

Emotional support doesn't even have to come from other people. It can also come from pets. Numerous studies show that people who have pets are relatively less prone to stress, and less vulnerable to stress-related diseases. One recent study indicated that heart-disease patients who owned pets were significantly less likely to die than heart-disease patients who didn't own pets. Another study showed that among heart-disease patients, owning a pet was an even better predictor of survival than having a spouse.

An experiment with dog owners showed that when these people were given a stressful task, their biological markers for stress increased *only* if their pets were not present. If their dogs were there, the people did not internalize their stressors as stress.

Pets are an effective buffer against stress simply because pets *love their owners.* Similarly, love from *any* source is extremely valuable in overcoming the physical effects of stress. In one revealing study of the power of love—a survey of ten thousand men with heart disease—it was discovered that patients who perceived their wives as loving and supportive experienced 50 percent less severe chest pain (angina) than patients who did not perceive their wives as loving and supportive.

One of the best ways to increase your perception of *being* loved is to *act* lovingly toward others. The stress pioneer Dr. Hans

Selye found this phenomenon to be so powerful as an anti-stress mechanism that he described it as "altruistic egoism."

In a purely practical sense, it "pays" to love others, simply because they will probably love you back. As the old aphorism goes, "To have a friend, be a friend."

But there is a benefit to love that extends beyond practicality. Love that is *not* returned can also lower stress. In one study of coronary heart disease, physicians discovered that patients who were self-centered had far lower survival rates than did loving, altruistic patients, even if the altruistic patients had no one to love them back.

Perhaps this phenomenon exists because of something as simple as the fact that *love feels good.* Or perhaps it's because if we love someone else, it takes our focus off our own problems. Or perhaps there is a more ethereal component to the healing force of love, such as the power of God.

Only one thing is certain: Love stops stress. Love heals.

The Regenerative Power of Stress Release

Release, along with *control* and *support*, is the third crucial anti-stress coping skill. When you can't keep a stressor from becoming stress, the best you can do is *release* the stress you feel.

The stress response originally evolved to create a *physical response*—a *reaction*—to a stressor. In the distant past, people almost always responded to stress with physical actions that released the stress. Physical action protected our distant ancestors from the accumulation of stress. When our forebears ran from saber-toothed tigers, they didn't "bottle up" very much stress.

These days, though, when we're confronted with a stressor, we're usually supposed to sit quietly and figure out how to solve the problem. Unfortunately, this doesn't release the stress. Instead, it allows stress to build up, until it begins to destroy our bodies and brains.

Many animal experiments have shown that if animals have no outlet for stress, it causes them to suffer severe physical damage.

In one series of experiments on rats, one group was subjected to a mild shock, but was given an outlet for stress, such as a treadmill. The other group of rats was also shocked, but was given no way to release stress. The group that had no outlet quickly developed much higher levels of cortisol than the other group, and developed significantly more stress-related illnesses.

Humans also need outlets. People who habitually hold in stress—psychologically repressing it instead of releasing it—commonly suffer from physical ailments that are at least partly related to stress. In three different studies of chronic diseases—rheumatoid arthritis, ulcerative colitis, and cancer—a common denominator among a majority of patients was their inability to express anger effectively. This doesn't mean anger caused those diseases, but it does indicate that the degenerative disease process is probably exacerbated by lack of emotional release.

There are three primary ways to release stress. The first is to release it with *physical action*, such as exercise or hard physical work. The second is to *verbally vent* your emotions, by talking, crying, yelling, or otherwise expressing your frustrations. The third is to *displace* your stress, by finding a practical, real-world release for it.

Physical action. This is wonderfully effective at releasing stress, for an obvious reason. The stress response evolved specifically to stimulate physical action.

If you "burn off" stress with physical activity, you're dealing with it in exactly the way it was *meant* to be dealt with. The elements of the stress response—e.g., increased heart rate, higher blood pressure, slowed digestion—mesh perfectly with the demands of exercise. Therefore, exercise is extremely efficient at returning your body to its normal, relaxed, resting state.

One of my patients, who wanted to exercise but was pressed for time, adopted the habit of working out on a stair-stepper machine in his business office. He was able to ready reports, make phone calls, and conduct other aspects of his business while simultaneously exercising. He soon discovered that he felt a very satisfying sense of emotional release from combining work with exercise. His work was naturally stressful, but when he immediately "burned off" that stress through exercise, he enjoyed much higher levels of focus, relaxation, and energy. Further, the latest research on cognitive development indicates that when exercise and mental enrichment are engaged in simultaneously, the cognitive benefits of both activities are multiplied.

Even more effective at releasing stress than smooth, rhythmic exercises are physical activities that allow short bursts of aggressive physical movements, such as kicks, lifts, or thrusts. This type of action allows you to punctuate your workout with movements that harmlessly mimic aggression. Therefore, this style of exercise offers a more liberating release of pent-up frustrations.

One of the best forms of "aggressive" exercise is hard physical work. One of my younger patients found that doing rigorous landscaping in his yard released his stress much more effectively than did smooth, rhythmic exercises, such as jogging. He told me that when he was digging up a boulder, or chopping brush, he was able to focus his stress release into a few hard, aggressive actions, which drained his tension amazingly well. In addition, he said, he got a sense of satisfaction from the work that he couldn't get from "nonproductive" exercises, such as running.

When you exercise, you not only release stress you've already experienced, but also help make yourself resistant to future stress. Exercise creates a form of the relaxation response that lasts long after the exercise is over. Furthermore, when you exercise, you gradually develop a lower resting heart rate, and a lower resting heart rate helps prevent easy triggering of the stress response.

Also, exercise actually *helps the brain grow.* It's so physically beneficial to the brain that it's one of the four basic elements of my brain longevity programs. All of chapter 16 is devoted to exercise.

Verbal venting. This is probably the most common way of releasing stress. You do this by talking, crying, yelling, or voicing your stress in some other way.

It's generally not wise, or kind, to vent your frustrations directly *at* someone else. Venting is just as effective if no one else is present. If you direct your frustrations at another person, you're likely to create conflict, and cause even more stress. If someone *is* present when you vent your emotions, make sure that person knows you're not directing your displeasure *at him or her.*

Crying is a simple and natural form of verbal release. It allows you to focus directly upon the source of your stress, and to "speak from your heart." Often, when you allow yourself to become vulnerable enough to cry, you're able to strip away the protective intellectual "shields" that you place around your hurt, and to "zero in" on *exactly* what's bothering you. Crying discharges "hurt feelings," releases stress-tightened muscles, and relieves tension.

In addition, recent research indicates that tears may, in themselves, offer some release from stress. This belief stems from the research of William Frey, Ph.D., a psychiatric biochemist.

Dr. Frey first became interested in tears when he studied the work of researchers who discovered, in 1949, that children who were physically unable to release tears, because of a genetic disorder, were extremely sensitive to stress. Children with an inherited disorder that made their tear glands nonfunctional could not tolerate even mild stressors. When subjected to stressors, their blood pressure skyrocketed, they salivated and sweated excessively, and they broke out in red splotches.

These children were able to express their unhappiness in every way except for secreting tears when they cried.

Dr. Frey theorized from this that tear secretion somehow helped people release emotional pain. Underlying this theory was Frey's knowledge that all other human excretory functions serve a biological purpose; if tear secretion serves no biological purpose, it is unique among human excretory functions.

Dr. Frey began to study the composition of tears. He found that tears produced by emotional upset were different from those that were caused by eye irritants, such as wind. "Emotional" tears, he found, were significantly higher than "irritant" tears in their concentrations of various hormones, endorphins, and neurotransmitters. Especially abundant in emotion-caused tears are stress-related neurotransmitters, including adrenaline.

Dr. Frey remains uncertain about the exact biological function of tears, but he is convinced that they help people to release stress.

Just as crying can help release stress, so can laughing. Recent experiments have shown that the act of laughing actually helps deactivate stress hormones, and increases production of the antibodies of the immune system.

Having a good sense of humor also appears to help some elements of cognitive function. For example, in one study, 84 percent of personnel directors said that employees with good senses of humor tended to be creative, and adept at problem-solving.

Humor also helps people get along. A recent study at the University of Oregon showed that spouses who both had good senses of humor were significantly more likely to remain happily married than spouses with poor senses of humor.

Unfortunately, though, we tend to lose our sense of humor as we age. Children, on average, laugh about three hundred times per day, but adults generally laugh only fifteen times per day.

Other forms of verbal emotional release have also been proven to drain stress. It helps to talk about your problems—even if you're just talking to, say, a tree. It enables you to focus on what's really bothering you, and also allows you to "let off steam." Just *saying* how you feel—even if you don't get any advice or help—will make you feel better.

As a rule, the more animated you can become in verbally discharging your stress, the more cathartic the experience will be. If you're uninhibited enough, it can help to kick and yell and punch a pillow. This kind of "overreaction" may seem extreme to you, but if you do it, you will probably feel better. Of course, this is "undignified" behavior, so you will probably want to be alone when you do it.

Displacement. Dr. Robert Sapolsky found that the cortisol levels of stressed-out lab animals declined when they displaced their frustration by attacking other animals. Obviously, *people* shouldn't do this, because it isn't morally or socially acceptable. Nonetheless, it is possible to displace stress without hurting someone.

For example, you can take out your frustrations on inanimate objects. If you get a flat tire and it makes you angry, kick the tire. Call the tire names. You'll feel better.

You can also displace stress by consciously shifting your worry to a *less difficult* problem. This may seem contrived, but it's highly effective. For example, if you're worried about your sick daughter, you could shift your concern to finding her the best possible treatment. This will lower your level of stress. It will also rechannel your stress into a more constructive outlet.

Sports fans commonly employ displacement when they "worry" about the outcome of a sports event. They know it doesn't *really* matter if their team wins or loses—and this is precisely what prompts them to invest their emotions in the game. The fans are displacing their own real worries.

All of the best strategies for achieving emotional release—physical action, verbal venting, and displacement—will help you to keep from accumulating neurotoxic levels of stress.

You should use each of these strategies virtually every day. If you do, you'll save yourself from emotional wear and tear—and you may also *save your brain.* Your current cognitive function will be considerably enhanced, and you'll be far more able to attain brain longevity.

As you can see, there are a number of coping skills that you can use to resist damage from the stress response, and from the general adaptation syndrome. The best of these coping skills boil down to just three categories: *control, support,* and *release.*

If you incorporate control, support, and release into your life, you will be well on your way to putting mind over matter. As noted early in this chapter, though, there is a mental exercise that will work wonders for your stress management program: meditation.

For controlling stress, meditation is a virtual "magic bullet."

A Case in Point

The Last 10 Percent of Improvement Can Be the Hardest 10 Percent

J.R., seventy-five years of age, was the kind of man who is easy to envy. Even though he was well past middle age, he had the demeanor of a young and vital man. An avid sportsman and tennis player, he was extremely physically fit; "his muscles had muscles." He was about six feet two inches tall, weighed 190 pounds, and had silver hair and a healthy tan. He was a multimillionaire, and was still working as an important executive. He and his wife, who was about twenty years younger than he, were still very much in love.

When J.R. first came to me, complaining of mild age-associated memory impairment, I told him, "Most people would *kill* to be like you."

"That may be," he said, "but I want to stay like this. Or to get even better."

J.R. had always lived life to the fullest, and he intended to continue doing so, regardless of his age.

He had previously consulted with a neurologist, who had confirmed that J.R. was suffering from age-associated memory impairment. But, according to the patient, the neurologist had told him not to worry about his mild cognitive decline. J.R. told me his physician had said that his small decline in cognition was "not important."

But it was important to J.R. Therefore, it was important to me. I've never believed in ignoring any patient's needs, just because other patients may have seemingly greater needs. If a patient wants to improve, I think that deserves respect.

I ran a lab test on J.R.'s DHEA levels, and they were relatively low, so I put him on DHEA replacement therapy. I also prescribed deprenyl for him.

In addition, I helped J.R. to refine his supplementation program. He was already taking a relative abundance of nutritional supplements, but like many people, he was taking some supplements he didn't need, and was not taking some that he did need. He was also taking too many of his supplements at the end of the day, instead of in the morning. I recommended that he "front-load" his supplements early in the day, so that he could get more energy from them during his workday.

J.R. enjoyed doing the mind/body exercises. He had never tried anything quite like them before, and was open to anything new that might, as he put it, "take me to the next level." In the beginning, however, he had some difficulty coordinating the movements of the kirtan kriya. I thought this might be indicative of a mild deficit of dopamine, which I hoped would be corrected by the deprenyl.

After his first three months on the program, J.R. said that he only felt "about 1 percent better." I reminded him that, because he'd been in very good physical and mental condition to begin with, he could only hope to improve by about 10 percent. If he *did* achieve that 10-percent improvement, he would be at the absolute height of cognitive function for someone his age. I told him not to be discouraged.

He said that he wasn't discouraged, and I believed him.

J.R. redoubled his efforts, and followed his program very conscientiously. Slowly he gained momentum.

After a few more months, J.R. called me again, and said that he had mastered the kirtan kriya. He told me that his overall muscular coordination was better, and that he'd even made some improvements in his tennis game. He also said that his energy level seemed to be on the rise, and that he no longer seemed to be forgetful. The last time I talked to J.R., he was doing even a little better. He said he felt terrific. His progress never was quick or easy. But none of J.D.'s major achievements in life had been quick or easy.

I would estimate that J.R. has achieved most of the improvement that is possible for him. He is at an extremely high level of physical and mental fitness. He's probably in better physical and mental condition than most people in midlife, or younger.

Even so, J.R. is still happily working away—still intent upon becoming "younger" with each passing day. And, so far, he's *achieving* it.

15

The Magic Bullet of Stress Management

When I was an intern, I lived the typically harried life of a young doctor. I worked in the hospital until the point of exhaustion, hanging on by my fingernails until my shift was over. Then I would gulp a gallon of coffee and work *another* shift. After that, I'd stagger out of the hospital—and head straight for the perpetual party that always seems to exist among groups of young physicians.

After the party ended, I'd drag home and get some sleep. Sometimes I'd get as much as four or five hours. Then I'd run back to the hospital, and do it all over again. I *loved* the adrenaline rush of the hospital and couldn't get enough of it.

But after about a year of that routine, I was the Cortisol Kid. My adrenals were exhausted, my brain was "running on empty," and my immunity was so low that I knew both of my white blood cells, by name. My eyes were little red dots. I needed a *lift*.

For help, I turned to transcendental meditation. I knew the Beatles had done TM, and to a young doc like me in the mid-1970s, that was like the *Good Housekeeping* Seal of Approval.

I tried it—and the most amazing thing happened. I became so suffused with vitality that huge expenditures of energy—like a ten-hour shift followed by a five-hour party—no longer phased me. I simply did what I *wanted* to do, and somehow seemed to have even more energy than I needed.

Some of my colleagues at the hospital said they were "in awe" of my energy. They thought I had some kind of secret weapon. At night, around 2:00 A.M., I'd go up to my sleeping quarters and meditate for ten to twenty minutes. Then I'd return to the wards, and skate through the rest of my shift. My supervisor, a hard-charging New Yorker who was famous for his frenetic energy, was amazed that I could keep up with him, because no one else had ever been able to. Before long, I was named chief resident of my anesthesia program.

Then, gradually, an even more beneficial effect of TM began to take hold: I lost my need for a harried lifestyle. I kept my abundant energy, but my vigor became bound together with a serene calmness. I no longer relied on my work to give me a sense of purpose—*or* a brain full of adrenaline. Nor did I have to go to parties to feel alive and exhilarated. For me, meditation opened the door to the inner world, and I found this world to be so rich and fulfilling that I never again really needed all the rewards and the tumult that the material world can offer. I had something better. I had discovered a way to help prevent my stressors from becoming stress.

Once I became relatively stress-free, I no longer wasted as much of my energy on worry, regret, and frustration. I was able to live in the here and now, which, for me, was a heavenly place to be.

After my internship, during my anesthesia residency, I could not help noticing the role that stress played in the lives of my patients. Often it seemed as if stress played a greater role in their diseases than did any microbe or biochemical disorder. Therefore I began an earnest study of stress medicine. Eventually I wrote a ground-breaking research paper about how high levels of stress affect a certain type of heart surgery.

As part of my study of stress, I pored over the works of

Charles Garfield, Ph.D., and Hal Zina Bennett, Ph.D., the primary investigators of human "peak performance." I also devoured the research of Dr. Herbert Benson, the creator of the "relaxation response."

I was particularly impressed by the brilliance of Dr. Benson's work, because of its elegant simplicity. So I went to Harvard for a postgraduate training course under Dr. Benson.

I began to apply the techniques of Garfield and Benson to the patients in my clinical practice. As I started to specialize in the treatment of pain, I found that patients who were suffering from chronic pain—and the stress this pain caused—responded very positively to the techniques of Garfield and Benson. Used in combination with other naturalistic modalities, these techniques literally achieved miracles in some patients.

For example, I had one pain patient, named Victor, who had broken his back in a fall from the top of an oil rig in the North Sea. Five operations later, Victor was still in excruciating pain, and was addicted to painkillers. Because of the constant stress caused by his pain, as well as the cumulative effects of the narcotics he was taking, Victor suffered from severe cognitive decline, and from acute depression. His decision-making ability was poor, and his reasoning skills were badly impaired. In addition, he had become impotent, and was about sixty-five pounds overweight. He told me that he had "no reason to live."

I put Victor on a fledgling version of my brain longevity program, one that stressed meditation and relaxation.

He quickly began to feel better, mentally and emotionally. He said that the meditation and relaxation techniques gave him a drug-free refuge from his pain, and made him "feel in control again." His cognition and mood improved dramatically. He began to lose weight, and to use far fewer painkillers.

As he lost weight, his mobility increased and he was able to more effectively exercise his back muscles. Soon his sexual function returned, his cognitive abilities became fully normalized, and his pain diminished to a very manageable level. He told me that the meditation and relaxation techniques had saved his life.

I don't think he was exaggerating. Were it not for the meditation and relaxation techniques he'd learned, I doubt that Victor would be alive today. These techniques were the foundation of his recovery.

I soon discovered that meditation—which elicits the relaxation response—not only helped people recover from serious problems, but also helped *healthy* people to achieve optimal cognitive function. I found this out when I began to teach a course to doctors studying for their board exams. I showed all of them how to meditate, and how to apply the mental training techniques of peak performance. This gave most of them as big a lift as it had given me. As I mentioned earlier, the doctors taking my course had over a 90-percent pass rate, compared to the national average of about 50 percent.

When I began to study kundalini yoga, and became a Sikh, I gained a complete appreciation of the power of the mind and spirit. I saw that the mind and spirit can heal.

I also discovered, after years of studying meditation, that *the space between our thoughts*—what the Asian healers call "the sacred space"—is where most spirit-directed healing originates.

Within this sacred space, which can be reached only through meditation, lies the heart of all spiritual healing.

Perhaps this heart consists of the purest essence of the human spirit. Or perhaps, as I believe, this heart is the *divine* spirit.

Whatever it is, it is one of the most potent healing forces you possess. I believe that most healing "miracles"—recoveries that seem scientifically impossible—stem from this force.

But you do not need to wait until you need a miracle to experience the power of the sacred space. You can tap into this power today. And you can do it for just a simple, mundane purpose—to gain relief from your stress.

How to Meditate

Connecting directly with your inner spirit, through meditation, is probably far simpler than you think.

Part of the genius of Dr. Benson was that he *demystified* meditation, and welcomed the common person into the realm of the spirit. He did not jump on the bandwagon of any particular style of meditation, and did not reinvent himself as a spiritual master. Instead he endorsed several styles of meditation, all of which, he said, elicited the relaxation response.

The relaxation response, as I've mentioned, is the opposite physical and mental condition to the stress response. It is a condition characterized by a lowered metabolic rate and a calm state of mind.

The relaxation response is created when the "thinking" neocortex "tells" the amygdala and hippocampus—in the "emotional" limbic system—to relax. The amygdala and hippocampus then relay the message to the hypothalamus, which begins orchestrating the release of a flood of calming neurotransmitters and hormones. Soon the entire body, as well as the brain, shifts into a soothing state of relaxation.

When you meditate, and elicit the relaxation response, your mind stops racing with thoughts, and there are longer spaces between your thoughts. The space between thoughts usually feels "timeless."

How you *use* this space between thoughts—this sacred space—is up to you. You can use it to tune in to your own spirit, or to tune in to the divine spirit.

If you use it in either of these ways, you may well experience an increase in your sense of consciousness. As T. S. Eliot wrote:

Time past and time future
Allow but a little consciousness.
To be conscious is not to be in time.

If you choose to do so, however, you can use the meditative state for nothing more mystical than giving yourself a break from stress, and lowering your cortisol level. Although this may not be the most esoteric use of the meditative state, it is still *absolutely valid.* After all, many religions employ meditation—but meditation, in itself, is not a religion.

Here are the general guidelines for eliciting the relaxation response, through meditation. Most of these guidelines reflect the methods used in simple, basic meditation.

• Find a quiet place, with as few distracting elements as possible. Avoid interruptions.

• Give yourself ten to twenty minutes to meditate, once or twice a day, preferably before breakfast and dinner, and don't stop until this time is up. Check a clock occasionally, but don't use an alarm, because it might startle you and ruin your relaxation.

• Sit comfortably, consciously relax all your muscles from the bottom of your feet to the top of your head, and close your eyes. Adopt a calm, passive attitude. Breathe slowly and deeply.

• Try not to think about all the things that are on your mind. Stop your "internal dialogue." Stop thinking in words. Don't make plans, or recall memories.

• To help you to stop thinking, and to help you calm down, silently repeat a word or phrase to yourself. This is called a *mantra*. Make it a calming, positive mantra, such as "peace," or "love." Or use words that have religious significance for you, such as, "The Lord is my shepherd," or "Shalom," or "One."

A *poor* choice of mantras might include "tax audit," "cancer," or "alimony."

• Don't be concerned when thoughts intrude, because they inevitably will. When this happens, simply say to yourself, "Oh well, Self (your name), relax, *One* (or your mantra)." Then inhale, and go back to meditating.

• When you finish, sit quietly for a minute or two, and try to merge your calm state of mind with your normal, nonmeditative outlook.

That's all there is to it.

If it sounds simple, that's because it is.

Now I'll tell you how to do a more advanced form of meditation. Even though this form generally elicits a more powerful response, it's still very easy to do.

Deep Meditation into Thoughtlessness

• Sit with your legs comfortably crossed and your spine straight. Put your hands together in your lap, with your palms up, and your right hand resting in your left, thumbs touching.

• Close your eyes, and let go of absolutely all tension throughout your body. Imagine watching all the tension flow out of your body.

• Focus all of your mental energy on the point between your eyebrows, at the top of your nose.

• Silently chant the mantra *Whahe Guru*, breaking it into four syllables: *Wha-he-Gu-ru*. This mantra has the effect of bringing your mind to a state of clarity.

• Continue this for eleven minutes. If you become distracted, try to ignore the distraction and return to your meditation.

• Then inhale deeply, hold the breath for fifteen seconds, exhale, and relax.

The value of this meditation is that it allows you to experience a continuous flow of energy. This happens because your mind becomes very still. It is a quick way to achieve a profound state of deep relaxation and stress relief.

Other mental techniques that also elicit the relaxation response are just as simple. The two most popular of these are "autogenic training" and "progressive relaxation."

Autogenic training is a mental exercise that shifts the mind and body to a relaxed state. To do autogenic training, (1) lie down in a quiet room, adopt a passive attitude, close your eyes, and imagine a feeling of heaviness in your arms and legs; (2) imagine your limbs are becoming warm; (3) imagine that you are slowing down your heartbeat; (4) concentrate on deep breathing; and (5) imagine that your forehead is becoming cool.

People who practice this method assiduously can actually create the physical conditions that they are imagining.

Progressive relaxation is just as simple. To do this, lie down, close your eyes, adopt a passive attitude, focus on a particular group of muscles, and try to relax those muscles as much as possible. Keep shifting your focus from one muscle group to another.

People who practice the progressive relaxation technique learn to detect even minuscule muscular tensions.

Both autogenic training and progressive relaxation focus more on the body than meditation does, but much of the purpose of this focus is to shift your attention away from your thoughts. Therefore, like meditation, these techniques effectively create a meditative state.

Although the techniques that create the relaxation response are extremely simple, they have profound effects.

Meditation has been very carefully studied by the medical profession for the past twenty-five years. Those studies have shown that meditation is a virtual "magic bullet" for eliminating the physical effects of stress.

How Meditation Affects Your Body and Brain

Virtually all of my patients who try meditation for the first time are astonished at how good it makes them feel.

One of my patients told me that if he meditated for ten to fifteen minutes before he left for work in the morning, it was "like putting on a suit of armor against stress."

Another of my patients, a middle-aged man with age-associated memory impairment, received considerable benefit from doing his meditation at the *end* of his workday. Before he had started meditating, he told me, he had needed two or three cocktails to relax after work. But when he meditated, he said, he had no desire for alcohol. After meditating, he told me, alcohol just made him "feel dull."

Several experiments have shown that meditating allows people to reach a condition of slowed metabolism, which is also called a *hypometabolic* state. Only two other activities commonly create this state. One is sleep, and the other is hibernation (which humans, of course, do not engage in).

During the hypometabolic state, there is a significant decrease in the body's consumption of oxygen. When we sleep, our oxygen consumption drops by about 8 percent. But during meditation, it drops by 10 to 20 percent. This decreased use of oxygen reflects the deeply relaxed state that meditation creates, and also reflects the rest that is given to the entire physical system. This temporary decrease of oxygen use accounts, in part, for the increased physical energy imparted by meditation.

Another physical effect of meditation is a decrease in *blood lactate*. Lactate is a substance secreted by the muscles, and it contributes to feelings of anxiety. In a fascinating experiment, one group of patients with anxiety disorder was injected with lactate. Another group, with the same disorder, was injected with a placebo. Almost every patient in the group that got the lactate quickly experienced an anxiety attack. None of the people in the placebo group experienced such an attack.

In a related experiment, people with *no* history of anxiety disorder were injected with lactate, and 20 percent of them experienced an anxiety attack.

During meditation, though, blood lactate levels drop significantly, generally within ten minutes.

Other physical effects of meditation are decreases in heart rate, blood pressure, and respiration rate. Studies indicate that heart rate slows by an average of about three beats per minute during meditation.

Even the "sleep hormone" melatonin is increased by meditation. In a study at the University of Massachusetts Medical Center, researchers found that meditators regularly produced significantly more melatonin than nonmeditators.

Of significance to brain longevity patients is the fact that meditation also causes a decline in cortisol production. This decline usually persists long after the period of meditation ends. Furthermore, among people who meditate regularly, cortisol levels tend to remain low, day after day.

This medley of physical effects caused by meditation creates lifelong health advantages. Meditation has been shown to slow the aging process significantly, and to increase not just lifespan but "health span."

In one important study of meditation, researchers found that it had a powerfully positive influence on three important biological markers of aging: blood pressure, hearing ability, and vision of close objects. This study showed that if people had meditated for five years or less, they had "biological ages" that were about five years younger than their chronological ages. If they had meditated for more than five years, their biological ages were about *twelve* years younger than their chronological ages.

In another study, two thousand meditators showed a uniform superiority over nonmeditators in thirteen major health categories and disease conditions. The meditators, for example, had 80 percent less heart disease, and 50 percent less cancer.

Another important marker of aging that is improved by meditation is the level of the steroid hormone DHEA (dehydroepiandrosterone). As cortisol is secreted throughout life, the body's supply of DHEA gradually becomes depleted. By the end of a person's life, he or she often has only about 5 or 10 percent as much DHEA as he or she did at age twenty-five. Thus, people's DHEA levels indicate *how much stress* they have endured during their lives. A study of meditators, however, showed that men over age forty-five had an average of 23 percent *more DHEA* than nonmeditators, and women had an average of 47 percent more.

In another fascinating study, researchers found that another significant marker of aging—a chemical that corresponds to free-radical production—was lower in subjects aged sixty to sixty-nine who meditated than in an age-matched control group who did not meditate. This marker was even lower in a group of subjects aged seventy to seventy-nine.

In a study of nursing-home residents, one group meditated, and a control group did not. After three years, none of the meditators had died, but 33 percent of the control group had.

Other studies have shown that by using meditation, 75 percent of insomniacs were able to sleep normally, 34 percent of people with chronic pain were able to reduce their analgesic medication, and 35 percent of women diagnosed with infertility were able to become pregnant.

Still another benefit of meditation is that it apparently decreases the need for mood-enhancing substances, such as drugs and alcohol. In one study of beginning meditators who tended to be recreational drug users, use of marijuana declined precipitously. When they began meditation, 78 percent of the group used marijuana, but after six months of meditation, only 37 percent used it. Further, the *amount* of marijuana those meditators consumed dropped tremendously. In the beginning, 28 percent used marijuana every day, but at the end of the six months, only .001 percent used it daily.

Obviously, meditation can help eliminate negative conditions. But it can also create positive conditions. It can, for example, significantly heighten learning ability and creative problem-solving.

It does this, in part, by altering brain waves.

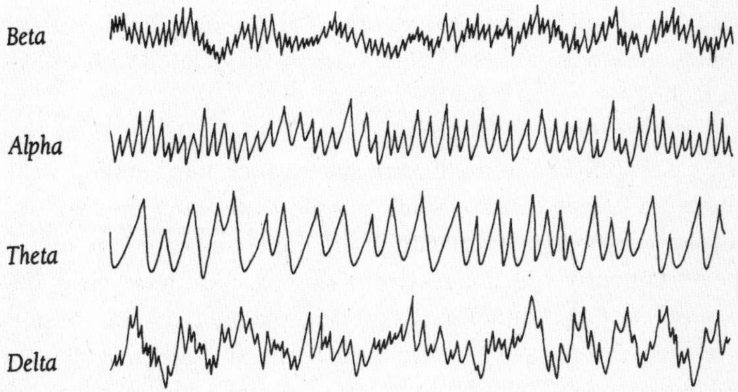

Figure 8
Your brain has four types of bioelectric waves. The most powerful waves for learning and relaxation—theta waves—can be consciously created through meditation.

Meditation and Theta-State "Super Learning"

As you know, your brain is powered by electricity. Every second, trillions of neurons in your brain are firing their electrical impulses. Like most regular, repeated impulses in nature, these neuronal firings naturally organize themselves into rhythmical patterns, or *waves*.

Like all other waves, brain waves occur at varying speeds, or "frequencies."

There are four frequencies of brain waves:

• *Beta waves* are the most common brain waves, and they occur at the highest frequency. We experience beta waves during our waking moments, when our eyes are open and our minds are racing with thoughts. These waves are associated with normal cognition, and also with anxiety.

• *Alpha waves* are slower in frequency, and occur when we are in a state of mild relaxation. A *lack* of alpha-wave activity usually reflects anxiety and stress. These waves are associated with a pleasant feeling.

• *Theta waves* are about two to four times slower than beta waves, and reflect the meditative state, which lies between wakefulness and sleep. Often, when people experience theta waves, they have access to information in their subconscious minds. They frequently see images from the past, or have vivid daydreams. They also sometimes experience deep personal insights. They frequently have creative ideas, and are adept at creative problem-solving. Theta brain waves combine a pleasant, relaxed feeling with extreme alertness.

• *Delta waves* occur when you fall asleep. They are the slowest brain waves.

As you can see, the brain waves that offer the most potential for enhanced cognition are theta waves, the waves that come from meditation.

One researcher has illustrated the power of theta waves by likening them to the power of a group of soldiers marching across a bridge. As you may know, when troops march across a bridge, they do not do it in normal, rhythmical cadence, because this can create strong, slow, rhythmic vibrations that can collapse a bridge. Theta waves have this same power. Because they are the slowest of waking brain waves, their "peaks and valleys" are significantly farther from the baseline than those of other brain waves. This powerful pattern of organization allows the brain to operate at a higher level of efficiency. It amplifies the bioelectric power of "memory traces," the chains of neuronal firings that combine to form complete memories.

Theta waves are not strictly confined to periods of formal meditation. Theta waves can occur at various moments throughout the day. Experienced meditators frequently experience periods of theta waves even when they are not meditating. For the most part, the more a person practices meditation, the more adept he or she becomes at producing theta waves at will. Many meditators are able to shift to theta waves just by focusing on them.

You have probably experienced this shift to theta waves yourself, during moments of insight or creative breakthrough. Experiments show that when someone is grappling with a mental problem, and then suddenly understands it, his or her brain waves shift to the theta pattern. This is partly why you feel a sudden release of tension when you solve a problem.

Further, part of the reason you are able to solve problems is that you instinctively know how to "psych yourself up" to the theta-wave condition.

Conversely, when you have felt "stuck" or "blocked" by a problem, you were almost certainly in the beta-wave condition. This condition is generally associated with a sense of flat emotional affect, or with anxiety.

In one study of brain waves, a researcher gave his subjects a complex problem that demanded creative thinking. Invariably, when the subjects began to approach the solution to the problem, their brain waves shifted to the theta condition.

Other researchers have found that stimulating theta brain waves enables people to enhance their learning abilities vastly. One European psychiatrist developed a method of teaching that employed the elicitation of theta waves. With this method he was able to teach people typically as many as five hundred new foreign-language words per day (with some people learning as many as three thousand words per day). The retention rate for this learning was an average of 88 percent after six months.

One reason for this enhanced learning ability is that theta waves naturally encourage long-term potentiation. As you may recall, LTP (which I described in chapter 7) is the phenomenon that makes information *biologically easier to remember* each time you're exposed to it. Each exposure adds to the memory exponentially—that is, if you see something five times, you won't be only five times more apt to remember it, but about *twenty* times. This happens because the "path" of the memory becomes "beaten down." Powerful theta waves have a similar ability to "beat down" the paths of memory traces.

Occasionally my patients will add various elements of their brain longevity programs one at a time, and will delay their participation in meditation. Sometimes they put off meditation for a week or two, because it seems exotic to them, particularly if they are older people who have never meditated. But when they *do* finally begin to meditate, they invariably report to me that the meditation "took them to a new level." Meditation is really that powerful.

Besides enhancing cognitive performance, the meditative state is also highly conducive to achieving excellence in *physical* performance. Most great athletes enter into a meditative mental state during their athletic events. Some of them refer to this state as "the zone of altered consciousness," or just as "the zone."

Dr. Steven Undgerleider, one of the world's premier researchers on the psychology of athletics, maintains that many elite athletes enter into a theta-wave "dissociative state" during their events. This theta-wave state, he says, frees them from pain, fatigue, and fear of failure.

One athlete who commonly achieves this dissociative state

during games is Michael Jordan. Jordan creates a theta state that is so powerful that he visualizes it as a "ball of power" that surrounds him. Once Jordan discussed this "ball of power" with Cameron Stauth, who also has studied the psychology of athletics. Jordan told Stauth that he could not "get into the ball of power *intellectually*. To get into it, I've got to *stop* thinking. I've got to be *aware*, but without *thought*."

The great runner Roger Bannister—the first man to break the "psychological barrier" of the four-minute mile—said that during his record-breaking run, he was "no longer conscious of my movement. I discovered a new unity with nature. I had found a source of power and beauty, a source I never dreamt existed."

Obviously there is great power to be gained from the meditative state. It can help make you stress-free, and can help you to accomplish extraordinary mental and physical feats.

Now let's look at one last form of meditation, probably one you have already tried. It's a fascinating form of meditation, and sometimes it can be absolutely electrifying, because—more than any other mental activity—it merges the power of psychology with the power of spirituality.

This form of meditation is prayer.

The Healing Science of Prayer

If you believe in God, and in a God who answers prayers, then you probably already believe that prayer can heal.

But even if you do not believe in God—or do not believe in a God who answers prayers—you may still end up believing that prayer can heal, after you read the following material.

If you do believe in the power of prayer, you are in the majority. Prayer is extremely popular today in America. Recent surveys indicate that about 89 percent of all Americans pray regularly. There is an even higher percentage of religious involvement now than among Americans who lived at the time of the Revolutionary War. More Americans now pray than do the people of any other Western country except Ireland. In the

United States and Ireland, 80 percent of all people surveyed said they prayed at least once a week. In Italy and New Zealand the figure was 70 percent. In Spain, Australia, and Germany it was between 60 and 70 percent. In England, Denmark, and France it was 40 to 50 percent.

In America, 57 percent of those surveyed said they prayed daily. Women prayed more than men, older people more than younger people, blacks more than whites, and less-educated people more than well-educated people.

A recent Gallup poll showed that four out of five respondents believed that prayer could cure disease. Nearly half said they had been healed by prayer.

A Time/CNN poll in 1996 indicated that 82 percent of all people polled thought that prayer could help them recover from an illness, and 73 percent believed they could help someone else recover from an illness by praying for them.

The most popular form of prayer is the "colloquial conversation" type, in which people talk to God in their own words about a variety of matters. The other most common types are "petitionary prayers," in which a person asks God for something; "ritual prayers," which employ a prepared script; and "meditative prayers," which focus on feeling the presence of God.

Technically, only meditative prayers involve meditation, but virtually any type of prayer can elicit the meditative state, and the relaxation response.

It appears, however, as if the formal meditative prayer—which involves *listening* to God more than *talking* to Him—is the most effective style of prayer for creating a subjective perception of closeness to God. Survey respondents were twice as likely to feel a "strong relationship with God" if they used the meditative style instead of one of the other three styles. The style that *least* elicited a subjective sense of connection to God was the petitionary style.

The emotion that was most associated with feeling a connection to God was "a deep sense of peace and well-being." Another common feeling was of having "deeper insight into spiritual truth."

This sense of peace, well-being, and spiritual understanding appears to be of tremendous value to those who experience it. One major study of prayer found that people who have a subjective sense of connection to God get more psychological support from that connection than from any other element in their lives, including their material possessions and their spouses. The people who *most* value this connection are people with a high number of stressors in their lives.

Engaging in prayer, however, improves more than just the subjective sense of well-being; it also improves objective measures of physical health. This is quite understandable, of course, since a subjective sense of well-being virtually always contributes to physical health.

It is conceivable that the power of prayer reflects nothing more than the placebo effect. It may be that prayer improves health merely because people who pray *think* it will improve their health.

If this is true, it still reinforces the power of prayer. Many doctors are contemptuous of the placebo effect, but I most certainly am not. I support virtually any phenomenon that helps people to achieve health, including the placebo effect. I agree with Dr. Herbert Benson, who once wrote, in the *Journal of the American Medical Association,* "The placebo effect, in most instances, enhances the well-being of the patient, and this is an essential aspect of medicine."

The placebo effect is so strong that, for some illnesses, a placebo drug achieves about a 30-percent rate of effectiveness. Therefore, even if prayer is merely a placebo, it is still of value. The placebo effect is a sterling example of a technique that has the power to put mind over matter. As such, it should be celebrated, not disdained.

If prayer is a placebo, it's apparently a powerful one. Numerous studies, including a recent Dartmouth University study of 232 heart surgery patients, indicate that people with a strong religious faith are more resistant to major illnesses, and recover faster from surgery, than people with no religious faith.

There is some scientific evidence, however, that the power of prayer does not depend upon the placebo effect. One remarkable study of prayer was performed by Randolph Byrd, M.D., who studied 393 coronary-care patients over a ten-month period. This study was a controlled, double-blind study, and the placebo effect was not a factor in it.

In Dr. Byrd's study, half of the 393 patients were prayed for by an outside prayer group. The prayer group was given the first names of the patients, their diagnoses, and a brief description of each patient. None of the doctors or nurses treating any of the patients knew who was being prayed for. The prayer group prayed for the patients each day. Each patient who was prayed for had five to seven people praying for him or her.

At the end of ten months, the patients in the group that was prayed for had fared significantly better than the other group. They were 500 percent less likely to have required antibiotics, and 300 percent less likely to have developed the common, serious problem of pulmonary edema. None of the patients who were prayed for required artificial ventilation, but twelve of those who were not prayed for did. Also, fewer of the patients who were prayed for died (though this number was not large enough to be statistically meaningful.)

This study captured the attention of many rationalistic physicians, including Dr. William Nolen, who had written a book critical of faith healing. Dr. Nolen noted, "If this is a valid study, we doctors ought to be writing on our order sheet, 'Pray three times a day.' If it works, it works."

Another recent experiment also reflects the possible power of prayer. In this experiment, sixty-one volunteers focused their mental energies upon members of a group of 271 healthy subjects. The sixty-one volunteers tried to mentally project either a "calming influence" or an "activating influence" upon the subjects. They did this in thirty-second "influence periods," twenty times per session.

Astonishingly, the mental influence of the volunteers was in many cases somehow *communicated* to the subjects. Some subjects responded in ways that were objectively apparent and statistically meaningful. The responses of the subjects, the researchers noted, were "consistent, replicable, and robust." In fact, specific images were sometimes transmitted. For example, a volunteer one day mentioned that the personality of a particular female subject reminded him of the precision of the musical group Kraftwerk. During that day's session, the *subject* reported that the group Kraftwerk had entered her thoughts.

This could, of course, have been a coincidence. If so, it was a highly improbable one. I believe this incident is relatively more likely to have been a result of some form of extrasensory perception. Of course, extrasensory perception *always* seems unlikely, but in this case it seems relatively more likely than coincidence.

Thus it's possible that the power of prayer might in some way be related to extrasensory perceptual abilities. Maybe a person who is prayed for somehow *senses* another person's concern. If this were to happen, it's possible that the person who sensed another person's caring attitude would benefit psychologically, and would then transform this psychological boost into physical healing.

If you do not believe that a divine spirit answers prayers, perhaps you might believe that some prayers can be perceived through extrasensory perception.

I believe that the mystery of the power of prayer has an explanation that is simpler than this ESP interpretation, but far more profound. I believe that we all can "tune in" to the divine spirit, or God. And I believe that when we do, we can affect the realities of our lives.

Therefore, when I pray for my patients, I believe that I am actually helping them to connect with the divine spirit, and that I am evoking the loving, healing energy of God. As a physician, I feel that I *owe* my patients my prayers, just as much as I owe them my scientific expertise. I *care* about my patients. If doctors don't personally care about their patients, they may still be doctors, but I don't think they are truly healers.

I believe medical care should be just that: medical *care.*

And providing the services of science is only part of caring. The other part is to provide the power of prayer.

A Case in Point

Every Brain Longevity Program Is Unique

E.M., fifty-nine, came to me as an apparent victim of abuse, which had resulted in her sustaining serious head injuries. E.M., who came from the Middle East, told me that she had been treated very badly by her fiancé, who was an American medical professional. He had reportedly beaten her frequently, and one beating, she said, had culminated in his banging her head repeatedly into a wall. E.M. told me that her fiancé had knocked her unconscious, and had then taken her to a hospital emergency room.

E.M. came to me because she had a lifelong interest in complementary medicine, and had heard about my work at a conference she'd attended.

When she first consulted with me, E.M. suffered from extreme vertigo. She could not drive on busy streets or highways because of her dizziness, and was unable to do things that required proper balance and visual perception, such as walking across bridges. In addition, she experienced very frequent nausea. She also had significant cognitive dysfunction, including memory impairment and concentration difficulties.

Partly because of her injuries, she felt very insecure, and tended to be passive. It seemed to me that this psychological trait had probably, to some extent, predated her injuries, and had caused her to stay in the abusive relationship.

She began a complete brain longevity program. Like almost all of my patients, certain aspects of her program were formulated uniquely for her. One unusual element was her use of a homeopathic medication for vertigo. She also received medical acupuncture, which I do not administer to all my patients.

She responded almost immediately to the homeopathic vertigo medication. Like other medications, homeopathic remedies don't always work for everyone, but when they do work, they often elicit a response that's fast and dramatic.

She was overjoyed with her quick response, partly because she said her own physician had told her that her vertigo problems would take months or years to treat, and might never go away. His advice to her, she said, had been to let her healing occur "at its own pace."

The first week that she began taking the homeopathic medication, she was able to walk normally. Soon she was able to do a full range of exercises, including mind/body exercises, with no interference from her vertigo. Within about a month she was able to drive on the freeway.

I will always remember the day she came to a consultation after she had walked across a pedestrian bridge. On that day, a look lit her eyes that I can describe only as pure, unalloyed joy.

In less than six months, virtually all signs of her brain injuries were gone. Her memory was sharp, and it was easy for her to concentrate. She ran a small business, and was active from morning until night.

Furthermore, she gained a deep sense of self-confidence and personal strength from her journey through the healing process. Most encouraging of all, she eventually got emotionally strong enough to confront her fiancé— her *ex*-fiancé, that is. She told me that she met with him one final time—in a court of law, where she sued him. Now, *that's* healing in action.

16

Exercise and Brain Regeneration

A seventy-year-old woman named Mary drowsed in her hospital bed, lapsing in and out of a dim, twilight consciousness. Her mind, ravaged by Alzheimer's, was almost gone. She had virtually no remaining memory, or any vestige of an individualistic personality. But her doctors held out hope. They told Mary's husband that an experimental procedure might rescue her from the "living dead."

The physicians at the Karolinska Institute, in Stockholm, Sweden, believed that Mary might respond to a bold, new neurological treatment.

They drilled a tiny hole into her skull, and inserted a catheter directly into her brain. Into the catheter they slowly dripped a solution containing nerve growth factor.

Nerve growth factor stimulates neurons to grow new dendritic branches. Mary's doctors hoped that it might revive enough of her neurons to bring her mind back to life.

Mary had to lie in bed constantly to receive the treatment, but she was accustomed to inactivity, because for many years she had been very sedentary.

For three weeks the physicians bathed Mary's brain in the substance. But nothing happened.

One day, however, the doctors noticed that her expression had become more lucid. Gradually, Mary began to be more aware of her surroundings. The improvements gained momentum. She began to speak.

Then, on a day when her husband was in her room, she began to talk quietly to him about their life together. Her memories began flooding back. Her husband wept.

When the procedure was concluded, Mary retained some of the advances she had made. However, when the tube was removed, much of her cognitive improvement began to fade.

When I heard about this procedure, I was struck by two emotions. First, I was happy that her doctors had been so innovative and aggressive. In that kind of seemingly hopeless situation, it would have been easier to remain passive. But I also felt a twinge of frustration, because this patient had been inadvertently deprived of producing her own supply of nerve growth factor *throughout* her old age. She had been deprived of it simply by her own lack of knowledge: she had not known that *everyone* can produce nerve growth factor, every day.

How? Just by exercising.

Exercise has been proven repeatedly to produce abundant amounts of nerve growth factor. Because of this phenomenon, and because of other benefits of exercise, it is one of the "fountains of youth" that can keep your brain young, vital, and regenerative throughout your entire life.

Besides producing nerve growth factor, exercise protects and stimulates your brain in two other extremely important ways. Exercise greatly enhances neuronal metabolism, and it is also a powerful tool for stress reduction.

Because of its critically important benefits to the brain, exercise is one of the "four pillars" of my brain longevity programs (along with nutritional therapy, stress management, and pharmacology).

As I will demonstrate in this chapter, much of the cognitive decline that we commonly ascribe to aging actually results from our sedentary lifestyles.

Because many older people are sedentary, we tend to accept inactivity as a normal part of growing old. But, as with many other aspects of our modern lives, just because inactivity is common does *not* mean it's normal. Our bodies and brains have been programmed by evolution to require physical activity, and old people need this activity just as much as, or more than, young people.

In fact, regular exercise can help the brains of active old people to be sharper than the brains of sedentary young people. In one classic study of exercise and cognition, the mental acuity of a group of fifty-to-seventy-year-old men who played racquetball at least three times a week was tested against the mental acuity of a group of sedentary men in their twenties. The older, active men were not only more physically fit, but were also more "mentally fit," than the younger men. The older men performed better on tests of fluid intelligence.

Throughout history, it has been generally accepted that physical fitness benefits the mind. Plato said, in 400 B.C., that a healthy body was necessary for a healthy brain. Thomas Jefferson noted that "no less than two hours a day should be devoted to exercise." President Kennedy, in establishing physical goals for America's children, responded to Jefferson's view of exercise by stating, "If the man who wrote the Declaration of Independence, was Secretary of State, and twice President, could give it two hours, our children can give it ten or fifteen minutes."

What, specifically, does exercise do for the brain? As mentioned previously, it (1) supplies the brain with nerve growth factor, (2) reduces stress, and (3) enhances neuronal metabolism.

The most wide-reaching effects are those dealing with *neuronal metabolism*. Exercise increases the amount of oxygen and glucose the brain gets. It expedites the removal of necrotic debris from brain cells. It tones some neurotransmitter systems, increasing the output of such neurotransmitters as norepinephrine and dopamine. It increases the availability of brain-related enzymes, such as coenzyme Q-10. It increases output of some neuropeptides, including endorphins. It decreases low-density lipoprotein, which clogs brain circulation. It decreases cortisol output by placing a physical "governor" on the stress response. It decreases depression. It lowers blood pressure. And it helps stabilize blood sugar levels (thereby helping to stabilize mood and energy).

Exercise also improves endocrine function, boosting immunity and speeding up the metabolism. It also burns calories, increases muscle mass, and strengthens bones.

From a purely psychological perspective, exercise enhances body image and contributes to self-confidence.

Quite obviously, exercise is a godsend to the brain and body.

In addition, there are two types of exercise that are critically important to the brain: mental exercise and certain yogic mind/body exercises.

Very recent research has shown that getting mental exercise is as important to your brain as getting physical exercise. Mental exercise does far more than just increase your knowledge. It actually changes the brain *physically*. It increases the brain's size, and increases the number of dendritic connections among brain cells. The eminent brain researcher Dr. Arnold Scheibel has noted that mental exercise "sets off dendritic fireworks."

Specific yogic mind/body exercises are also tremendously beneficial to the physical health of the brain. They can literally help you to "build a better brain."

Chapter 17 will describe the benefits of mental exercise. Chapter 18 will discuss mind/body exercises. Right now, we'll take a look at the value of physical exercise. Let's start with the bad news: Currently, millions of Americans are not exercising enough.

And for that, many of them are paying a high price.

The Lamentable State of Exercise Today

The current perception that America is now a nation of fitness-obsessed joggers is notably false. It is a media-created fairy tale that serves only to salve our collective conscience and to sell hundred-dollar sneakers.

In reality, Americans are *less fit* now than they have been at any other time in the nation's history, just as Americans are—not coincidentally—fatter than they have ever been before. Currently, one-half of all Americans engage in *no* physical exercise at all on any given day.

Our modern lifestyle is simply not conducive to exercise. This current sad state of affairs is in stark contrast to former times. In chapter 11, I pointed out that the American diet deteriorated drastically at approximately the turn of the century, as an indirect result of increased industrialization. At that time, Americans began to be victims of their own economic success. The same phenomenon applies to physical activity. In 1900, about 40 percent of all Americans worked on farms, and human labor accounted for approximately 80 percent of all energy expended in farm production. During that same era, millions of people in cities worked vigorously in industrial jobs. The automobile was not yet in common use, and most domestic labor-saving devices did not yet exist.

Thus physical activity, in the early 1900s, was a natural and unavoidable aspect of life for most people. Most people were at least moderately active for five to ten hours each day.

If you ever reach a point where you're doing a daily two-hour workout, as Thomas Jefferson recommended, remember that the majority of your *very recent ancestors* did about a five-to-ten-hour workout almost every day of their lives, as a matter of course. They expended almost as much energy in their regular, daily jobs and chores as you would if you walked a twenty-six-mile marathon every day.

By the 1920s, however, the shift toward industrialization had begun to decrease radically the level of physical activity in this country, and in other Western countries. Also in the 1920s, the American cardiovascular disease "epidemic" began. By the 1960s, physical activity had declined markedly, and since then it has declined further.

Unfortunately, it's not just adults today who don't get enough exercise. Only thirty percent of all children from first grade through high school get even thirty minutes of exercise daily at school. Exercise among teenagers declined by 10 percent in the last ten years alone. Partly because of this, 40 percent of children as young as five years of age already have at least one risk factor for cardiovascular disease (such as obesity or high blood pressure).

Some of the blame for this inactivity belongs not just to shifts in work patterns, but also to shifts in recreational habits. People are far less active these days during their leisure time, mostly because so much leisure time is spent watching television. The average American, including the average American child, watches up to eight hours of television per day. This astronomical amount of television watching naturally decreases physical activity. As you can see, too many people today are physically sedentary.

If you are currently too sedentary yourself, you may be surprised to know how much your brain and body can be helped by just a little physical activity.

Let's take a look at what happens when you get off the couch and start moving.

Exercise "Lights Up" the Brain

For many years the neurological effects of exercise were largely ignored by the scientific community. Like other lifestyle elements, such as nutrition or stress management, exercise just wasn't "sexy" enough to capture the attention of a broad section of the neurological research community. Like researchers in other medical areas, neurological researchers have long been primarily preoccupied with discovering the pharmacologic "magic bullet" that will solve problems like Alzheimer's, Parkinson's disease, and stroke. During the past ten years, though, this attitude has begun to change. Recently, several researchers revealed stunning evidence that powerfully supports the efficacy of exercise in achieving and maintaining optimal mental function.

For example, one study showed that vigorous exercise can make young, intelligent people even smarter than they already are. A group of cross-country runners was tested for cognitive ability during their off season, and were then tested again at the end of the season, during which they had run at least thirty miles per week. They tested significantly higher at the end of the season.

In an experiment with young, healthy monkeys, one group of monkeys was kept sedentary, while another group was given a running wheel, and another group was given an intricate series of ropes and bridges to play on. Both groups that exercised showed heightened cognitive abilities; they grew more capillaries to their neurons, and these capillaries delivered more oxygen and nutrients to the monkeys' brain cells.

However, the monkeys with the complex play structures grew the largest number of dendritic connections. This indicates that exercise is most valuable when it is combined with thinking.

Many studies show that exercise is particularly effective at improving memory. One study compared the memories of a group of elderly people who were put on a walking program with the memories of a group of sedentary elderly people. Over a period of several weeks, the group that exercised showed significant improvement in memory skills, while the sedentary group remained the same.

Studies and experiments indicate that an exercise program does not have to be long-term to yield dramatic cognitive benefits. One study showed the thirty-two subjects improved significantly in fluid intelligence, learning ability, and mood from just a ten-week program. In another study, a group of patients with an average age of sixty years walked or jogged six to ten miles per day, for only twenty-six days. At the end of that period, their average test scores were markedly higher on measures of verbal fluency, concentration, and abstract reasoning.

Studies also show that exercise does not have to be very strenuous to yield positive results. Many of the most prominent researchers believe that only about thirty minutes of brisk walking per day is enough to produce satisfactory cognitive results. Many of my patients do even less than this, and still report subjective perception of cognitive improvement.

I've already mentioned briefly why exercise is so helpful to the brain, but now let's dig a little more deeply into the subject. I believe that if you fully understand why exercise is such a powerful stimulator of brain power, you will be even more motivated to do it. If you're already exercising regularly, the following short section will help you to appreciate just how much good you are doing for yourself.

How Exercise Increases Brain Power

As mentioned previously, exercise achieves three primary benefits for the brain: (1) it stimulates production of nerve growth factor; (2) it is a powerful tool for stress management; and (3) it enhances neuronal metabolism.

Let's take a quick look at each of those three benefits.

Nerve growth factor. A virtual wonder drug for the brain, nerve growth factor, or NGF, is similar to a brain hormone that also stimulates regeneration of the brain: *brain-derived neurotrophic factor,* or BDNF. NGF and BDNF are both produced most abundantly when the body is physically active. In all likelihood, these important brain chemicals were created by the evolutionary process to support the brain as it withstood physical challenges.

Of prime importance to brain longevity patients is the fact that the greatest effects of exercise on both NGF and BDNF are in the most plastic areas of the brain, including the hippocampus (the brain's primary memory center). This regional concentration accounts for much of the improvement in memory experienced by patients who begin to exercise. NGF and BDNF, however, also support neurons *throughout* the brain, in the following ways:

• They transport BDNF to the forebrain cholinergic neurons, a major site of degeneration in Alzheimer's disease, and in age-associated memory impairment.

• They "rescue" damaged neurons from imminent death.

• They increase the production of the important neurotransmitters acetylcholine and dopamine, and increase the number of dopamine receptors.

• They increase the activity of neuronal free-radical scavengers (thereby protecting brain cells).

Unfortunately, stress decreases BDNF, because stress-produced cortisol destroys BDNF. Exercise can help to *restore* the BDNF that cortisol destroys, however. Exercise also helps reduce chronic cortisol oversecretion.

NGF has shown the ability in animal experiments to increase animals' intelligence significantly. In one experiment, one group of rats was injected with nerve growth factor, and another group was not. Then both groups were tested in a "Morris maze," a tank filled with murky water that contains a platform the rats cannot see. Eventually, all the rats found the platform. Then the two groups were tested again. The group that had received NGF remembered where the platform was. The other group did not.

When I tell some patients about NGF, their first question is, "Where can I *buy* some?" These patients are missing the point. If your own body can manufacture this substance in abundance, without producing any side effects, it is ludicrous to seek an artificial source.

Besides, when you exercise, you do a great deal more for your brain and body than just produce NGF and BDNF. One of the other things you achieve is the enhancement neuronal metabolism.

Enhancing neuronal metabolism. This means improving the total energy exchange between your brain cells and the outside environment. This energy exchange includes the exchange of oxygen, nutrients, and cellular waste debris. These three aspects of neuronal metabolism are improved considerably by exercise, primarily because exercise improves blood circulation to the brain.

Improving your brain's blood circulation is one of the best things you can do for your cognitive power. Again, "what's good for the heart is good for the head." Even though your brain makes up only about 2 percent of your body's total weight, it uses about 25 percent of your total blood supply. In children, the brain sometimes uses up to 50 percent of the total blood supply.

Exercise is inarguably effective at improving circulation. It does so by increasing the strength of the heart, lowering blood pressure, contributing to the elasticity of blood vessels, and reducing levels of low-density lipoprotein and cholesterol.

Innumerable studies have proved that exercise greatly improves the cardiovascular system. For example, one recent, large study indicated that men who exercised were 32 percent less likely to die of heart disease than men who were sedentary, even if the men who exercised ate a poor diet and smoked cigarettes. Another study showed that a sedentary lifestyle increased the risk of stroke by 400 percent. This increased risk of stroke is particularly ominous for brain longevity patients, because multiple minor strokes represent the second most common cause of dementia in elderly people. Only Alzheimer's causes a greater number of cases of dementia. In addition, elderly people sometimes suffer from *simultaneous* Alzheimer's and multiple minor strokes. When this happens, the symptoms of each condition exacerbate those of the other.

Another crucially important cardiovascular benefit of exercise is that it increases your body's ability to absorb oxygen efficiently. Your ability to inhale oxygen, and then to transport it throughout your body (via your bloodstream) is called your VO_2 *max*. In general, a sedentary person's VO_2 max reaches its peak during his or her teen years, then begins to decline at about 1 percent per year. If you exercise regularly, however, your VO_2 max will decline much more slowly. Further, if you have been sedentary, but then begin to exercise, it is possible to improve your VO_2 max by the equivalent of about fifteen to forty calendar years.

If you improve your VO_2 max, it will almost certainly increase your cognitive function. In one recent study, a group of sedentary people, aged fifty to seventy, engaged in a four-month exercise program. During that time, their VO_2 max figures increased, and so did their scores on cognitive function tests. They showed particular improvement in cognitive processing speed, and in ability to focus.

Reducing stress. This is the third major way that exercise helps improve cognitive function. To find out how much exercise might help you to deal with stress, take the quiz below.

This quiz can help you determine if you tend to have primarily physical reactions to stress, or primarily psychological reactions. If you are mostly a *physical reactor*, stress will tend to affect primarily your body, and you will tend to cope with it through physical responses, such as pacing. If you are mostly a *psychological reactor*, stress will tend to affect primarily your mind, and you will tend to cope with it with mental responses, such as denial or rationalization.

If you *are* mostly a physical reactor, exercise will be particularly valuable for you as a coping mechanism, because it will help you to let go of the physical tensions that stress can create.

YOUR COPING STYLE

When I encounter stress, the following often occurs
(mark the applicable traits):

1. _____ I get "butterflies" in my stomach.
2. _____ I find it hard to concentrate.
3. _____ My pulse rate increases.
4. _____ I start to worry about things I can't control.
5. _____ I feel as if there's not enough time to solve my problems.
6. _____ I feel warm, and frequently begin to sweat.
7. _____ I get a burst of energy, but soon feel hungry and weak.
8. _____ My mind races with thoughts.
9. _____ I get depressed.
10. _____ I develop intestinal problems, such as diarrhea.
11. _____ I have trouble sleeping.
12. _____ I get mental images of the worst things that could happen.
13. _____ My feet get cold.
14. _____ My sex drive declines.
15. _____ I talk to myself about my options.
16. _____ My body feels almost "paralyzed."
17. _____ I escape mentally, by focusing on happy thoughts.
18. _____ I relieve tension with pacing, jiggling my leg, or engaging in some other "nervous habit."
19. _____ I become coldly logical.
20. _____ My hands tremble, and I feel shaky.

The questions in the quiz that reveal primarily *physical* reactions to stress are numbers 1, 3, 6, 7, 10, 11, 13, 14, 16, 18, and 20. If you marked more than five of those eleven questions, you have a relatively strong tendency to be a *physical reactor.*

Even if you are mostly a psychological reactor, however, you can still benefit by using exercise for stress release. In fact, many people are primarily psychological reactors specifically *because* they exercise regularly, because *exercise decreases the physical stress response.* The more fit you are, the less you will tend to have a strong physical reaction to stressors. Cardiovascular fitness puts a natural "governor" on the stress response. When you have a low resting heart rate, as a result of exercise, it prevents your adrenal glands from overreacting to stressors, and oversecreting cortisol.

For example, in one study, a physically fit subject had a resting heart rate of sixty-five beats per minute, and his heart rate increased to only sixty-seven beats per minute when he was subjected to a stressor. However, a sedentary subject, with a resting heart rate of seventy-five beats per minute, showed an increase to ninety-five beats per minute when subjected to a stressor.

Many of my patients who are *not* physically fit exhibit relatively more signs of a heightened stress response. I often notice this when I do their intake testing. The intake testing of all my patients is naturally stressful for them, because they are worried about the results. More physically fit patients, though, often show fewer signs than sedentary patients of the stress response. The sedentary patients are more prone to become flushed, to perspire, to breathe shallowly, and to fidget nervously.

Few of my patients, though, are notably fit. For the most part they are well-educated, older people who have put a great deal of energy into their careers, but not enough energy into their fitness programs. Ironically, if they had remained more fit, they might well have been even more successful in their careers. At the very least, these people might have avoided hitting a midlife, career-stunting "wall" of cognitive impairment.

Exercise does more for the psyche, though, than just put a governor on the stress response. It also markedly enhances mood, creating a feeling of tranquillity. This well-documented "tranquilizer effect" lasts long after the exercise period ends. Most studies show that exercise's tranquilizer effect lasts about four hours. Remnants of the tranquilizer effect may remain for up to twenty-four hours.

To achieve the tranquilizer effect, you must do neither too much exercise nor too little. In one study of joggers, those who jogged twenty-four miles per week, or about thirty to forty-five minutes per day, experienced the greatest degree of the tranquilizer effect. Those who jogged significantly less (fifteen miles per week), or significantly more (fifty-two miles per week), experienced less of the tranquilizer effect.

One of the primary reasons the tranquilizer effect occurs is that exercise releases endorphins. These "feel good" neuropeptides—the body's own opiates—begin to be produced in abundant quantities after about fifteen to thirty minutes of exercise. After they are secreted, they remain active for about five hours—approximately the same length of time that the tranquilizer effect lasts.

Endorphins, which are about two hundred times more potent than morphine, increase approximately five hundred percent during relatively vigorous exercise. They are at their highest levels during the first thirty minutes after an exercise period.

Exercise is also extraordinarily effective at reducing depression. Numerous studies have shown that for most forms of relatively mild depression, exercise is as valuable a treatment as traditional psychotherapy. This does not, of course, negate the value of psychotherapy, but underscores the importance of exercise.

In one classic study, depression patients were placed in three groups. One group was given psychotherapy for a limited number of weeks. Another group was given psychotherapy for as many weeks as the patients desired. A third group received no psychotherapy, but participated in a jogging program. At the end of the experiment, the patients in the jogging program had the lowest incidence of depression, while those in the unlimited psychotherapy program had the highest incidence.

In another study, depression patients jogged either five days a week, three days a week, or not at all. Those who jogged five days a week had significantly less depression at the end of the ten-week study. Those who jogged three days a week fared almost as well. Those who did not jog at all did not improve.

Exercise reduces depression for a number of reasons: It releases stimulating catecholamine neurotransmitters; it stimulates endorphin production; it increases oxygen flow to the brain, and helps remove neuronal debris; it stimulates the nervous system; it provides a powerful boost to self-esteem; it improves body image; and it increases feelings of personal power.

Finally, as mentioned in chapter 14, exercising is an excellent way to "burn off" stress that has already been internalized. Physical activity is often as good a release for stress as verbal release activities, such as talking or crying. One study of exercise and anxiety showed that even fifteen minutes of exercise decreased anxiety.

Many of my patients love to exercise at the end of a stressful day. They say it brings them "back to earth."

Exercise even appears to be effective at combating phobias. Studies have shown that psychotherapy programs for such problems as claustrophobia and fear of flying are more effective when exercise is added as a component of therapy.

Exercise, of course, is every bit as beneficial for the body as it is for the brain. It encourages health, longevity, and immunity, and thus adds considerably to quality of life.

Exercise and Quality of Life

When I began working with Alzheimer's patients, I quickly discovered what their most common fear is. It is not fear of death, or the fear of the death of a spouse, or the fear of running out of money. What scares them most is *loss of personal independence*. They want to be able to take care of themselves physically. This independence, however, is often terribly compromised by illness, and by loss of physical function. But exercise can help prevent illness and loss of physical function.

As a rule, the general physical health of my patients improves considerably when they begin their brain longevity programs, and I am certain that exercise contributes to this improvement.

Exercise increases your immunity to disease by boosting your immune system's number of "natural killer" cells, and by increasing your production of immunoglobin-A, an antibody that is one of your first lines of defense against infection. It also boosts immunity to disease by lowering stress.

Many studies show that exercise decreases incidence of illness. One such study revealed that people who exercised missed 18 percent fewer workdays than sedentary people, and required 12 percent less hospital outpatient care and 30 percent less hospital inpatient care.

A study of ten thousand Harvard graduates, aged forty-five to eighty-four, showed that those who exercised had a 29-percent lower death rate than those who did not. Another study, of people over age sixty, found that those who exercised were 44 percent less likely than their sedentary peers to die during a given five-year period.

Exercise also powerfully promotes longevity, because it helps prevent the diseases that kill 75 percent of all Americans: cardiovascular disease (which kills about half of all Americans) and cancer (which kills about one-fourth of all Americans). As mentioned previously, being physically fit reduces your chance of heart disease by over 30 percent, and reduces your chance of having a stroke by about 400 percent. Also, studies indicate that exercise reduces the incidence of one of the most common deadly forms of cancer, colon cancer, by about two-thirds. It also reduces incidence of breast cancer by 200 percent, and of cancers of the reproductive system by 250 percent.

The benefits of exercise are so far-reaching that they even extend to organs that we do not usually associate with physical fitness, such as the eyes. Exercise significantly reduces pressure against the eyeball, which causes glaucoma and frequently leads to blindness. Exercise even optimizes the eyesight of people with no vision problems. A study of regular exercisers with 20/20 vision revealed that they had visual skills that were far superior to those of sedentary people who also had 20/20 vision.

Clearly, exercise is absolutely vital to physical fitness and cognitive fitness. But how much exercise do you need? And how should you get it? Let's take a look at the "nuts and bolts" of a physical training regime.

How to Exercise for Optimal Cognitive Function

When I first told W.R., a seventy-three-year-old female patient, that she should start exercising, she flatly refused. She said, "You mean go to a health club and dance around in a swimming suit? I'd rather be senile."

I quickly told her that all she needed to do was take a walk every day, or every other day. But even that sounded hard. She had mild coronary heart disease, with occasional chest pains and heart palpitations, and she had been sedentary for about twenty years. She feared that exercise would give her a heart attack.

I told her, however, that her inactivity had almost certainly contributed to her heart problem, and that if she exercised wisely, she could use exercise to help her recover from her heart disease.

I also told her that exercise would probably help alleviate the age-associated memory impairment that had prompted her visit to me. W.R. had poor short-term memory, and had difficulty concentrating. She frequently struggled to remember words, and often forgot details.

At the same time that she began the other elements of her program, she also began taking a daily walk around her block. At first it was hard for her to complete the walk; she had to rest on a bus bench halfway around the block. When she returned home, she told me, her face would be flushed, and she would be breathing deeply.

I told her that the flushing of her face was a good, healthy sign. It meant more blood was pumping to her brain. Hearing that encouraged her.

Within a few weeks, she began to enjoy the feeling of exertion. She realized that a short walk would not kill her, and was beginning to notice positive effects from the exercise. She fell asleep at night more easily, and her appetite was better. She also reported that the daily walk improved her mood. She said that her "constitutional," as she called it, made her feel "more awake, but more relaxed."

Gradually her walk increased in length. She began walking around not just her own block but also the adjacent block, and then she began to take longer walks through her neighborhood, stopping to rest if she became tired. Once in a while she would walk a little too far from her house, and would call a taxi to bring her home. She enjoyed it when this happened; it gave her a feeling of freedom and independence.

In less than a year her heart problem was vastly improved. She no longer had chest pains. In addition, her cognitive ability had improved considerably. She rarely forgot words or details. She was much more animated, and was better able to concentrate.

Even after W.R. became moderately fit, she rarely took a walk that was longer than about thirty minutes. But that seemed to be enough exercise for her, especially when it was combined with the other elements of her program.

Many of my patients never do more than about a thirty-minute walk, and it seems to be sufficient. From my observations of my own patients, and from the studies I have read, I have come to believe that it is acceptable to be only moderately fit. Achieving a relatively high level of fitness can help people to achieve optimal mental function, and moderate fitness seems to be enough to keep the brain and body healthy.

Dr. Dean Ornish, one of the most influential cardiologists of this era, has found that walking thirty minutes per day reduces mortality from cardiovascular disease almost as much as running thirty to forty miles per week. This was indicated in a well-known study that Dr. Ornish often cites. In this study, about thirteen thousand people were assigned to five different groups, according to their fitness levels. After eight years, the fittest group (which ran thirty to forty miles weekly) had a death rate approximately 300 percent lower than the least fit group (which was sedentary). However, the group that was *next-to-last* in fitness had a death rate almost as low as the most fit group. The only exercise of the group that was next-to-last in fitness was walking thirty minutes per day.

Thus, according to this study and others like it, a person's primary goal should be simply to become moderately fit.

A moderate level of fitness is not only adequate for proper neurological function, but might even be healthier, for some people, than an extremely high level of fitness. There is some evidence that people who engage in strenuous exercise over long periods actually damage their bodies. This damage, theoretically, comes from the assault of free radicals, which can be produced by strenuous exercise.

If one of my patients already engages in a form of exercise that he or she enjoys, I encourage him or her to do it for about thirty minutes daily. The most common exercise activity among my patients is just to walk about fifteen minutes away from home, then turn around and walk home. Some of my patients walk in shopping malls when the weather is bad, some ride exercise bikes, and some work out on stair-step machines. Others swim, or play tennis or golf. One patient of mine walks her three dogs every morning, one after the other. This provides her with fun, good exercise, and fresh air.

Some of my more frail Alzheimer's patients can't really get out for a walk, so they walk around their own homes and yards.

It's very important that you find a form of exercise that you *enjoy*. Exercise should be as playful as possible. If you don't enjoy it, you will be much less likely to do it regularly. Also, if it's not fun, it will not release stress as effectively. If possible, find a game or sport that you enjoy, and make that the focus of your program, even if you can't do it as often as you'd like. For example, if you love tennis, but can only play about once a week, you can motivate yourself throughout the week by "training" for your upcoming game.

Don't hesitate to set fitness goals for yourself, even if those goals fall far short of what you could have accomplished ten or twenty years ago. You're not in competition with your "younger self," and the beauty of sports goals is that the goals themselves don't really matter—they're just a good way to motivate yourself, and to keep track of your progress.

One thing that does matter is that you achieve the "training effect" during your exercise. The training effect is the temporary stress on your cardiovascular system that makes your heart beat faster, and speeds up your metabolism. You can use one of the following formulas to tell you when you have achieved the training effect:

• Determine your maximum pulse rate—your heartbeat during extreme exertion—and then multiply it by 60 percent. When you hit this pulse rate, you have achieved the training effect. (If your maximum pulse rate is 150 beats per minute, multiply 150 by 60 percent; your training-effect pulse rate would be 90 beats per minute.)

• Subtract your age from 220, and then multiply by 70 percent. (If your age is 50, subtract 50 from 220, which is 170. Then multiply 170 by 70 percent; your training-effect pulse rate is 119.)

• Multiply your *resting* pulse rate by 150 percent. (If your resting pulse rate is 74, multiply 74 by 150 percent; your training-effect pulse rate is 111.)

To maintain the training effect, you must do your exercise *continuously*. If you stop frequently, you will be much less likely to achieve the training effect.

If one of your goals is to lose weight, you should definitely try to achieve the training effect. If you fall short of it, you will not stimulate your metabolism, or burn many calories. If you exceed it, your body will stop converting fat into energy. Thus it's better to jog than to sprint. Sprinting will build muscles and strengthen your heart, but it's not an effective weight-loss strategy.

If losing weight is one of your primary exercise goals, don't be discouraged if your weight loss is gradual. If you jog or walk briskly for one mile, you will burn only 100 calories; therefore, a week of three-mile jogs burns only about 2,100 calories. However, it takes about 3,500 calories to burn one pound of fat. Thus, every week you might lose only about two-thirds of a pound of fat.

Bariatric physicians, though, who specialize in weight control, generally consider half a pound to one pound per week to be a good, safe rate of weight loss. If you do lose weight at this rate, you will lose about thirty-five pounds in a year.

You may lose weight at a somewhat faster rate than this, though, because exercise does more than just burn calories. It also increases your rate of metabolism, and this increase endures for several hours after you finish exercising. In addition, exercise builds muscle, and muscle burns calories more efficiently than fat does.

For my brain longevity patients, I recommend aerobic exercise—the type that taxes the heart and lungs, and creates a sustained, elevated pulse rate. A useful adjunct to aerobic exercise, however, is anaerobic exercise, which exerts the muscles, but does not create sustained, elevated pulse rate. The most common form of anaerobic exercise is weight training.

The renowned medical philosopher Deepak Chopra, M.D., has noted that weight training can benefit even the frail and elderly. According to Dr. Chopra, a group of eighty-seven-to-ninety-six-year-old patients, some of whom were not even ambulatory, benefited greatly from a weight-training program. Within eight weeks their average muscle mass increased by 300 percent, their balance and coordination improved, and some of the nonambulatory patients regained their ability to walk.

Even if you are already in relatively good physical condition, you will probably gain substantial benefit from a program of weight training. If you do a moderate weight-training program every two to three days for about ten weeks, you should be able to increase the amount of weight you can comfortably lift by about 150 percent.

As your strength and fitness levels begin to rise, though, it's important not to become too enamored of your improving body image. Remember that your goal is to achieve brain longevity—*not* to be an action movie hero. It's easy to get hung up on body image, though, since we are constantly bombarded by the media with visions of flawless, powerful bodies.

Cameron Stauth once had occasion to lift weights with a famous movie star at a gym in Venice Beach, California. What particularly struck Cameron about the experience was that the star was in superb condition—but he did not appear to be exploding with muscle, as he sometimes is when he gets "pumped up" with weight work to shoot a scene in an action movie. Onscreen, as a larger-than-life icon, he is no longer just himself; he's ACTION MOVIE HERO.

Moral of the story: Not even a movie star is always ACTION MOVIE HERO.

As you can see, physical exercise is a vital ingredient to a brain longevity program. But, as noted, there are two other kinds of exercise that are just as important, and I'll tell you about them in the next two chapters.

One is mental exercise, which is so powerful that it can physically change your brain. The other is mind/body exercise. For the past five thousand years, people have been using simple but potent mind/body exercises to achieve heightened cognitive power. In my opinion, these mind/body exercises are the "gold standard" of cognition-enhancing activities. They will help you to tap mental powers that you didn't even know you had.

A Case in Point

Beware of the Cognitive Side Effects of Medications

M.C., seventy-two years old, was a patient whom I was essentially unable to help, because her condition had deteriorated severely before I heard about her. I will tell you what happened to her, however, so that you can possibly keep it from happening to someone you love.

A late-stage emphysema patient, M.C. had been placed on the steroidal hormone prednisone by her doctor. Administration of steroidal hormones to emphysema patients is a valid therapy. But long-term use of steroids can cause damage to the brain similar to that which the stress hormone cortisol causes.

Prednisone was administered to M.C. in high dosages over several months, and apparently triggered the sudden onset of cognitive decline.

She went through several stages of cognitive decline. Her mental deterioration was similar to that of patients who suffer from chronically high levels of cortisol, but she went through these stages very quickly. In effect, she went through the various stages of hormone-related cognitive decline in "fast forward."

Long-term administration of a steroidal hormone such as prednisone has been reported to cause dementia, and M.C. had evidently suffered a grossly accelerated version of the "chronic stress effect."

When M.C. initially took the hormone, it had a positive effect. Prednisone generally decreases inflammation in the bronchial tubes, and this helps prevent the bronchial tubes from going into spasm. Bronchospasm— which is much like an asthma attack—is common among emphysema patients, and it can result in death.

The prednisone also initially improved M.C.'s quality of life. It gave her more energy, and improved her mood.

After several months, however, the steroid began to harm M.C.'s cognitive function. Her short-term memory became impaired, and her cognitive processing skills diminished. She would sometimes become suspicious and distrustful, and she experienced mood swings.

Over the next six to eight weeks, her condition deteriorated rapidly. During the first few weeks of her quick decline, she battled bravely against the fog of dementia that was enveloping her. She tried to follow current events on television, tried to keep reading, and tried to keep having meaningful conversations with her caregivers and family. She focused hard on what people told her, and took careful notes about things she considered important.

But the prednisone was quickly destroying her brain. She began to become delusional, believing that things happening on television were happening to her. Sometimes she would forget that she was bedridden, and would try to climb out of her bed. Once when she did this, she injured herself.

Her caregivers were gentle and tolerant, as are most of the thousands of women and men whose profession is to help take care of Alzheimer's patients and other chronically ill patients. But neither her caregivers nor her family could protect her from the pain of losing her emotional stability and her intellectual acumen. She often felt humiliated, afraid, and angry. She feared dementia even more than she feared death.

Her sons became very concerned about her deteriorating mental condition, so they consulted her doctor about it. According to one of her sons, the doctor told them that her mental deterioration was a result of hypoxia, or lack of oxygen to the brain.

Her sons, however, also consulted with an expert on emphysema and were informed that the degree of hypoxia that M.C. was experiencing would *not* cause such pronounced mental symptoms.

At that point, one of M.C.'s sons, whom I knew professionally, contacted me. I advised him to ask the doctor to withdraw M.C. gradually from the prednisone. The doctor agreed to discontinue the steroid. Unfortunately, though, the damage to M.C.'s brain had already been done.

Her mental symptoms improved somewhat as she was weaned from the drug. But she remained in a mental fog until she died. Sometimes she was coherent, and sometimes she was delusional.

The decline of M.C.'s cognitive function at the end of her life was a tragedy that could possibly have been avoided.

If someone you care about is taking a powerful pharmaceutical medication, I advise you to become familiar with all of the potential cognitive side effects of that medication. If our current medical system were perfect, your vigilance would not be necessary. But the system is not perfect, and we are *all* responsible—patients as well as doctors—for making the system as efficient as possible.

When M.C.'s son last spoke to me, he said, "When Mom's mind started to go, it was like we lost her even before we lost her. It was one of the worst things that could have happened."

The moral: *Be careful* with medication. It can heal—but it can also harm.

17

How Thinking Enlarges and Regenerates the Brain

In a recent conversation I had with Dr. Marian Diamond, the prominent and esteemed brain researcher, she made a remark that I considered profoundly astute: "The brain decides its own destiny."

By this, she meant that the more we choose to *use* our brains, the better our brains will function throughout our lives.

Dr. Diamond, who is in the forefront of research on the physical results of thinking, has proved that the more we think—regardless of our age—the bigger our brains become, and the better they function.

Dr. Diamond once commented upon the ability of brains to keep growing throughout life, when she wrote, "The nervous system possesses not just a 'morning' of plasticity, but an 'afternoon' and an 'evening' as well. Dr. Diamond believes that a healthy older brain—one supported by a healthy lifestyle, and by ongoing mental activity—can function virtually as well as a healthy *young* brain.

Of course, as you know by now, keeping your brain healthy

throughout midlife and beyond is easier said than done. *But this can be achieved.* That point has been proven by my many successful brain longevity patients.

To achieve brain regeneration, though, my brain longevity patients have found that they must do more than just keep their brains healthy with nutritional therapy, physical exercise, stress management, and appropriate pharmacology. They also must carefully nurture their brains with vigorous *mental exercise.*

In this chapter I'm going to tell you how to use mental activity to help achieve brain longevity.

Before I go into the how-to aspects, though, I would like to tell you why mental activity is so important. I never just tell my patients *what* they should do; I also tell them *why* they should do it—and you deserve the same courtesy.

The Secret of Einstein's Brain

In the mid-1980s, Dr. Diamond, former head of the prestigious Lawrence Hall of Science at UC Berkeley, was chosen to dissect and study the brain of Albert Einstein. The neurological community hoped that Dr. Diamond could answer an old and puzzling question: Are the brains of geniuses physically different from those of average people?

To help answer this question, Dr. Diamond used a clue that Einstein himself had left. Einstein once remarked that when he was deep in thought, words played no part in his mental deliberations. Instead, he said, his thoughts were a combination of "certain signs and more or less clear images." In other words, his most productive thoughts were primarily a result of deeply abstract, visually related cognitive function.

Therefore, Dr. Diamond decided to examine carefully the areas of Einstein's brain that were most intricately involved with imagery and abstract reasoning: the superior prefrontal and inferior parietal lobes.

As Dr. Diamond studied Einstein's brain, she compared it against a control base of eleven other human brains, harvested from intellectually average men who had died at approximately the same age as Einstein, i.e., seventy-six.

What Dr. Diamond discovered was that there was no discernible physical difference between Einstein's brain and the other brains—with one notable and exciting exception.

That exception was that Einstein had significantly more of a certain type of cell in one special area of his brain. That area was Area 39, which is located in the inferior parietal lobe (a part of the neocortex located in the upper, rear part of the brain).

It was very revealing to Dr. Diamond that Einstein had an enhanced Area 39, because she and other researchers believe Area 39 is the most highly evolved site in the brain. When people have lesions in Area 39, they have great difficulty with abstract imagery, memory, attention, and self-awareness. They are largely unable to read, recognize letters, spell, or do calculations. They also have much difficulty integrating visual, auditory, and tactile input. In short, if Area 39 is damaged, a person loses most of his or her higher intellect.

The special type of *cell* that was in abundance in Area 39 of Einstein's brain was the *glial cell.* To Dr. Diamond, this was extremely significant.

Glial cells are very common in the brain, but they are, in effect, "housekeeping" cells, and not "thinking" cells. Their job is to *support the metabolism* of the "thinking" neurons.

Einstein had only a measurable excess of "housekeeping" cells, and *not* a measurable excess of "thinking" cells. To Dr. Diamond, this meant Einstein's "thinking" cells in Area 39 needed a great deal of *metabolic support.* Why would they need so much support? Because they were doing a tremendous amount of work: a lot of *hard thinking.*

This abundance of glial cells had significantly *enlarged* Einstein's Area 39.

It appeared as if Einstein had probably been born with an excellent brain, rich in fluid intelligence. Fluid intelligence, as you'll recall, is the measure of how *efficiently* the brain works, rather than how many facts are stored in it. It was apparently *not* just Einstein's God-given fluid intelligence, however, that had made him a genius. His genius was probably more a result of what he had *done* with his brain. He had enlarged the most important part of his brain by *mentally exercising* it to the maximum possible degree. In effect, Einstein was a "mental athlete" who had "trained hard" all his life.

If it was true that thinking had actually enlarged Einstein's Area 39, Dr. Diamond reasoned, the same phenomenon should apply to animals. To test this theory, Dr. Diamond built two very different cages for rats. One was just a small bare box, in which Dr. Diamond placed one female rat and her three offspring. The other was large, and filled with interesting, thought-provoking "toys." In the large, "enriched environment" cage, Dr. Diamond placed three female rats, with three offspring each.

At death, the brains of all the rats were examined. In the rats that had lived in the interesting, thought-provoking environment, Area 39 was 16 percent larger than in the other rats—owing to an increased abundance of glial cells. In addition, other areas of their brains had *also* increased in size, by about 10 percent.

Then Dr. Diamond did the same experiment with "elderly" rats. Again, the challenging, enriched environment enlarged their brains. It particularly enlarged each rat's Area 39.

In a related experiment, Dr. Diamond deprived pregnant rats of protein. When their offspring were born, they had signs of mental deficiency. Dr. Diamond then rehabilitated one group of offspring with nutritional therapy, and another group with nutritional therapy plus an enriched environment. She found that the group with the enriched environment developed larger brains than the other group. Thus it appears as if intellectual enrichment can actually compensate for some forms of physical damage.

Dr. Diamond even discovered that the brains of rats could actually shrink if the rats were deprived of thought-provoking toys and enriched environments. When a group of rats was raised in a mentally impoverished environment, one part of their cortex (the dorsal cortex) shrank by 9 percent. Also, a part of the rats' brains that was closely associated with memory (the entohorinal cortex) shrank by 25 percent. From this experiment, researchers inferred that age-associated memory impairment in humans could be partly caused by lack of intellectual stimulation.

Another fascinating finding of Dr. Diamond's was that the rats' more mature, highly developed neurons responded even better to intellectual enrichment than less-developed neurons. As you probably remember, neurons gradually develop throughout life by reaching out to other neurons with branchlike dendrites. As you learn new information, your dendrites keep sending out new branches. Then each new branch sends out other branches. Dr. Diamond found that the *first* dendritic branch off a neuron did not grow any longer as a result of mental enrichment. Nor did the second branch, or the third, fourth, or fifth. The *sixth* branch, however, clearly increased in length in response to mental enrichment. This finding reinforced Dr. Diamond's belief that it's never too late in life to learn. Learning, it appears, is most valuable for older people, who tend to have relatively more six-branch dendrites than young people.

In fact, Dr. Diamond has written, "Whether we are young or old, we can continue to learn. The brain can change at any age. We began with a nerve cell, which starts in the embryo as just a sort of sphere. It sends its first branch out to overcome ignorance. As it reaches out, it is gathering knowledge and it is becoming creative. Then we become a little more idealistic, generous, and altruistic; but it is our six-sided dendrites which give us wisdom."

Dr. Diamond also made another important discovery: She found that it was not just the "thinking" neocortex that physically responded to environmental enrichment, but also the "feeling" limbic system.

To stimulate the development of her research animals' limbic systems, Dr. Diamond provided the animals with emotional enrichment—that is, tender loving care. Dr. Diamond found that when she lavished attention upon her experimental animals, they showed physical signs of improved function of their limbic systems.

Therefore, according to these animal experiments, mental enrichment can endow us with a greater physical capacity for intellectual intelligence, and emotional enrichment can endow us with a greater physical capacity for "emotional intelligence." And *this* type of intelligence, as Daniel Goleman indicated so eloquently in his excellent book *Emotional Intelligence*, is often even more important than intellectual intelligence.

But do all the findings that apply to animals also apply to humans? Apparently they do.

Dr. Diamond's basic premise—that mental enrichment increases fluid intelligence at any age—has been proved in large-scale, long-term human studies. The most convincing of these was a thirty-year study headed by the highly respected researcher Dr. K. Warner Schaie.

In 1956, at the beginning of his career, Dr. Schaie began to track the mental development of a large group of people in the Seattle area. By the mid-1980s, many of the people in his study had hit the "memory barrier" of their fifties and sixties, and showed symptoms of mental decline. In particular, they suffered from steep declines in inductive reasoning and spatial orientation, the mental abilities that are often among the first to erode during aging.

When his test subjects began to decline in cognitive ability, Dr. Schaie offered them a brief mental training program, consisting of five one-hour sessions. The sessions were aimed specifically at improving inductive reasoning and spatial orientation. In effect, the subjects were taught "how to think." As a result of these brief mental training sessions, the cognitive abilities of 50 percent of the subjects improved significantly. From this, Dr. Schaie concluded that "old dogs can be taught new tricks."

Many other researchers have corroborated the findings of Dr. Schaie. They strongly support his basic premise, that fluid intelligence in humans can be increased, at any age, with mental training.

Now I'll give you my own mental training program, similar to the program I offer to my brain longevity patients.

I'll start with a short section on "how to think." All of the ideas in this section are based on what you already know about how the brain works.

Then I will tell you the specific mental activities that I recommend to my patients.

Your Mental Training Program

This section is the only part of this book where I discuss memory aids, or *mnemonic devices*. I have no doubt that mnemonic device systems can work, and I encourage patients to use them as a small part of their multifaceted brain longevity programs. But I believe that mnemonic devices have been grossly oversold by some researchers as being the best way to develop a good memory. It's my opinion that, in the absence of a multimodality brain longevity program, mnemonic devices are of limited value. Far too often they simply squeeze the most out of a beleaguered brain. I believe it makes much more sense to *physically improve* your brain than to try to get more "mileage" out of an exhausted brain.

Nevertheless, from this book you have learned some valuable facts about *how the brain works*, and it makes sense to take practical advantage of this knowledge.

So here are some "thinking strategies" that will make it easier for you to *remember* and to *learn*.

Multiple associations. This is an excellent way to remember things. Multiple associations, of course, are multiple memories about a single subject. As you know, each of your memory traces has many other memories that are physically attached to it, by the dendrites of other neurons. The more associations you have with each memory, the more dendritic "paths" you will have to that memory. Richly encoded memories, which have many paths leading to them, are much easier to reach.

For example, let's say that you, like many other people, suffer from anomia, the frequent inability to remember names. When this happens to you, you probably focus hard on the memory of the name, only to come up blank. But focusing on just the name is a poor strategy, because you may only have one memory trace that leads directly to the name. A better strategy is to remember something else about the person—an associated memory—such as his wife's name, his job, the color of his car, or his hometown. You may know a dozen facts about this person, and *many* of those facts will be associated in your memory with his name. If you retrieve one of those memories, you may well retrieve the name along with it. You'll reach the memory through a "side door."

Another way to use associations to trigger memories is to use *cues*—such as calendars, diaries, or reminder notes. For example, a single diary-type cue such as, "Tuesday, went to the park," may trigger a hundred memories that are associated with that outing. But if you have *no* cue, you may totally forget the whole thing.

Acronyms are an associative cue that all of us use. For example, the letters in *M.A.D.D.* remind us that the full name of the group is Mothers Against Drunk Driving.

Another very common cue that people use to trigger associations is rhyme. For example: A stitch in time saves . . . how many? Rhyming sounds are excellent associative cues. That's why so many ad slogans rhyme.

Attaching emotion. Here is another way to imbed a memory more deeply. As you know, the norepinephrine secreted during an emotional experience helps the brain to "ship" the memory of the experience to long-term storage. But you may not have known that even a minor emotional jolt can help cement a memory.

I have a friend who uses an emotional memory-imbedding device to help strangers find his house. He lives atop a hill on a long, curving street, and the best way to spot his house is to look for it right after you turn onto his street. If you don't spot it then, it's easy to miss. He has found, however, that people *forget* to spot his house if he just tells them, "After you turn onto my street, my house is the one that's straight ahead, up the hill." However, they invariably *remember* to spot his house if he says, "After you turn onto my street, my house is the one that's straight ahead, up the hill—so if you keep going straight you'll crash right into it." Just that one whimsical remark, which conjures a highly charged image, creates enough emotion to make people remember.

Therefore, to keep from forgetting things, attach appropriate emotions to them. For example, if your wife asks you to get three things from the store, and tells you it's important, focus on how disappointed she'll be if you forget. This attachment of emotion will engrave the memory even better than a mnemonic device.

Another example of using emotion to solidify memory comes from the actor Christopher Plummer. Plummer, like many other actors, learns the *meaning* and *emotion* in his lines before he memorizes the words. The emotion of his lines then becomes the framework that holds together his left-brain, linguistic memories.

Multiple encoding. Encoding memories with more than just one of your five senses is also a good strategy. This is something that we all commonly do. All of us, for example, tend to say phone numbers aloud when we read them out of a phone book, so that we will have both a *visual* and an *auditory* memory of the number. Often, of course, we say the phone number under our breath, but this "subvocal rehearsal" triggers the same auditory memory mechanism as actually saying the number aloud.

Multiple encoding increases the number of sites in which a memory trace exists. Therefore, if you want to remember something, make *visual images* of things you *hear*, and make *verbal notes* about things you *see*.

You can also strengthen a memory by adding a kinesthetic association. If you touch something, or do something—and remember how it *feels*—you'll be much more likely to remember it. That's why "hands-on" learning works so well—especially for children, whose language centers are less developed than those of adults. Many adults, though, also have powerful kinesthetic memories. The actor John Barrymore, who had a poor memory for language, remembered his lines by placing cues at particular spots on the stage. Being in a specific *place* triggered his memory of the line.

Also, taking note of how things *smell* is a good way to powerfully encode memories. As you'll recall, the sense of smell goes directly to the hippocampus, without passing through the hypothalamus, like other sensory input. Because of this, smell is especially evocative of memory.

Chunking. Breaking down memories into "bite-sized pieces"

is also a smart memory strategy. Most people, as noted earlier, are able to recall readily only about seven individual bits of memory at any one time. That's why phone numbers are only seven digits long.

To most successfully move short-term memories to long-term storage, transport them in *chunks*. If, for example, you have to remember fourteen names, learn them seven at a time.

Break down long, complex pieces of information into short chunks. Break things into sections. Make outlines. Do an overview of the main points before you dive into details.

Review. Another thinking strategy that pays huge dividends, review is valuable because of the phenomenon of long-term potentiation. As mentioned earlier, because of long-term potentiation, remembering information becomes physically easier every time you're exposed to it. In other words, if you see something five times, you won't be only five times more likely to remember it, but about *twenty* times more likely. Every time a neurotransmitter travels down a memory "path," the path gets "beaten down," and the "trip" becomes physically easier.

Therefore, if you're trying to learn new information, you should be concerned about not just how hard you study it, but also how *often*. Three quick reviews will probably cement the memories better than one long, hard review.

Conscious forgetting. This is another good cognitive strategy. It's wise to consciously forget trivial details, because they clutter your mind. In fact, some memory researchers think that a person's memory is essentially finite—that there's only so much you can keep in your mind at one time. A theory of age-associated memory impairment says that one reason older people are forgetful about new information is that their minds are already crammed full. There is even laboratory evidence of this "congested brain theory"; older rats have much less space between their brain cells than younger rats, indicating a shortage of "room" for new memories.

Working memory, in particular, always seems to have a shortage of "shelf space." Therefore, try to spare your memory from as much triviality as possible. Create a few simple memory *systems* that will keep track of details. *Write things down*, so that you can forget about them until you need to remember them. Try to keep your life well organized, so that you won't have to stuff your memory with logistical details. Write down your schedule. Keep things in their proper places—especially the things you constantly need, like your keys and wallet. Use reminder notes. Make lists. Keep files.

If your mind is uncluttered by daily details, you'll be amazed at how much more clear it will feel.

Concentration. This is also critically important for efficient thinking and for memory. If you do not concentrate carefully on information, you probably won't remember it. Many brain longevity patients come to me thinking that they have a memory disorder, when in fact they have a concentration disorder.

As I've mentioned several times, brain longevity programs *physically improve* concentration, just as they physically improve memory. Being able to achieve a high level of concentration is largely a result of having a healthy brain, full of physical energy.

To some extent, however, concentration is also a result of willpower. You must make an effort to concentrate. You must try to keep other thoughts from breaking your concentration. You must learn to avoid interruptions. Many people *welcome* interruptions, as an escape from the hard work of concentration.

Needless to say, all of these thinking strategies can be synergistic. Combine them as much as possible, and they will help you to reach new heights of cognitive power.

Now let's take a look at the mental exercise regime that I recommend to my patients.

When I mentioned to my seventy-two-year-old patient T.I. that she should stay mentally active, the first thing she said was, "I'm *not* going to do crossword puzzles." Her hometown doctor had recommended that, and so had several friends. They all thought it would sharpen her mind, which had become dulled by age-associated memory impairment. "I *hate* crossword puzzles," she said. "And I *won't* do them."

"I won't, either," I replied. "I can't stand 'em." I asked her what she *did* like to do. Almost *all* mental exercise, I believe, should be fun. If it's drudgery, patients won't do it. And even if they do, it will harm them as much as it will help them, because drudgery will induce unhealthy levels of stress.

"When I still felt like myself mentally," T.I. said, "I liked to play the piano and to paint. But I gave all that up, because I can't remember how to read music anymore, and I don't paint as well as I used to."

I reminded her that she was not in a contest with her "younger self," as so many people seem to feel they are. I encouraged her to again play the piano and paint.

"If you keep playing and keep painting," I told her, "you'll be able to burn in those dendrites, and rebuild those memory traces. I'm sure it will be hard, but I know you can do it."

She agreed to try. To help keep her from being stressed by it, I suggested that she repeat a mantra whenever she began to get frustrated. I didn't call it a mantra, though, because that would have sounded too hippie-dippy to her. I just called it a "soothing phrase." The one she chose was "Hail Mary, full of grace."

I also suggested that she try to play her music from memory, instead of reading the music. That would employ more of her kinesthetic memory, which is invariably the last type of memory to fade. I advised her to pick a few of her favorite pieces, and to play them over and over, every day. If she did that for about an hour a day, I told her, she would probably be able to learn the songs.

But even if she couldn't play them perfectly, I said, the practice would still strengthen her cognitive function.

She began to play again, and to paint. But she did it with a new, less critical attitude; she focused more on the *process* of her work than on the product, because she knew that just *doing* it would help regenerate her brain. Her mantras were also very helpful. They enabled her to stick with her work, instead of becoming frustrated and quitting.

Before long she had memorized several of her favorite songs, and she took great pleasure and pride in playing them.

Within several months a significant degree of her cognitive function had returned. I have no doubt that her entire, synergistic brain longevity program—and not just her mental exercise—was responsible for her improvement. But I think it was her return to the piano, and to painting, that most made her feel "whole" again.

Another person who is a good example of someone who uses mental activity to stay cognitively young is my own mother. She is eighty-nine-years old, and her mind is still razor-sharp. For many years she has been on a brain longevity program. But she has always been so remarkably bright and aware, and so mentally active, that I have had little occasion to prescribe any cognitive-enhancement drugs for her.

My mother helps keep her brain strong and youthful with a number of mental activities. She avidly follows current events, plays canasta with her friends, and is active in organizations. She's also a big fan of the game show *Jeopardy*, and often impresses her friends by beating the contestants to the answers. She also uses her own form of meditative technique to keep her mind clear and relaxed.

My mother is a good example of someone whose mental activity program is uniquely suited to her own personal interests. Pursuing your own natural interests is the best form of mental exercise.

Almost any mental activity will fulfill the brain's needs, but the brain especially needs exercise in the areas of language, numbers, inductive and deductive reasoning, and spatial organization. Among the most productive exercises for these areas are reading, writing, drawing, playing word games, playing board games, building, conversing, and engaging in stimulating hobbies.

The important thing about mental activity is not *what* you do, but merely *that* you do it.

The most common mental-activity mistake that people make is to watch too much television. As I've mentioned, the average person watches about four hours daily. Unfortunately, although TV provides us with a great deal of information and entertainment, most TV programs allow the brain to be passive, and this erodes cognitive skills.

A few specific types of TV shows, however, encourage viewers to think, and not to be passive. One type is the quiz show with which viewers often "play along." Another type is news or documentary programming, which prompts viewers to engage in critical thinking as they watch. Unlike sitcoms, documentaries will build your brain instead of rotting it.

Researchers now believe that excessive television watching is particularly harmful to the development of right-brain, spatial intelligence in children. Children who watch long hours of television tend to avoid traditional childhood hobbies—such as art projects, building, or sports and games—which require three-dimensional, spatial reasoning skills. Partly as a result of this, spatial intelligence has been declining among school children for several decades. In one recent study, high school seniors achieved the same level of scores on right-brain, spatial intelligence tests that high school *freshmen* had achieved twenty years earlier.

Another terrible effect of television, and also of our hectic lifestyles, is that too few people today take time to read. Reading, many neurological researchers believe, is uniquely beneficial for the brain. Much reading matter, of course, is intellectually enriching, but the mere act of reading, regardless of content, is highly beneficial. Reading requires active engagement of the mind and imagination, and it powerfully stimulates both hemispheres of the brain, as well as the limbic system. Only about 20 percent of the population reads from a book on most days.

I advise my brain longevity patients to spend at least one or two hours a day doing mental exercise. That's not very much at all. Consider that you would get about *four* hours of mental exercise just by reading the newspaper, talking about current events with a friend, playing along with *Jeopardy* and *Wheel of Fortune*, and then playing a game of Scrabble.

That doesn't sound like too tough of a day, does it?

Dr. Arnold Scheibel, the highly respected director of UCLA's Brain Research Institute, believes that it's especially beneficial to the brain to challenge it with *novel* tasks—anything new and different. He advises people to do things they've never done before. He himself recently took up sculpture.

Other researchers agree that *novelty* is very biologically stimulating to the brain. Some recommend travel as a good way to coax the brain into making new dendritic connections.

What you should mostly avoid is simply doing *nothing*. One influential researcher, Dr. Carl Cotman, recently noted, "There's a study that looks at retired couch potatoes, and the retired active. Over a period of years, the ones who remain active better preserve cognitive function and brain metabolism."

Clearly, then, mental exercise is vitally important for brain regeneration. Now let's look at one final type of exercise that will help you achieve optimal mental function. This type of exercise has been used for thousands of years to facilitate brain regeneration.

In my opinion, this type of exercise—mind/body exercise—is one of the best things you can do for your brain.

A Case in Point

The Brain Is Just Another of the Body's Organs

H.K., forty-seven, was an ambitious and intelligent young woman who had been struck down by a tragic disease. In the early 1990s, H.K. was one of a number of people who ingested tryptophan tablets that may have been contaminated. She contracted, possibly from these tablets, "eosinophilic myalgic syndrome," which is characterized by chronic flu-like symptoms. (Because of this incident, tryptophan supplements were banned by the F.D.A.)

Her only interest was in getting well again.

H.K. faced a difficult battle. Eosinophilic myalgic syndrome is generally considered incurable. Symptoms can wax and wane, but there is no therapy that is considered to be curative.

Her symptoms included chronic muscle aches, fevers, night sweats, and extreme fatigue. In addition, her mental energy was very low, she had a tendency toward depression, she experienced a chronic sense of emotional malaise, and her memory and cognitive function were impaired.

Because of this constellation of mental symptoms, and because, as a hospital administrator, she had heard about my work, she consulted with me.

During our first consultation, I told her that her brain longevity program would not reverse the general course of her illness, but that it might reduce her mental symptomatology.

"That would be a blessing," she said, "because the mental part of this thing is the *worst* part. Half the time I can't think clearly, and I feel like I'm in a bad mood all the time. It feels like my depression has a mind of its own. It comes over me even when I'm not thinking about any of my problems."

I told her that I thought her eosinophilic condition was contributing to a neuropeptide disorder, and that the neuropeptide disorder was probably a primary cause of her depression and cognitive impairment.

I had noticed a similar phenomenon in other patients. These patients had chronic fatigue syndrome. They, too, had experienced severe mental lassitude and mood disorders. In fact, researchers have found that the IQs of people with chronic fatigue syndrome can decline by up to fifty-five points.

I had found that when I placed chronic fatigue patients on brain longevity programs, they still suffered from many of the *physical* symptoms of the disease, but their *mental* symptoms were substantially relieved.

Sometimes it seemed odd to these patients that their mental symptoms could improve while their overall physical condition remained about the same. But, to me, this did not seem particularly unusual. The brain is, after all, just another organ in the body, and the brain's health can often be improved even when the patient's overall physical health cannot be significantly improved.

H.K. became very actively involved with her brain longevity program. She modified her diet, started taking relatively high dosages of supplements and natural medicinal tonics, and began doing mind/body exercises. She meditated, did some mild aerobic exercise, and tried to manage her stress as effectively as possible.

In addition, she took two pharmaceutical medications. I had her DHEA level tested, and it was very low, so I prescribed DHEA hormonal replacement therapy. I also prescribed daily ingestion of 2,400 mg of piracetam, which is a relatively high dosage.

Over a matter of months, she began to improve markedly. The first thing she noticed was that her mood improved. She became much more buoyant and optimistic, which was how she had generally felt before she'd become ill. Her depressive symptoms subsided drastically, and she no longer brooded about being sick. Her memory normalized, and she regained the same high level of fluid intelligence and cognitive processing speed that she'd had before her illness.

Her primary physical symptoms did seem to improve somewhat. Nonetheless, she still suffers from eosinophilia. She is able to withstand her physical ailments, though, she said, as long as her own mind doesn't, as she put it, "drag me down." She told me that she felt "like a new person."

H.K. is a courageous woman. Many patients with her problem would have just given up. She did not—and now she is reaping the rewards of her courage.

18

Mind/Body Exercises: The Ancient Art of Brain Regeneration

Like all human beings—like all matter in the universe, in fact—you are physically composed of electrons, protons, and neutrons, all of which are moving constantly and consistently within your thirty trillion cells. Your body is, in effect, thirty trillion "dancing cells of light."

Thus you possess a high degree of energy potential at the cellular level.

You can more efficiently harness this energy potential by using a fascinating array of mind/body exercises. These exercises employ specific muscular contractions, powerful breathing techniques, energy-channeling body positions, and "primal sound" mantras. They stimulate health and regeneration not just on a macrocosmic level, but also at the *cellular* level.

The mind/body exercises can shift tremendous amounts of energy to your brain and nervous and endocrine systems, and enable you to use that energy more efficiently. They can also help balance the energy of your brain and your nervous and endocrine systems. Therefore they can help you to function at a consistently higher level, without exhausting your mind and body.

Many of my patients have told me that they believe their mind/body exercises have proven to be the single most beneficial element of their brain longevity programs. My personal belief is that the mind/body exercises are among the most powerful tools we possess for brain regeneration.

I carefully chose the mind/body exercises that I recommend to my patients. Over the past seventeen years I have studied more than two thousand yogic exercises. From these exercises I have selected about forty that were specifically developed to stimulate cognitive function. Many of these forty exercises have been used by yogic masters for thousands of years.

Out of these forty exercises I have selected just a few that are not only extremely powerful, but are also relatively easy to perform. These are the exercises I most often recommend to my patients.

For the most part, the evidence that supports the efficacy of the mind/body exercises is empirical—based on observation rather than on formal research. Thus the mind/body exercises are more of an art than a science. Many practitioners of Western medicine, however, including myself, have formulated clear theories about exactly *why* these mind/body exercises achieve the results they do.

There is absolutely no doubt in my mind that the exercises work. Their effect is quite profound, and very clinically evident.

Each of the exercises I most often recommend is part of a *kriya*, the name given to a set of exercises that has been tested and used by master practitioners over time. A kriya is a combination of movement, breathing, a posture, a mantra, and a positioning of the fingers.

Each kriya is designed to increase blood flow and energy flow to the brain, to the nervous system, and to certain glands of the endocrine system.

As you know, increased blood flow has a powerful effect. It gives an immediate boost to cognitive function, by supplying abundant amounts of oxygen and glucose. It also improves the long-term health of the brain, by enhancing neuronal metabolism.

The mind/body exercises are even more efficient than strenuous cardiovascular exercise at increasing cerebral blood flow. This is partly because these exercises were specifically *designed* to channel blood flow directly to the brain. One way they do this is by temporarily impeding cerebral blood flow, to build pressure. When this pressure is released, it powers blood to the brain.

Mind/body exercises also channel energy to the brain and endocrine system. From the Western perspective, this is energy derived from and transported by the nervous system. From the Eastern perspective, this is not *just* nerve energy, but is also the "life energy" that is central to Oriental medicine. In traditional Chinese medicine, this life energy is called *ch'i*. In the Indian yogic tradition, it is called *prana*, and the energy that it releases and channels *in the body* is called *kundalini*. The body's kundalini energy is stimulated by kundalini yoga exercises, such as the mind/body exercises that are part of brain longevity programs.

This vital energy, according to the Eastern perspective, inhabits not just your body, but also the entire cosmos. Thus it is sometimes referred to as "cosmic energy."

Many Western analysts conceive of ch'i, or kundalini, as *bioelectric* energy, much like the bioelectric energy that powers your neurons. Like any form of electricity, this life energy must be *flowing* in order to exist. When it is blocked, or slowed to a point of "stagnation," it becomes as defunct as an electric power line with a short circuit.

As you probably know, electricity is created by positive and negative polarity. Similarly, ch'i is created by the action of the forces that Eastern philosophy refers to as *yin* and *yang*. The complementary opposites of yin and yang are believed to "move" ch'i, and this movement is believed to provide physical and mental energy.

The yin quality is essentially characterized by darkness, passivity, a yielding nature, contraction, cold, dampness, and femininity. The yang quality is essentially characterized by lightness, activism, resistance, expansion, heat, dryness, and masculinity.

Neither quality is superior to the other, nor could either exist without the other. Every living organism possesses both.

In Eastern philosophy and medicine, the key to wellness and happiness is simply to balance yin and yang, thereby producing a greater abundance of ch'i. Lao Tzu, a Chinese philosopher, wrote, more than three thousand years ago, "The ceaseless intermingling of heaven (yang) and earth (yin) gives form to all things."

From the Eastern perspective, the universe and all things in it are constantly moving from yin to yang and yang to yin, and back again, in a continual cycle of change. Eastern philosophers, therefore, see change as cyclical, while Western philosophers tend to see it as linear.

According to Eastern medicine, health is best achieved when we do not resist the cycles of change, but move in accord with them.

Eastern medicine, therefore, places a tremendous emphasis on adaptation and flexibility. One example of this comes from Asian herbal medicine. The most celebrated Eastern medicinal tonic, ginseng, is considered an *adaptogen*. Ginseng is believed to endow those who use it with greater ability to adapt to life's changes, rather than to rigidly resist them, and then become stressed by them.

This Eastern interpretation of ginseng's value is paralleled by the Western view. According to Western nutritionists, ginseng is a powerful adrenal tonic—and your adrenals, of course, are vitally important in enabling you to respond to stressful change in a positive way. Strong adrenal function helps you to deal with stress by "bending without breaking."

Just as we cannot see or technologically measure yin and yang, we are also unable to see or technologically measure ch'i, or kundalini. Therefore it has not been scientifically proved that the qualities of ch'i and kundalini exist.

Nonetheless, from the empirical perspective—the view based purely upon *experiences*—ch'i certainly appears to exist. As a medical acupuncturist, I have noted the flow of ch'i thousands of times. I am quite capable of locating and manipulating this flow in an orderly and predictable manner. Countless times over the past decade, I have used the manipulation of ch'i powerfully to stimulate the health of many patients.

Some Western practitioners who doubt the existence of ch'i argue that acupuncturists achieve their clinical successes by placing their needles into nerves, and manipulating nerve energy. As a Western physician with a strong background in anatomy, I am virtually certain that the effects I achieve do not result from contact with nerves.

These effects are almost certainly a result of contact with ch'i, which flows through the body in energy "meridians." These meridians can be visualized as being much like nerves—except that they are not *physical* entities, as nerves are. In a sense, they are like the channels through which rivers flow: they exist as space, rather than as a solid entity.

The mind/body exercises that I recommend manipulate the energy that flows through these meridians, and through other subtle energy channels. The exercises manipulate this vital energy in somewhat the same way that acupuncture does.

Through this action, the mind/body exercises are able to balance and stimulate vital energy in the body, brain, and the nervous and endocrine systems.

As I mentioned, the mind/body exercises increase blood flow, and also increase the flow of the kundalini. Thus they are a unique element in the science of brain regeneration.

From my own clinical experience, and from extensive research done by others, I have come to believe that the mind/body exercises can have specific influences on the *biochemistry* of the brain. This occurs partly because of the exercises' effects upon blood flow and energy flow to the brain, and also because of the exercises' effects upon the release of specific brain chemicals, including neuropeptides and neurotransmitters.

Ever since Dr. Candace Pert and her associates discovered receptors for the neuropeptide endorphins, it has been accepted that every feeling and mood is influenced by neuropeptides. There are more than one hundred neuropeptides and neurohormones in the brain, and each has a profound, specific influence upon mood and emotion. Certain neuropeptides, for example, are intricately associated with anger, and others are closely linked to fear, love, and happiness.

Research on the effects of acupuncture has shown that stimulating particular energy meridians with acupuncture stimulates the release of particular neuropeptides and neurotransmitters. This is especially possible when mild electric currents are attached to acupuncture needles.

Because acupuncturists can stimulate the release of neuropeptide endorphins, they can completely block pain in patients undergoing major surgery. This practice is common in the East. Acupuncturists can also trigger the release of neurotransmitters such as acetylcholine, serotonin, and norepinephrine.

The mind/body exercises can achieve a similar result. When you perform the various movements of the mind/body exercises, in combination with the prescribed breathing techniques, you will be able to influence your brain biochemistry. You will help balance your brain biochemistry, stimulate cognitive function, and achieve a stable, positive mood.

Although many medical authors have presented basic yogic exercises, no such author yet has described how to potentiate optimal neurological function with yogic mind/body exercises. Perhaps, because these exercises are so new to the medical profession and to the general public, some people will be skeptical of their validity. I do not object to this skepticism, because rational skepticism is a valuable tool for scientific inquiry.

I am certain, however, that if you try these mind/body exercises yourself, your possible skepticism will soon blossom into enthusiasm, for a very simple reason. They work.

If it were my sole objective to have my brain longevity programs immediately embraced by all segments of the Western medical community, I might not mention these mind-body exercises, because some conventional practitioners may consider them inappropriate for a medical program.

But universal acceptance is not my ultimate goal. My ultimate goal is to *help patients*.

And this can best be achieved by presenting these exercises.

* * *

Recently, I had a long conversation with one of my patients, S.L., the female patient whom I told you about in chapter 1's "Case in Point." As you may remember, S.L. was in an auto accident, and suffered severe brain damage. After the accident, she had great difficulty concentrating. She also suffered from severe vertigo, partial paralysis, and a seizure disorder. But she made a remarkable, full recovery, and credited the mind/body exercises for much of her comeback.

I asked her, in the beginning of our recent conversation, about her first impressions of the mind/body exercises.

"To be totally honest," she told me, "when you first mentioned them to me, I didn't have any expectation that they would work for me. But I was willing to try anything, because my neurologist had told me that I probably wouldn't ever again be able to function at a high intellectual level."

"What was it that you had been doing before the accident?" I asked.

"I was a regional manager for a federal agency. Before that, I was a CPA."

"But you were unemployed when you began your program, weren't you?"

"Yes, I was incapacitated, mentally and physically."

"How long did you remain incapacitated after you began your program?"

"Within the first month, I improved physically. My ability to use my left side, which had been paralyzed, began to return, and my coordination got better. Also, my vertigo began to improve."

"What did you notice in terms of cognitive improvement?"

"At first, not much. I was really mentally scattered; I couldn't focus. And my short-term recall just wasn't functioning. When I'd think of something, I'd have to write it down. But I'd go to find a piece of paper, and I'd forget what I was looking for. After about two months I began to make a lot of progress. I was able to focus my mind, and I could just feel the energy in it moving around."

"After that, did your memory improve quickly?"

"Yes, but part of that was just because my concentration improved. First I regained the ability to learn things. *Then* I could retrieve them."

"Do different exercises give you different effects?"

"They sure do. It feels like the blood and energy are moving to different parts of my body and brain when I do different types of exercises. Some of them give me energy, some of them calm me down, and some help me to focus."

"Which ones are stimulating?"

"Breath of Fire. Definitely. Also the Pineal Gland Kriya."

"Do you do your meditation at the same time you do the mind/body exercises?"

"I think of it all as one package. Wherever you're trying to go with the mind/body exercises—stimulation, relaxation, or whatever—the meditation goes right with it."

"What effect did acupuncture have on you?"

"It helped with my vertigo, and that helped me do the mind/body exercises. And it made me feel more centered, although that feeling is hard to describe."

"So, summing up, what was the net effect of the mind/body exercises?"

"I wouldn't be where I am without them. They opened up new worlds for me. I can concentrate. I can focus my energy. I'm much more flexible. I just feel a whole lot better, all the way around."

The mind/body exercises are a form of yoga. Virtually all forms of yoga seek to unite body and mind. The word *yoga* is derived from the same source as *yoke*, meaning "to join."

The mind/body exercises that I recommend to my brain longevity patients come primarily from the ancient practice of kundalini yoga, a comprehensive system of physical exercises, meditation, and a carefully balanced diet. It originated near Amritsar, and is very popular in northern India, particularly among the Sikhs.

Kundalini yoga is a relatively challenging form of yoga that yields dramatic results. Not all kundalini exercises are difficult, though. I recommend *easy* exercises to my brain longevity patients, because I don't want them to become discouraged. Also, many of my patients are older people who can't perform difficult exercises.

The essential goal of kundalini yoga is to *channel and move energy*, via the nervous system and via the meridian system. Kundalini yoga transports energy from the body's "lower" energy centers (in the pelvic region) to the "higher" energy centers (in the brain). Similarly, it transports nerve energy from the base of the spine to the brain.

Yogi Bhajan, the master of kundalini yoga, has said, "You experience the effects of kundalini when the energy of the glandular system combines with the power of the nervous system, to produce such a heightened sensitivity that your brain can function at its optimum capacity. You become totally and wholly aware."

What that means to me as a physician is that the practice of these mind/body exercises is excitatory, neuroprotective, memory-enhancing, and also anti-aging.

When applied properly, the mind/body exercises offer a transcendent experience. Yogi Bhajan believes that all people "have the ability, sleeping within them, to be totally intuitive, creative, and effective." However, he thinks that people are generally unable to tap into this ability, because of the barrier of suboptimal neorological function. But he believes that the mind/body exercises "can remove that barrier, and with time, take people to a state where nothing is lacking."

As someone who has practiced this form of yoga for many years, I can assure you that it is a safe and realistic approach to the rejuvenation of your brain, and to the achievement of your highest potential.

Besides kundalini yoga, the other primary component of the mind/body exercises is *naad yoga*. Naad yoga, like kundalini, is an ancient yogic art that has been practiced by many millions of people for thousands of years.

Naad yoga is a form of chanting or *mantra* yoga. To do it, you simply say specific sounds, generally while you are exercising and meditating. Naad Yoga is different from other forms of mantra yoga, though, in that it employs the chanting of exclusively "primal" sounds—sounds that are considered most basic and central to human speech, and that are believed by yogic masters to resonate throughout the cosmos. The best known of these primal sounds is *Om*, or *Um*.

The fascinating thing about these primal sounds is that they appear to invigorate specific endocrine glands, as well as the brain itself, apparently through simple vibration.

The mind/body exercises also involve regulation of the breath. The breathing techniques help to control the flow of blood and of kundalini energy.

In addition, the mind/body exercises employ a careful system of positioning of the hands and fingers. From the Western study of anatomy, we know that the hands and fingers are "highly represented" in the cortex of the brain; that is, there is a relative abundance of area in the cortex that is dedicated to the control of the hands and fingers. We also know that certain movements of the hands and fingers seem to help the brain to "pattern" physical coordination. Thus, positioning the hands and fingers apparently has an effect upon cognitive function.

From the Eastern perspective, the hands and fingers have a more profound significance. According to yogic masters, each area of the hand "reflexes," or helps to control, a particular area of the brain. Eastern medical practitioners believe that it is possible to influence the brain by stretching the fingers, crossing them, or touching the fingertips to the thumb or to another part of the hand. Therefore, many of the mind/body exercises include specific finger positions, which the yogis call *mudras*.

All of these elements—movements, breath, mantra, and mudra—combine to form a mind/body exercise kriya. Each kriya is designed to achieve a particular effect. Later in this chapter, I will introduce you to several kriyas, and tell you how to perform them. When you perform them, you will more fully appreciate the specific, individualistic powers of each kriya. First, though, let's take a little closer look at *naad yoga*, since it's probably a new concept to you.

Brain Regeneration and Naad Yoga

Recent research into the effects of *vibrational sound currents* on cells has yielded fascinating results. In one experiment, cancer cells were subjected to different continuous tones from the musical scale (the notes D, C, and E), and then monitored technologically. Each note appeared to create different changes in the "energy fields" of the cells. Each of the three notes also had the fascinating effect of decreasing the malignant reproductive rate of the cells.

This experiment indicates the considerable power that sound current possesses. In the future, perhaps sound current, or ultrasound, will be used to combat cancer and other diseases, just as ultrasound is now used to break up gallstones and kidney stones, and to take internal "photographs."

Another interesting experiment on the effect of sound currents was recently done at the University of Arizona. Using a PET scan that recorded the activity of an isotope of glucose, a researcher looked for changes in the cerebral function of a subject who chanted primal naad yoga mantras, such as *Sa Ta Na Ma* and *Wha He Guru*. The PET scan recorded a strong shift in function during chanting. During chanting, the primary activities of the brain were transferred from the left hemisphere to the right frontal and parietal regions. This shift is indicative of a strong enhancement of mood, and of an increase in alertness.

Other research has shown that the chanting of primal tones stimulates the *vagus nerve*, the large cranial nerve that travels throughout the thoracic and abdominal areas, servicing the heart, lungs, intestinal tract, and back muscles. The vagus nerve supplies the motor and sensory fibers that regulate pancreatic and gastric secretions, and also carries the inhibitory nerve fibers that service the heart. Thus the vagus nerve is considered by many anatomists to be the most important single nerve in the body. It is reasonable to expect that the vagus nerve would be stimulated by chanting, because it passes through the larynx, or voice box.

From the Eastern perspective, the power of naad yoga does not stem solely from its effects upon nerve energy, but also from its ability to raise the kundalini energy.

According to Eastern medicine, there are seventy-two energy meridians that flow throughout the body. There are also three *central* kundalini energy channels, which flow up the spine into the brain. Each of these meridians and channels is believed to be in a continual state of vibration.

At various points along these meridians are *reflex points*, which are points of accessibility, rather like bus stops along a bus route. According to yogic philosophy, eighty-four of these reflex points are located in the upper palate of the mouth alone.

The chanting of primal sounds is believed to stimulate the re-flex points in the mouth, and to change subtly the vibration of the energy meridian upon which the reflex points lie. The tongue, in particular, directly strikes many of these reflex points during naad yoga. The striking of these points by the tongue has been likened to striking a computer keyboard with the fingers, in that the mere act of striking is very simple, but the results can be far-reaching.

Even if you are skeptical of the *intrinsic* value of naad yoga, you probably still recognize the value of repeating mantras during meditation. As you learned in the chapter on meditation, one of the primary values of repeating mantras is that they "silence the internal dialogue," and give your mind a few moments of peace.

The quieting of the mind can have extremely important effects. The poet Alfred, Lord Tennyson, who practiced mantra yoga, once described the effect of chanting a simple mantra: "Individuality seemed to dissolve and fade away into boundless being; and this is not a confused state, but the clearest of the clear, and surest of the sure, the weirdest of the weird, utterly beyond words—where death was an almost laughable impossibility."

Of course, the effects of chanting are usually not this dramatic. Even so, mantras almost always "turn off" your worries and reduce your stress, simply because your mind is preoccupied with your mantra. Thus, because they help manage stress, mantras can be a valuable element of a brain longevity program.

I know that some of these concepts may seem odd to you, especially if you were raised in the culture of the West, which has traditionally emphasized a strictly physical approach to health and healing. As Western medicine has become increasingly advanced, however, it has adopted many of the formerly mysterious tenets of Eastern healing. For example, acupuncture is now commonly used as an adjunctive therapy in Western medicine, and many substances from the Asian herbal pharmacopeia are also now commonly employed by Westerners. As Western medicine has progressed, it has increasingly embraced the philosophy that the mind can control the body—a philosophy that largely originated in the East. As Western medicine grows ever more sophisticated, I expect it to merge even more fully with Eastern medicine.

As I've said, much about the brain remains a mystery. Things that are mysterious today will be clear tomorrow. For example, thirty years ago, a mysterious concept called *transcranial electrical stimulation* was introduced. According to its creators, if electrodes were placed on the scalp, and electromagnetic current was supplied, neurotransmitter levels would be influenced. At the time of its introduction, this modality was considered somewhat bizarre. Now, however, the neurological community has a more complete understanding of the bioelectricity of the brain, and transcranial electrical stimulation is generally considered to be orthodox.

I believe that mind/body exercises will be similarly embraced by the medical community in the future, after researchers have had time to test them objectively, and to quantify their effects.

So now let's take a look at specific mind/body exercises, and I'll tell you exactly how to do them.

How to Do Mind/Body Exercises

After you have practiced the techniques of the mind/body exercises just a few times, you will begin to experience their effects.

You should practice the exercises on an empty stomach, as you would a cardiovascular exercise, and do them at a time of day when you have few distractions. For many people, the best time is shortly after waking in the morning, before breakfast.

At the end of each exercise, relax briefly. In this short relaxation phase, breathe deeply, and enjoy the new feeling you have created. This will allow your energy to circulate freely, and to be fully integrated into your brain.

To perform these exercises, you will have to know how to activate your body's energy "locks," which help to harness the energy that you will be transferring. These locks—or *bhandas,* as the yogis say—are similar to "switches" that direct the energy that has been generated. To achieve a lock, all you have to do is tighten specific muscles.

There are three locks, called the *root lock,* the *diaphragm lock,* and the *neck lock.* All three locks, applied together, constitute the *great lock.*

The *root lock* is activated by tensing the muscles at the base of your pelvic region, including the anus and sex organs. To apply this lock, pull your abdomen toward your spine, and tighten the muscles in your pelvis region. This lock is used to channel energy up from the pelvic region to the diaphragm area. For many centuries, Eastern yogis have used this lock to increase sexual energy. Currently, most Western sexual therapists advocate periodic tightening of these muscles to increase control over orgasm.

The *diaphragm lock* is applied by lifting your diaphragm toward your chest, and pulling your upper abdominal muscles toward your spine. This can be visualized as "sucking in your gut." This lock channels energy farther upward, to the neck region. Applying it generally stimulates mental energy. As a rule, it is applied as you exhale.

The *neck lock* is applied by pulling the muscles of your neck and throat back toward your spine. When you apply this lock, your chin remains level to the ground and slightly pulled back. Try not to tilt your head forward. This lock will straighten your neck, and optimize the blood and energy flow to your brain. Yogis believe that the neck lock also optimizes the function of the thyroid and parathyroid.

The *great lock*—applying three locks at once—generally creates a pleasant sensation of increased mental and physical energy. The effect of the great lock is heightened when you roll your eyes toward the middle of your forehead, and focus your mental energy on your frontal lobe.

Now let's look at some specific mind/body exercises.

Long, Slow, Deep Breathing

The long, slow, deep breath is the most basic form of yogic breathing, and is part of each kriya.

When you are stressed, your breath is rapid, shallow, and irregular. To correct that, simply inhale through your nose, and try to fill the base of your lungs. Let your belly come out first, then allow the breath to come up to the mid-portion of your lungs. Finally, hold the breath briefly at the top of your lungs. Breathe out slowly in reverse order, through your nose. Focus on your breath as you perform this exercise. If you mind wanders, focus again on your breath.

Besides helping to relieve and prevent stress, this technique is important for brain longevity because it helps to increase the capacity of the lungs. Thus it supplies more oxygen to all the cells in your body, including those in your brain.

The Breath of Fire

The Breath of Fire is a powerful exercise that almost always increases energy. The yogis believe that the Breath of Fire is the "spark" that will "kindle your personal flame." Just three minutes of Breath of Fire will increase your physical and mental energy.

From a Western perspective, the Breath of Fire—which employs quick abdominal breaths—is believed to be effective because it stimulates the *splanchnic nerves* in the abdominal cavity. Stimulation of these nerves causes the release of epinephrine and norepinephrine.

Sometimes the Breath of Fire will cause mild perspiration on your forehead. Yogis believe this is caused by the generation of psychic heat, or *tapa*. You may have to practice this exercise several times before you are able to generate tapa.

To do the Breath of Fire, breathe through your nostrils rapidly—more that one inhalation per second. Do not pause between inhaling and exhaling.

You should inhale by bringing your diaphragm down, instead of up. Breathe from your diaphragm, and keep your chest relaxed. Focus your mental energy on your navel area.

This exercise may cause a mild feeling of lightheadedness, which may feel like hyperventilation (a decrease in blood carbon dioxide), but this is probably not the case. Clinical studies have indicated, in fact, that while the carbon dioxide level in the blood remains normal, the oxygen level actually increases during the Breath of Fire. Other studies indicate that the Breath of Fire produces alpha rhythms in the brain. This is probably why the exercise is able to simultaneously create increased calmness and increased alertness.

Yogis—and also some Western researchers, including myself—believe that the Breath of Fire also increases oxygen delivery to the brain. Because of this increased delivery of oxygen, neuronal metabolism is improved. Neurons are "cleansed" and rejuvenated.

One of my oldest friends, Gerry Greenhouse, M.A., a special-education teacher for the Albuquerque school system, uses the Breath of Fire periodically for quick energy, the same way some people use a cup of coffee. He says that going through his day without the Breath of Fire is like "trying to drive my car without starting the engine."

The Basic Spinal Energy Series

This is a powerful exercise for creating energy, increasing the flexibility of the spine, and enhancing cerebral circulation.

From the Eastern perspective, spinal flexibility is crucial. Yogis often *measure age* in terms of spinal flexibility instead of chronology. This measure of age has a metaphorical meaning as well as a practical one. As a metaphor, spinal flexibility represents one's ability to adapt, to "bend without breaking." In a practical sense, spinal flexibility determines one's potential for successfully moving energy throughout the body.

A study done at the University of California at Davis showed that the basic spinal energy series strongly affected EEG patterns. It significantly increased the amounts and strengths of alpha and theta waves.

To begin the basic spinal energy series, or any of the mind/body exercises, you start by "tuning in." To do this, sit comfortably on the floor, with your legs crossed. Yogis call this the "easy pose." Or you can sit in a chair. The most important thing is to make sure your spine is straight.

To tune in, bring your hands up to the level of your heart, with your palms together and the knuckles of your thumbs pressing against your breastbone. Yogis call this the "prayer pose." Then inhale deeply and chant the mantra *Ong Namo Guru Dev*

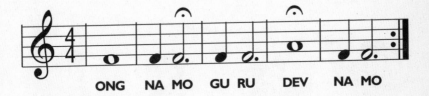

ONG   NA MO   GU RU   DEV   NA MO

Figure 9
To "tune in," chant this mantra, vibrating the sound current loudly, from the back of your nose and throat:

Ong Namo Guru Dev Namo
"I bow before my highest consciousness."

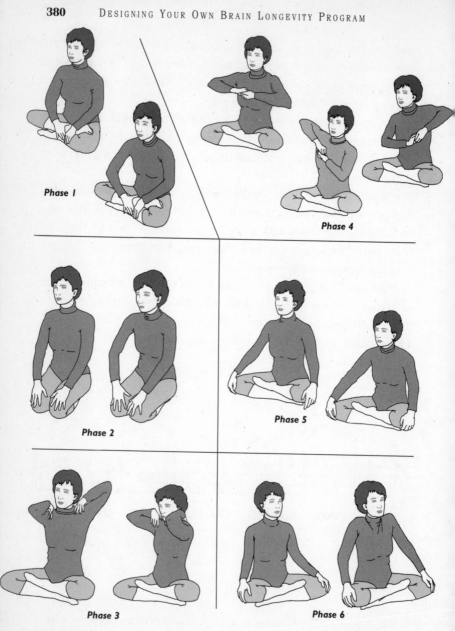

Figure 10
This set of exercises—the basic spinal energy series—increases both your mental and physical energy and is a great way to start your day. Remember to breathe powerfully through the nose only in each exercise.

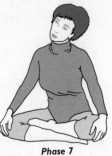

Phase 7

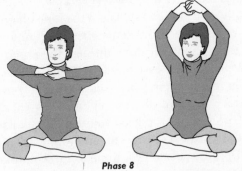

Phase 8

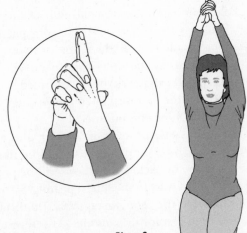

Phase 9

Namo. This means, "I bow before my highest consciousness." Vibrate this sound current loudly, from the back of your nose and throat.

Doing this allows you to release any distractions, and to concentrate on doing the exercises. Yogis believe that this also links you to a "golden chain" of teachers—the yogic masters who have taught these exercises throughout history.

After chanting this mantra three times, inhale deeply. Hold the breath and then relax. The next few minutes are an excellent time to visualize your goals, say your affirmations, or pray. As your mind becomes still and calm, it is very receptive to your direction. After tuning in, you are ready to begin the nine-phase basic spinal energy series (Figure 10). Remember that unless otherwise stated, breathing should be done through the nose.

Phase 1. Stay in the easy pose, grab your ankles, and inhale deeply. If you're in a chair, place your hands on your knees. Flex your spine forward, and lift your chest. Then exhale, and flex your spine backward. Try to keep your head level. Each time you inhale, say the word *Sat* to yourself, and with each exhale say the word *Nam.* Do this repeatedly for one to three minutes. Then inhale, relax, and focus on your breath for one minute. *Sat Nam* means "my true identity."

Phase 2. Fold your legs under you and sit back on your heels. If you're in a chair, stay in an easy pose with your palms on your thighs. Put your palms on your thighs. Then flex your spine forward and inhale, as you say the word *Sat* to yourself. Then flex your spine backward and exhale, as you say the word *Nam.* Do this repeatedly for one to three minutes. Then inhale deeply, rest, and meditate on your breath for one minute.

Phase 3. Sit in the easy pose, or in a chair, and grasp your shoulders with your hands. Your fingers should be in front and your thumbs should be in back. Your elbows will be pointed outward. Inhale deeply and twist to the left, repeating *Sat* to yourself, then exhale and twist to the right, saying *Nam.* Do this for one to two minutes, and then rest for one minute. As you rest, meditate with long, slow, deep breaths. Feel the energy you are creating.

Phase 4. Sit in the easy pose, or in a chair, and clench your hands together, with your fingers locked (as if you were doing an isometric exercise). Raise your hands to the level of your heart. Then, while the hands remain in place, lift your right elbow and lower your left elbow. This will create a seesaw motion. As you lift your right elbow, inhale; as you lift your left, exhale. Breathe powerfully with the movement. Repeat for one to three minutes, then exhale in the center, pull on your locked fingers, and relax for one minute.

Phase 5. Sit in the easy pose, with your legs crossed, and grasp your knees. If you're in a chair, just keep your hands on your knees. Keeping your elbows straight, flex your spine. Inhale as you pull your spine forward, and exhale as you thrust it back. Say *Sat* to yourself as you inhale, and *Nam* as you exhale. Do this repeatedly for one to three minutes. Relax deeply for one minute as you meditate.

Phase 6. Sit in the easy pose, or in a chair, and shrug your shoulders upward as you inhale deeply, and downward as you exhale. Do this for one to two minutes, then inhale and hold your breath for fifteen seconds, with your shoulders pressed upward. Then relax your shoulders, and rest for one minute.

Phase 7. Sit in the easy pose, or in a chair and roll your head slowly to the right, all the way around. Do this five times, with long, slow, deep breathing. Then repeat the motion, rolling your neck to the left five times. Inhale, hold your breath, pull your neck straight, and bring the energy up. Exhale, and relax for one minute.

Phase 8. Sit in the easy pose, or in a chair, and lock the fingers of your two hands, as you did in Phase 4. This time, though, do it at throat level. Then raise your hands, still locked, above your head. Inhale, and apply the root lock. Exhale, and apply the root lock as you bring your hands down to the throat level. Repeat this cycle two more times, then relax for one minute.

Phase 9. Fold your legs under you and sit on your heels, or remain in your chair. If you can't sit on your heels, stay in the easy pose. Raise your arms over your head, and join your hands, with your two index fingers pointing toward the sky and the rest of your fingers locked together. Chant *Sat* out loud as you pull in your abdomen. Then chant *Nam* as you relax. Continue this for one to three minutes. Focus your concentration upward. Let the breath come on its own, naturally. Then inhale deeply, and apply the great lock as you squeeze energy and blood from the base of your spine to the top of your head. Hold your breath for fifteen seconds, exhale, and slowly sweep your arms down.

After the entire basic spinal energy series, relax on your back, legs apart, with your eyes closed, for five minutes. Place your arms at forty-five-degree angles, palms up. Cover yourself with a blanket to stay warm, and breathe deeply.

The spinal energy series is designed to bring the maximum amount of kundalini energy and blood to the brain. Therefore, you will almost certainly experience a sense of increased mental energy from it.

The Kirtan Kriya

The kirtan kriya meditation for creativity is excellent to do after the relaxation period that follows the basic spinal energy series. It celebrates the cycle of creation: birth, life, death, rebirth.

This kriya involves the chanting of the primal sounds that signify the stages of life. They are: *Sa*, which means "birth," "infinity," or "cosmos"; *Ta*, which means "life," or "existence"; *Na*, which means "death," or "completion"; and *Ma*, which means "rebirth."

Say each of these words repeatedly, in order: *Sa Ta Na Ma*. The *a* in these words is pronounced as a soft *a*, or *ah*.

Repeat this mantra while sitting with your spine straight, and your mental energy focused on the area of your brow, or forebrain. Yogis believe that this stimulates your pituitary. You can find this spot by rolling your eyes to the top, or root, of your nose.

For two minutes, chant in your normal voice, which yogis call the "voice of action." For the next two minutes, chant in a whisper, which yogis call the "voice of the lover." For the next three minutes, chant silently; the yogis call this "the divine language." Then reverse the order, whispering for two minutes and chanting the mantra out loud for two minutes, for a total of eleven minutes.

The *mudras*, or finger positions, are very important in this

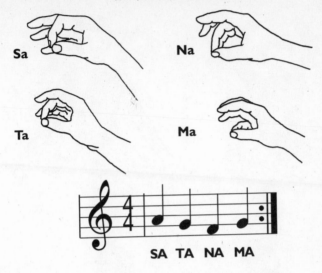

Figure 11
For the kirtan kriya, touching the fingertips in succession while chanting stimulates the brain and increases mental energy.

kriya. On *Sa*, touch the index fingers of each hand to your thumbs. On *Ta*, touch your middle fingers to your thumbs. On *Na*, touch your ring fingers to your thumbs. On *Ma*, touch your little fingers to your thumbs. (See illustration.)

To come out of the kriya, inhale very deeply, stretch your hands above your head, and then bring them down in a sweeping motion as you exhale.

In a short time, the kirtan kriya may well increase your intuition, creativity, and mental energy.

The Pineal Gland Kriya

Sit comfortably on the floor, with your legs crossed, or sit in a chair.

Raise your hands above your head, with your fingers locked. Try to pull the hands apart, while you take long, deep breaths, for one to two minutes. (See illustration 1, Figure 12.)

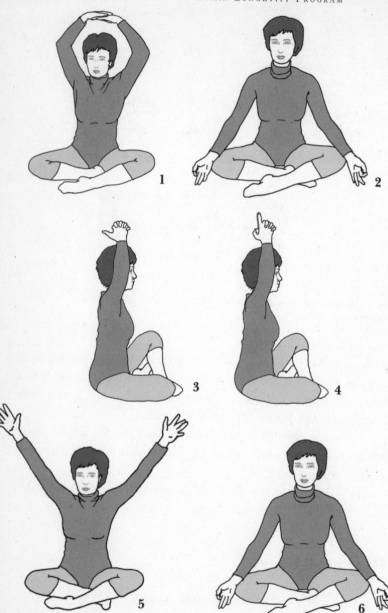

Figure 12

This kriya tonifies and activates the pineal gland. It produces an enhanced state of awareness, clarity, and the ability to focus.

Then bring your hands to your knees, and touch your index finger to your thumb, creating a small circle. This is called *Gyan mudra.* Extend your other three fingers, with your palms facing away from you. In this position, meditate for one minute. (See illustration 2.)

Raise your hands over your head, with your fingers intertwined and your thumbs apart (pointing behind you). Hold this position for one to two minutes, as you breathe deeply. (See illustration 3.) Then meditate for one minute with your hands again on your knees, in the same position as before.

Extend your arms over your head, with your fingers clasped and your two index fingers extended, pointing toward the sky. Pull your hands apart, but resist the pull. As you pull on your hands, breathe deeply for one to two minutes. (See illustration 4.)

Raise your arms at your sides, at about a sixty-degree angle. Spread your fingers wide apart and do the Breath of Fire for three minutes. (See illustration 5.)

Bring your hands to your knees, with your thumb and index fingers touching, your palms forward, and your other three fingers extended. Meditate by focusing out the top of your head for three to eleven minutes. (See illustration 6.)

An Exercise to Increase Blood Flow to the Brain

Yogis believe that this exercise (Figure 13) not only increases blood flow to the brain but also enhances overall cognitive function and stimulates proper function of the endocrine system. Musical conductors are known for their longevity, and practicing arm aerobics like the following is certainly a contributing factor.

Sit in the easy pose, or in a chair, with your arms out to your sides and your fingers pulled back from your palms and tensed, as if they were claws. Raise your arms and cross them over your head (alternating right over left, left over right), then bring them back down to your sides. Repeat this motion powerfully and rhythmically, as you begin to do the Breath of Fire, coordinating one inhale and exhale with each movement of your arms. Continue without stopping for three minutes, then thrust your tongue out

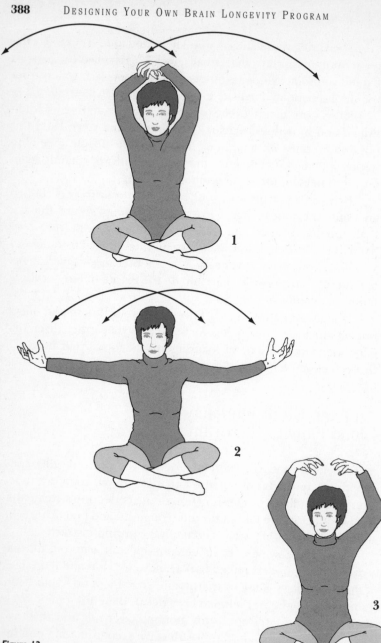

Figure 13
This exercise will help drive blood to the brain
and facilitate cognitive function.

as far as it will go and continue the movement for fifteen more seconds. Then inhale and hold your arms up at a sixty-degree angle for fifteen seconds. Exhale, and repeat. Then inhale again and hold the position for fifteen seconds. Exhale and relax by meditating or listening to music for three to four minutes. Then breathe long and gently for three to four minutes.

After concluding mind/body exercises, kundalini yoga practitioners usually recite, or sing, a simple poem:

> May the longtime sun shine upon you,
> All love surround you,
> And the pure light within you
> Guide your way on.

After you repeat this poem two times, inhale deeply and chant *Sat Nam* three times.

You have now learned the basic exercises that I most often recommend to patients. I am convinced that if you include any of them in your daily regime, they will become one of the foundations of your brain longevity program. Start with the basic spinal energy series and kirtan kriya.

There is only one element of your brain longevity program that we have not yet discussed: pharmacology. This is an exciting time in the field of neurology, because many new pharmaceutical nootropic drugs are now being introduced. Quite possibly, one of those drugs will help you to achieve optimal cognitive function and brain longevity.

A Case in Point

Anyone Can Benefit from Mind/Body Exercises

It may seem to you that the mind/body exercises would be more readily embraced by esoterically inclined patients who have already had experience with Eastern healing modalities. But this is not the case. Some of my most traditional, conservative patients have become the biggest supporters of the mind/body exercises.

S.M. is such a patient.

S.M., fifty-four years old, came to me complaining of severe short-term memory loss, and depression. She had to bring a tape recorder to her initial consultation with me, because without it she would have forgotten most of what I told her. Her memory had deteriorated to the point where her thoughts, as she put it, "went in one ear and out the other."

She was afraid she might have early-onset Alzheimer's, because her mother and her aunt had suffered from the disease. It was unclear, however, even after testing, whether her problem was indeed Alzheimer's or just severe age-associated memory impairment.

It was quite possible that S.M. did not have a genetic predisposition for Alzheimer's. Perhaps, instead, the illness of her aunt and mother had contributed to her memory loss by causing her a tremendous amount of stress. S.M. had served both her aunt and her mother as a caregiver, and that role can be excruciatingly stress-provoking, especially if the caregiver is deeply attached to the patient.

S.M. had also recently been hit by another stressor—her business. She helped manage a large farm in Florida, and had recently experienced two years of serious crop failure caused by freezing. According to S.M., the stress from this had exacerbated her mental decline.

She had been treated with antidepressants, but they had been of little help in alleviating her depression.

S.M. began an essentially standard brain longevity program. Her program, however, included supplementation with phosphatidyl serine, and administration of the hormonal agent pregnenolone. She also took 1 mg nightly of melatonin, for insomnia.

From the outset, she enthusiastically embraced the mind/body exercises. As a self-described "country girl," she found these exercises a new experience. She had never done any form of yoga, or participated in any type of "New Age" activity. Nonetheless, after I explained the exercises to her, she had no resistance at all to doing them. Her only interest was in feeling better. And the exercises *did* make her feel better, almost immediately.

After two months, she had no remaining clinical depression, even though she had discontinued use of her antidepressant. She told me that she felt "on top of the world." She also told me, "It's a new feeling for me to feel great all the time. Finally, at fifty-four, I love life."

Her memory improved dramatically after less than six months on her program.

Some of her improvement probably stemmed from her relief from depression, because clinical depression is often a major contributor to memory loss. Some of her improvement also probably came from her use of phosphatidyl serine and pregnenolone. But part of it—*much* of it—probably came from S.M. herself, who was wise enough not to reject the mind/body exercises just because they were a new concept for her.

19

The Pharmacology of Brain Regeneration

One dark night, R.L., forty-nine years of age, was supposed to meet her grade-school child on a street corner. But R.L., who had begun to suffer from age-associated memory impairment, couldn't remember which corner to go to.

By the time she finally found the right corner, her daughter had been standing there alone for half an hour.

The experience frightened R.L's daughter, and it frightened R.L. even more. As a single mother, R.L. knew that she could not allow her declining memory to compromise her parental responsibilities, but she did not know what to do about her memory loss. Her family physician offered no therapeutic program.

R.L.'s mother had died of Alzheimer's, and R.L. was afraid that she was beginning to experience symptoms similar to those of her mother. She could no longer hold seven-digit phone numbers in her "working memory," and she had to carry a very detailed list of her daily activities. If she lost the list, she was often unable to remember what she had planned to do.

Her memory loss was taking a toll on her self-esteem. Even

though she had worked as a professional all of her adult life, she had begun to see herself as unintelligent.

Shortly after the experience of forgetting where to meet her daughter, she heard about my work from another doctor, and began a brain longevity program under my supervision. One aspect of her program, which I believed was especially important for her, was use of deprenyl, to build higher levels of dopamine and "rescue" damaged neurons from further deterioration and death.

Pharmaceutical drugs compose the fourth and final pillar of my brain longevity programs. Many of my patients are unable to achieve full brain regeneration without pharmaceutical medication. R.L. was one such patient.

She responded quickly and dramatically to her multimodality program. She soon regained her ability to remember phone numbers, and she no longer needed a detailed list to remind her of her daily activities. Her self-esteem soared.

After about two years on her program, R.L. ran out of deprenyl, and chose not to refill her prescription immediately. She believed that she had fully recovered from her cognitive decline, and she thought that if she carefully adhered to the other elements of her program, she could easily get by for a few weeks without deprenyl.

She quickly discovered, however, that deprenyl was a vital component of her ongoing recovery. While on a short trip, she tried to call a close friend, whose number she had long before memorized. But she couldn't remember the number. Then she tried to call another number she had also previously memorized, and found that she had forgotten that number, too.

After discontinuing deprenyl, she later told me, her memory had become "generally a lot foggier."

When she got home from her trip, she refilled her prescription. Her memory problems improved almost immediately, and she once again became her "new self."

That was the last time R.L. ever neglected to take her nootropic medication.

*　　　*　　　*

Deprenyl: The Memory Drug

In the 1950s, during the initial blossoming of interest in medications for cognitive and emotional function, a Hungarian doctor who was experimenting with antidepressants developed deprenyl. The doctor, Jozsef Knoll, M.D., a university professor, referred to his new drug as a "psychic energizer."

Deprenyl, Dr. Knoll discovered, was capable of protecting dopamine, the important neurotransmitter that is needed for normal muscular control, for sex drive, for immunity, and for cognition. Deprenyl, as Dr. Knoll found, protects dopamine by interfering with the chemical that *breaks down* dopamine: monoamine oxidase-B. Deprenyl, a monoamine oxidase-B (or MAO-B) inhibitor, keeps the neurotransmitter from becoming depleted.

Deprenyl's ability to counteract MAO-B is valuable for Alzheimer's patients, because they almost always have higher amounts of MAO-B than other elderly people.

Deprenyl also stimulates the part of the brain where dopamine-producing neurons are especially abundant. Thus deprenyl not only protects dopamine that already exists, but also helps the brain to produce more of it.

Protecting dopamine is important for almost all older people, because dopamine commonly declines during the aging process. In most people, this decline amounts to about 13 percent per decade, beginning at age forty to forty-five. Even in healthy people, a decline of about 50 percent usually occurs by age eighty.

If dopamine declines at a significantly faster rate, however, the results can be disastrous. When dopamine levels fall to about 30 percent of the full, youthful levels, the result is Parkinson's disease. Parkinson's is characterized by an extreme shortage of dopamine. When dopamine levels fall to 10 percent of the youthful, healthy levels, the Parkinson's patient generally dies.

Even if dopamine levels never decline to the disastrous 30-percent level, which indicates Parkinson's, *moderately* low levels of dopamine can still reduce quality of life. Moderately low levels can cause a gradual loss of coordination, trembling, and the uncertain gait that is typical of many elderly people.

Slightly low levels of dopamine, even in otherwise healthy people, decrease sex drive, lower immunity to disease, and impair cognitive function.

Deprenyl, however, helps stop the decline of dopamine. Besides protecting dopamine, deprenyl also helps protect other neurotransmitters, including norepinephrine and phenylethylamine (both of which are important to the intellect and the emotions). It also aids neuronal metabolism, and helps repair damaged and dying brain cells.

Understandably, the first disease to be treated with deprenyl was Parkinson's. Some physicians believe that deprenyl increases the life expectancy of Parkinson's patients, and generally improves their symptomatology. Studies also show that when deprenyl is used relatively early in the progression of Parkinson's, doctors can usually delay prescribing the medication L-dopa, which acts as a synthetic replacement for dopamine.

As deprenyl became a popular treatment for Parkinson's, physicians noted that it not only improved the physical symptoms of the disease, but also improved cognitive symptoms, which strike about 25 percent of all Parkinson's patients. When Parkinson's patients with cognitive dysfunction took deprenyl, they generally suffered less memory loss, fewer concentration problems, and less depression.

After observing these improvements in cognitive and emotional function in Parkinson's patients, some doctors began prescribing deprenyl to their Alzheimer's patients.

Much of the clinical use of deprenyl for Alzheimer's disease has occurred in Europe, where physicians tend to be somewhat more knowledgeable about nootropic drugs. Many American doctors, however, have also prescribed deprenyl for Alzheimer's. Clinical studies indicate that deprenyl can be of significant value to Alzheimer's patients.

In one six-month, double-blind study of Alzheimer's patients, deprenyl showed the ability to increase verbal memory. On memory tests, including a "delayed recall" test, Alzheimer's patients on deprenyl did about 400 percent better than Alzheimer's patients taking a placebo.

In another study, conducted by the National Institutes of Health, Alzheimer's patients taking deprenyl showed improved memory, and improved ability to focus. Because of this improvement in focus and memory, these patients also experienced a significant increase in learning ability, and in ability to process complex information.

Another study showed that after just six days of treatment, deprenyl reduced MAO-B activity in the brains of Alzheimer's patients by 90 percent. This same study revealed that deprenyl not only deterred the destruction of dopamine, but also stopped production of the neurotoxin MPTP, which contributes to long-term brain degeneration. In this study, patients on deprenyl performed considerably better on tests that measured word fluency, recall, and ability to copy a drawing from memory, than did patients on a placebo.

A study presented at the Fourth International Congress on the Advances in Alzheimer's Disease showed that, over a five-year period, Alzheimer's patients treated with deprenyl degenerated at a much slower rate than an untreated control group.

As a clinician, I have found that medications that boost cognitive power in Alzheimer's patients generally have an even more dramatic effect on patients who suffer from only mild to moderate memory impairment. My Alzheimer's patients certainly appear to benefit from deprenyl, but the most obvious and profound effects are generally exhibited by my patients with mild to moderate age-associated memory impairment. Furthermore, in patients with mild to moderate memory loss, improvements in memory are often equaled or surpassed by improvements in concentration, cognitive processing speed, and ability to process complex information.

One of the important secondary benefits of deprenyl is its ability to improve sex drive. For many people, the common diminution of sex drive at about age fifty is as disconcerting as hitting the "memory barrier" at that age. When both problems strike at approximately the same time, it feels like the "end of youth" to many people.

Deprenyl increases sex drive primarily by enhancing levels of dopamine, which is a major biochemical factor in sex drive, particularly in males. It also increases levels of *phenylethylamine*, the stimulating brain chemical that is often at its peak when a person is in the first exciting stages of love. Phenylethylamine, or PEA, causes the classic symptoms of being "lovesick": loss of appetite, difficulty sleeping, and euphoria. Some researchers call PEA the "love hormone."

It's quite possible that increased levels of both dopamine and phenylethylamine contribute to the heightened sexual arousal that frequently occurs when people take deprenyl. In addition, deprenyl increases levels of stimulating norepinephrine, and this may also contribute to increased sexual vigor.

In fact, about twenty years ago, some of the first reports about deprenyl that appeared in the lay press focused on its effect upon sex drive. The first highly circulated article about the drug said that it caused an eighty-year-old Parkinson's patient to "chase his nurse around the bed."

A less sensational effect of deprenyl, but one that is much more important to many patients, is its ability to vastly improve symptoms of clinical depression. Deprenyl seems particularly effective for depression when the medication is administered in conjunction with phenylalanine, the nutritional precursor of norepinephrine.

One study showed that deprenyl and phenylalanine, used together, achieved a "full recovery" in 65 percent of patients who were suffering from clinical unipolar depression. Another 21 percent of patients achieved "moderate improvement." Only 6 percent did not improve.

In another study, 60 percent of patients diagnosed with "drug-resistant major depressive disorders" achieved complete relief from depression after less than one week on a course of deprenyl, phenylalanine (1,000 to 6,000 mg daily), and vitamin B6 (100 mg daily). These patients had been suffering from a variety of serious depressive illnesses, including bipolar type II depression, schizoaffective disorder, seasonal affective disorder, and re-current unipolar depression.

In my own practice, I have also observed mood-related im-provements in patients who did not have clinical depression, but who suffered from occasional, mild depressive symptoms, such as low energy, diminished willpower, and mild mood disorders.

I have also seen deprenyl have a very positive effect on the energy levels and moods of people with *no* depressive symptoms. Patients who are generally healthy, but who are suffering from mild memory loss, typically respond to deprenyl with *increased* en-ergy and vitality. Often they achieve remarkable levels of energy and zest for life. Their renewed levels of energy are similar to the energy levels of much younger people.

In fact, when administering deprenyl, I have found that the primary negative side effect of the drug is that it can create too *much* energy. If too much deprenyl is taken, the patient some-times experiences insomnia, and a sensation of being overstimu-lated. Some people, especially those with very demanding jobs, *like* this abundance of energy, but other people find it annoying.

Therefore, I generally start patients on very low dosages of deprenyl, and increase the dosage gradually. If the patient begins to feel overstimulated, I reduce the dosage. I often tailor the dosage to the patient's age, giving more to older people.

Frequently, if the patient is less than fifty years old, and has only mild memory impairment, I prescribe only 1 mg of deprenyl, to be taken twice weekly. This is a very cautious dosage, but, as you have probably noticed, I tend to prescribe very conservatively. I prefer to support the body's own natural functions, so that it can "solve its own problems." Furthermore, the other elements of my brain longevity programs increase patients' responses to medica-tions.

If my patient is fifty to fifty-five years old, and exhibits mod-erate symptoms of cognitive decline, I might prescribe 1 to 2 mg, three times per week. If the patient is fifty-five to sixty, with *ele-vated* cognitive impairment, I might prescribe 2 to 3 mg daily. If the patient has early symptoms of Alzheimer's, I often prescribe more aggressively.

In all three of the studies I mentioned, the Alzheimer's patients on deprenyl were receiving 10 mg daily. This dosage would be notably overstimulating to most young, healthy people, but it can easily be tolerated by most Alzheimer's patients.

Deprenyl is very safe, so there is little need to worry about side effects. In animal experiments, deprenyl's lethal dose (or LD-50) was found to be three hundred to five hundred times greater than the amount needed to *completely halt* production of MAO-B. Humans have tolerated up to 60 mg daily with no significant side effects. *More* deprenyl, however, is not necessarily better than *less* deprenyl. Like most drugs, it is most effective when used at the proper dosage, rather than the highest possible dosage.

As I mentioned, I tend to prescribe somewhat lower dosages of deprenyl and other medications, because the other aspects of my brain longevity programs increase the effectiveness of medications. For example, deprenyl has been proven to be more effective, at least for depression, when it is taken with phenylalanine. And, as you'll recall, I recommend adequate phenylalanine intake to all of my patients, as part of their nutritional therapy programs.

If a patient were to receive deprenyl as his or her *only* therapy, more of the drug would probably be needed. But I do not practice that type of single-modality medicine, because I consider it to be simplistic, lazy, and ineffective.

Deprenyl can be prescribed by any physician. However, the Food and Drug Administration has not approved it as a treatment for Alzheimer's or other memory disorders. Therefore, the drug company that makes it is prohibited from disseminating information to doctors about treating memory problems with it. Because of this, many physicians are still not very well informed about deprenyl as a treatment for Alzheimer's, as a treatment for other memory disorders, or as a general anti-aging medication.

Even though deprenyl, along with Vitamin E, is currently under investigation as a drug for preventing Alzheimer's, it is not likely that a major drug company will soon attempt to have deprenyl approved as an Alzheimer's treatment, because the testing necessary for this approval would cost about $200 million. The drug company that owns the patent on deprenyl has little finan-cial incentive to do this, because it already has the right to sell the product.

You should not be surprised if your family doctor knows very little about the use of deprenyl for memory disorders. Even many neurologists, I have found, are only casually informed about the use of deprenyl for improving memory.

DHEA: The Youth Hormone

I think the steroid hormone DHEA (or dehydroepiandrosterone) may soon be touted as society's new all-around "wonder drug." It is already being promoted as the hot new pharmaceutical "magic bullet" that will make you smarter, thinner, healthier, and forever young.

The hyperbole bothers me. DHEA is indeed a wondrous compound, and it deserves all the attention it can get. But to as-sume that it will do *everything* for you—and that you will no longer have to do *anything* for yourself—is misguided thinking. DHEA is no more a "magic bullet" than deprenyl is. But it can be an ex-tremely important and valuable weapon in your arsenal of brain longevity medications.

DHEA is called the body's "mother steroid hormone," be-cause it is a precursor steroidal hormone that can be converted into *other* steroid hormones, including estrogen and testosterone.

DHEA is the most abundant steroid in the bloodstream, and can be found throughout the body. DHEA is, however, 6.5 times more concentrated in your neurons than in your blood—pre-sumably because your brain needs the protection that the hor-mone offers.

Alzheimer's patients, however, invariably have much lower levels of DHEA than do non–Alzheimer's patients of the same age. One study indicated that Alzheimer's patients had 48 percent less DHEA than a matched control group.

Virtually all people achieve their peak levels of DHEA in their mid-twenties, and then their production begins to decline.

By the time you hit seventy, you will probably only have about 10 percent as much DHEA as you did in your twenties.

Because DHEA is an adrenal steroidal hormone, it is part of the body's response mechanism to stress. Generally, stress depletes DHEA. In fact, many clinicians monitor DHEA levels as a measure of long-term stress. If DHEA levels are low, it can indicate that the patient has suffered long-term, chronic stress.

As you know, stress usually causes an increase in the stress hormone cortisol. Thus, as a rule, if cortisol levels are high, DHEA levels are low.

Besides helping to maintain proper neurological function, DHEA appears to have a very broad range of positive effects. It is widely believed that DHEA slows the biological symptoms of aging, and helps protect the body from cancer, diabetes, arthritis, osteoporosis, obesity, viral and bacterial infection, and hypertension. Therefore it is understandable that many researchers regard DHEA as a "wonder drug."

In one impressive study, 242 men aged fifty to seventy-nine were monitored for their DHEA levels, and then their health was tracked for twelve years. Those with the highest levels of DHEA had the best long-term health, even if they smoked and had high cholesterol. For every 20-percent *increase* in DHEA levels in these men, there was a 48-percent *decrease* in heart disease, and a 36-percent decrease in death from *any* cause.

Besides helping to prevent disease, DHEA enhances the general quality of life. A great many of my patients who take DHEA in oral tablets tell me that they feel younger and more energetic than they did previously, and enjoy a generally improved mood.

This improvement in mood was reflected by a study done at a University of California medical school. In this study, 67 percent of men and 84 percent of women taking DHEA reported a substantial increase in perceived psychological and physical well-being. The subjects reported improved ability to handle stress, to sleep, and to relax. They also reported considerable increases in energy.

Many of my patients also report to me that DHEA has enabled them to lose weight. This probably occurs because of

DHEA's ability to stabilize blood glucose levels, as well as its ability to stimulate the thermogenic "burning" of fat, and to control appetite.

For women who are experiencing menopause—which can affect emotional well-being and cognitive function—DHEA can be helpful as a component of hormonal replacement therapy.

In the brain, DHEA acts as a growth factor, helping neurons to sprout new dendrites. It also helps the brain by controlling levels of cortisol.

Studies uniformly indicate that administration of DHEA improves memory and cognitive processing. However, the primary evidence that has persuaded me of DHEA's neurological efficacy has been the response of my own patients.

Dosage levels of DHEA depend largely upon the existing levels of DHEA in the patient's blood, prior to treatment. My approach is to prescribe a dosage of DHEA that will return DHEA levels to approximately the same levels as those of a healthy person in his or her mid-twenties. This dosage range can vary from 25 mg to 200 mg daily. The 200-mg dosage would be for an elderly person whose DHEA levels had been almost totally decimated, or for a person with severe chronic fatigue syndrome. A common dosage is 50 mg daily.

To determine what the dosage should be, I have existing DHEA levels determined by laboratory testing. Three different lab tests can determine the levels of DHEA—a twenty-four-hour urine test, a blood test, and a saliva test. I generally prefer to use the blood test (although I am investigating the use of the less invasive saliva test).

DHEA is an extremely safe hormone. Because it is a precursor to the steroid hormones, it has none of the many dangerous side effects associated with fully formed steroids, unless it is taken in gross excess over a long period of time. Up to 1,600 mg daily have been taken in short-term administration without side effects. In *extremely* high dosages over an extended period, however, DHEA can have a mild, temporary masculinizing effect upon females, causing increased growth of facial hair, and acne. Also, because DHEA elevates male hormones, it is not an appropriate drug for men who have prostate cancer.

Before you begin DHEA replacement therapy, you should consult your doctor. To determine your proper dosage, your doctor will want to have your current levels checked. You should also get a complete biochemical profile, including an assessment of your liver function. Men should also get a PSA blood test (which evaluates prostate function), and a prostate examination. (I recommend to my male patients over fifty that they consider taking saw palmetto berries, a prostate-protecting herb.)

Recently, low-strength formulations of DHEA have begun to appear in some health food stores and mail-order catalogs, but I believe it is unwise to use this medication without the supervision of a doctor. Currently, some young bodybuilders are taking over-the-counter DHEA indiscriminately. Because young people *already* have optimal levels of DHEA, this use poses a potentially dangerous risk.

Like deprenyl, DHEA may be somewhat unfamiliar to many doctors, even though it has been available for many years. It is not a product that can be patented, so drug companies do not have a significant financial incentive to inform doctors about it.

You should not be discouraged if the first doctor you consult about DHEA is poorly informed about it. Patients often seem to expect all doctors to know "everything about everything," but that is simply not a realistic expectation.

If you are diligent, you will be able to find a doctor who is fully conversant with DHEA. Perhaps some of the informational agencies listed in the "Resources and Referrals" appendix will help you to find a doctor who is knowledgeable about DHEA and other cognitive-enhancement medications.

Pregnenolone: The "Memory and Mood Hormone"

Pregnenolone, like DHEA, is a precursor hormone, one from which other hormones are derived. Pregnenolone, however, sits at the very top of the "hormonal cascade": *All* other steroidal hormones, including DHEA, are made from pregnenolone.

Pregnenolone is synthesized directly from cholesterol. Large amounts of pregnenolone are produced in the brain and the peripheral nerves. Because pregnenolone is produced by the brain, it's sometimes called a *neurohormone*.

Because pregnenolone is the source of other hormones, it is used by the body to fulfill the body's constantly changing hormonal needs. Therefore, it is often referred to as an *adaptogen*.

As you know, Eastern medicine places great value on substances that enable the body to adapt to change. Thus pregnenolone is somewhat similar to the highly prized Asian adaptogens, such as ginseng.

Because pregnenolone is used in various ways, according to the "wisdom of the body," it can have a wide range of effects. It can, for example, stimulate the brain—by increasing the uptake of glutamate—and it can also *calm* the brain, by activating the receptors of the sedating neurotransmitter GABA. Pregnenolone is used for whatever the body needs most, at the moment.

Pregnenolone, according to animal experiments, also has the ability to extend lifespan, increase resistance to some cancers (particularly breast cancer), and reduce the tendency to obesity.

In addition, pregnenolone helps protect against arthritis. In fact, pregnenolone was first developed as an anti-arthritis agent, in the 1930s. Gradually, however, it was replaced as an arthritis drug by synthetic anti-inflammatory steroids.

Pregnenolone also improves the transmission of impulses among neurons, and therefore has a positive effect upon memory and cognitive processing.

Many researchers believe that pregnenolone is the most powerful memory-enhancing hormone. Although only a limited number of studies and experiments have been done on its cognitive-enhancement properties, those that have been done support the efficacy of the substance. For example, in one experiment, mice treated with pregnenolone showed a dramatic increase in their abilities to navigate a maze.

In a human study, pilots given pregnenolone improved their abilities to control a flight simulator. In the first phase of this study, when the pilots were given a placebo, they achieved perfect scores on the flight simulator 20 to 35 percent of the time. In the second phase, when they were given pregnenolone, they achieved perfect scores on the flight simulator 35 to 50 percent of the time.

In a study of the relationship between pregnenolone levels and mood, it was discovered that patients with depression typically have low levels of pregnenolone. The average level of pregnenolone in one group of people with clinical depression was just one-half as high as the average level in a group of people with no depression.

In my own practice, I have observed improvements in both memory and mood when patients began taking pregnenolone. One elderly patient, who had begun her program without pregnenolone, but who added it later, told me that the hormone helped her to feel "happy again, like I did when I was young." Another very elderly patient credited pregnenolone with restoring her ability to maintain her train of thought.

Dosage levels vary from patient to patient. A reasonable starting point is 50 mg per day. If that dosage elicits no discernible response in three months, it can be increased, upon advice of your doctor, up to 75 mg daily. (Some patients take as much as 100 mg daily.)

Pregnenolone has no significant reported side effects of which I am aware. It may be purchased without a prescription but, like all powerful medications, it should only be used while under the care of a physician.

Piracetam:
The "Creativity and Learning Drug"

Piracetam is a fascinating and valuable drug that benefits not only cognitively impaired patients, but also people who have no cognitive dysfunction.

Piracetam helps improve the function of the brain's cholinergic system, the primary conduit of thought and memory. As you'll recall, the cholinergic system primarily employs the neurotransmitter acetylcholine. *All* of the modalities I've mentioned in this book that improve acetylcholine function are good for memory and thought.

Piracetam enhances acetylcholine function because it is derived from a substance called *pyrrolidine*, which boosts the metabolism of the neurons that manufacture acetylcholine. Another substance that also has this ability is the amino acid *pyroglutamate*, which is found in meat, vegetables, and dairy products. Piracetam is very similar to pyroglutamate in its chemical structure.

Because the primary function of piracetam is to stimulate the cholinergic system, it works best when it is taken along with other substances that also stimulate the cholingeric system. These substances include phosphatidyl choline (derived from lecithin), and DMAE, both of which I described in detail in chapter 13.

In addition, there are pharmaceutical drugs that increase the effectiveness of piracetam. These drugs, which also boost the cholingeric system, include lucidryl and Hydergine. Both are described later in this chapter.

Because piracetam stimulates production of acetylcholine, it helps to keep the brain from "cannibalizing" itself by digesting the choline in its own cells.

Piracetam not only increases the amount of acetylcholine that is produced, but also increases the number of cholinergic receptors in the brain. In one animal experiment, piracetam increased the density of cholinergic receptors by 30 to 40 percent.

Piracetam also helps the brain by enhancing general neuronal metabolism. It does this by increasing the amount of the energy-producing substance called ATP (adenosine triphosphate), which is found in all neurons.

One other beneficial effect of piracetam is that it improves neuronal glucose metabolism. This can be very helpful to people enduring chronic stress, because the stress hormone cortisol interferes with neuronal glucose metabolism.

Several studies indicate that piracetam is valuable for Alzheimer's patients. Piracetam significantly slows the *progression* of the disease. This, of course, can be extremely beneficial to Alzheimer's patients, because it can spare them the horrible final stages of advanced Alzheimer's.

One year-long study examined the effects of piracetam on a group of patients with early Alzheimer's. These patients were given a high dosage (8 grams daily), and were tested at the beginning and end of the year. A control group of patients, given a placebo, showed the usual evidence of mental deterioration during that year. The group taking piracetam, however, showed significantly less mental decline.

Because the researchers conducting this study were trying to determine the effectiveness of just piracetam, no other substance, such as choline, was administered to the patients along with the piracetam. It is probable that if adjunctive substances had been administered, the results would have been even more dramatic.

In another study, reported in the *New England Journal of Medicine*, choline *was* given to patients, along with piracetam. In this study, which lasted only seven days, ten Alzheimer's patients were given 4.8 grams of piracetam daily, along with 9 grams of choline. According to the researchers, three of the ten patients experienced "marked improvement." The three patients who improved scored 70 percent higher in verbal memory tests, compared to their test scores before taking piracetam.

This study seems to indicate that piracetam plus choline can not only slow Alzheimer's progression, but cause improvement. The study certainly does not *prove* this, however. Perhaps, over a longer period of time, the rate of improvement would have leveled off, or stopped.

In another fascinating study, researchers tested piracetam on elderly people who did *not* have Alzheimer's. They found that the subjects who took piracetam significantly improved their scores on tests of cognitive function, while subjects taking a placebo did not improve. This study indicates that piracetam can be of value to healthy older people.

Another study tested the value of piracetam on healthy *young* people. All of the test subjects were university students in excellent physical and mental health. The students took cognitive-function tests before the administration of piracetam, and then were tested again after two weeks of daily ingestion of 1,200 mg of piracetam. The students did significantly better after taking piracetam.

Piracetam has helped a wide cross-section of patients throughout the world. It has apparently been beneficial for some patients with early Alzheimer's, and also for patients who have only mild memory impairment.

The most unusual and intriguing aspect of piracetam is its apparent ability to better "connect" the two hemispheres of the brain. For reasons that are not clearly understood, piracetam seems to improve the function of the corpus callosum, the network of nerve fibers that coordinates the functions of the left and right hemispheres.

Here's how researchers determined that piracetam helps the corpus callosum. As you probably know, the right side of the brain controls the left side of the body, and vice versa. That's why a person who has a stroke on the right side of his or her brain may become paralyzed on the left side of his or her body.

Similarly, most information that you hear in your left ear travels to the hearing center in the right side of your brain, and most information that you hear in your right ear travels to the hearing center in the left side of your brain.

Language, however, is, for the most part, processed in the left side of the brain. Therefore, when language comes in through your left ear, it goes to your right hemisphere first, and then has to be relayed to the left hemisphere by your corpus callosum. But when language comes in through your *right* ear, it goes straight to your left hemisphere, and doesn't require the relay through the corpus callosum. When language has to go through the "relay," it's a harder task for the brain, and sometimes some of the message gets "lost in shipping." Because of this, most people prefer to talk on the phone with their right ear to the receiver. That way, what they hear is sent directly to their left hemisphere's language center.

Researchers have discovered that when people take piracetam, they have a markedly improved ability to process language that comes in through their "weak" left ear. This suggests that piracetam stimulates the corpus callosum, since most language that comes in through the left ear has to be relayed via the corpus callosum.

Apparently because of piracetam's benefit to the corpus callosum, it is an effective treatment for dyslexia, which is characterized by poor mental coordination between the two hemispheres. In one double-blind study of two hundred dyslexic children, aged seven to twelve, children receiving piracetam showed significant improvement in reading fluency, and in memory. Another study indicated that piracetam helped dyslexic children to improve their reading speed and writing abilities.

Because piracetam aids the "integrative action" of the two hemispheres, it is popular among creative people, such as writers and artists—particularly in Europe, where the drug is most widely used. Writers and artists who take the drug report that it increases their creativity. Conceptually this makes sense, because creativity is closely linked to effective coordination of the "logical left brain" and the "emotional right brain."

Piracetam has also been shown to be an effective treatment for hypoxia, or oxygen starvation of the brain. Therefore it might benefit people who smoke, or who have incurred hypoxia from some other cause.

The dosage range of piracetam depends upon the patient's age, and upon his or her mental status. The 8 grams given to Alzheimer's patients in the first study that I mentioned would be far too much for a healthy person. A healthy young person, seeking only to optimize his or her cognitive function, might do best at about 500 to 600 mg daily, or every other day. An older person with mild to moderate memory impairment might get the best results from a dosage of about 1,000 to 2,000 mg daily.

Piracetam is a very safe drug, with no known serious side effects. No toxic symptoms from piracetam have ever been reported. If a large dosage is taken, though, the patient may feel overstimulated, and may develop insomnia. If this occurs, the dosage should be scaled back until the insomnia goes away.

Despite its wide use throughout the world for many years, piracetam has not been approved by the U.S. Food and Drug Administration.

Under certain circumstances, it may be permissible to import medications that have not been approved in the United States, as long as you comply with all applicable laws and regulations, including federal, state, and local laws. Restrictions on the importation of unapproved drugs include, for example, requirements that the drugs be for personal use, that they be imported in relatively small quantities, that they not pose unreasonable or significant safety risks, and that they be for a serious condition for which there is no satisfactory treatment available in this country.

Remember that the FDA approves drugs on the basis of scientific data evaluating their safety and effectiveness, and such drugs are labeled with information designed to maximize their efficacy and minimize harmful side effects. Imported drugs may be of unknown quality and may have been subject to inadequate testing.

I recommend that you not take any drugs—especially non–FDA approved drugs—without the advice and supervision of a physician who is familiar with your particular health care needs.

Other Cognitive-Enhancement Drugs

Following are several of the other most promising drugs for increasing cognitive function.

Melatonin. A nonprescription drug, melatonin is the hormone secreted by the pineal gland that helps control sleep cycles. As I have mentioned, melatonin production declines with age.

Tests have shown that people taking melatonin fall asleep significantly faster than people who do not take it, and that they enjoy a longer and deeper sleep. Some studies indicate that melatonin is effective in up to 80 percent of cases of insomnia.

Melatonin is also an extremely powerful antioxidant, and helps prevent free-radical damage from fatty acids (which is a primary cause of brain aging).

Other studies indicate that melatonin boosts immune activity, and that it can help prevent a wide range of illnesses, including cancer.

Some melatonin advocates recommend dosages of 3 to even 20 mg each evening. Because I always take a conservative approach to medication, I advise my patients with insomnia to use only 1 to 3 mg. If insomnia is still a problem at this dosage range, the dosage may be increased. Many of my patients who meditate require lower dosages than people who do not meditate, because people who meditate produce more melatonin.

Melatonin boosts cognitive function by helping to regulate natural sleep rhythms. If sleep cycles, or *circadian rhythms*, are chronically disrupted, it can impair memory by interfering with the organization of memory, some of which is believed to occur during sleep. In experiments, subjects have suffered from amnesiac episodes when their circadian rhythms were systematically interrupted.

Furthermore, a good night's sleep is necessary for any high-level cognition.

Melatonin levels are generally lower in Alzheimer's patients than in age-matched healthy subjects. At this point, there is no definitive research indicating that melatonin is valuable therapeutically for Alzheimer's, but some research indicates that it does hold some promise for Alzheimer's patients.

However, melatonin can have a valuable indirect effect upon Alzheimer's patients because it can help restore normal sleep patterns, which better allows patients to function at their highest possible cognitive levels. Further, when patients sleep well, they do not disturb their caregivers with frequent late-night disruptions.

Recently, a number of books have been published that fully describe the powerful, wide-ranging effects of melatonin. The best of these, in my opinion, is *Melatonin: Your Body's Natural Wonder Drug*, by Russel J. Reiter, Ph.D., and noted medical author Jo Robinson.

Two other drugs are sometimes incorporated into brain longevity programs, but I do not have any clinical experience with either of them. One is **Lucidril** (known generically as *centrophenoxine*), a widely used nootropic that may reduce the accumulation of age-associated pigmentation deposits on the brain. These deposits, called *lipofuscin*, are essentially the same as the pigmentation deposits, or "age spots," that often form on the skin of older people (particularly on the backs of the hands).

It has been clearly established that lipofuscin deposits on the brain contribute to cognitive impairment. As a rule, Alzheimer's patients have elevated levels of lipofuscin.

In animal experiments, it has been shown that by decreasing lipofuscin deposits, cognitive ability can be increased.

In more than one experiment, the memories of laboratory animals were improved significantly through administration of Lucidril.

Lucidril also enhances uptake of glucose. Therefore it can help the brain to overcome the disruption of glucose metabolism that is caused by cortisol.

Thus far, no studies indicate that Lucidril is effective for the treatment of Alzheimer's.

In the body, Lucidril breaks down into DMAE. As you'll recall from the chapter on nutritional tonics, DMAE increases cholinergic function.

Because DMAE can be somewhat stimulating to the central nervous system, some patients find Lucidril to be mildly stimulating. If taken in excess, it can cause insomnia.

Dosages of Lucidril generally range from 1,000 to 3,000 mg daily.

The other drug is **Vinpocetine** (generically called *vincamine*), a powerful enhancer of cerebral blood flow. It also stimulates neuronal metabolism, by encouraging production of ATP in the energy centers of brain cells.

Vinpocetine is a prescription drug that is derived from the periwinkle plant. It appears to have the ability to increase blood flow to the head, without decreasing blood flow to other parts of the body.

Vinpocetine is often prescribed for neurological problems caused by impaired circulation, such as stroke. It can be particularly valuable for multi-infarct dementia, which is often characterized by symptoms very similar to those of Alzheimer's.

Vinpocetine is also helpful for less serious neurological disorders that are sometimes linked to impaired cerebral circulation, such as recurrent dizziness, or headaches.

In addition, Vinpocetine, like *Ginko biloba* (which also increases cerebral circulation), is notably effective for certain ophthalmological disorders. One study showed that Vinpocetine increased visual acuity in 70 percent of subjects. It's quite possible that Vinpocetine, like *Ginko biloba*, will prove to be effective in helping to prevent progression of macular degeneration, the leading cause of late-onset blindness.

Similarly, certain ear problems linked to poor circulation seem to respond to Vinpocetine.

In one study of 882 patients with neurological disorders (including stroke and insufficient cerebral circulation), 62 percent responded to vinpocetine with significant improvement in condition. This study indicated that Vinpocetine was also helpful for minor mood disorders, including irritability and depression.

In a study of subjects in good physical and mental health, Vinpocetine dramatically increased short-term memory. Subjects did almost twice as well on recall tests after administration of the drug.

It also appears to enhance concentration in healthy people, and to help normalize concentration in people who have difficulty retaining focus.

If taken in very high dosages, Vinpocetine may cause increased heartbeat in some patients, as well as dry mouth. The usual dosage range is about 5 to 10 mg daily, depending upon the needs and reactions of the patient.

Vinpocetine is not sold in the United States.

Again, I have no clinical experience with Vinpocetine, but some of the reports of it in the medical literature are encouraging and intriguing.

Human growth hormone. This may prove to be another valuable weapon in your arsenal of brain longevity medications. Several of my patients report that it has helped them to feel better, to lose weight, and to think more clearly. Synthetic hGH is, however, considerably more expensive than the other pharmaceutical drugs that help rejuvenate the body and brain.

Recently, numerous reports in the lay press have credited synthetic hGH as a "fountain of youth." It has restored energy, leanness, high-level cognitive power, and strength to a number of people.

In one interesting study, hGH helped emphysema patients to gain weight and to increase muscular strength, and it improved their oxygen intake by 30 percent. The synthetic hormone has also shown positive results in osteoporosis patients.

Some studies suggest that hGH may be an appropriate medication for early Alzheimer's, but the research in this area is still incomplete. The probable neurological effect of hGH is a stimulation of new dendritic growth.

Very few of my patients have used synthetic hGH, because of its cost, but those who have used it have responded quite positively.

Tacrine. Currently approved by the FDA as a treatment for Alzheimer's, tacrine has shown positive results in a number of studies. Tacrine stimulates the cholingeric system by inhibiting an enzyme (cholinesterase) that breaks down acetylcholine.

Recent studies indicate that tacrine is more effective when used in conjunction with a choline product, such as lecithin.

I have never prescribed tacrine, however, because it has been shown to be toxic to the liver in some patients and is very frequently ineffective. In my opinion, other pharmaceutical and nutritional agents can more effectively achieve stimulation of the cholingeric system, without tacrine's negative side effects. A number of new drugs with greater benefit than tacrine and less toxicity are in various stages of development.

A new drug that was recently approved for Alzheimer's, called **Aricept,** may have fewer side effects. Like tacrine, Aricept inhibits the breakdown of acetylcholine.

Hydergine. Shown in a number of studies to be a somewhat effective treatment for slowing the progression of Alzheimer's, Hydergine, an extract of a fungus called ergot, has been used for many years to treat a wide range of senile dementias. It seems to be particularly effective for multi-infarct dementia.

Hydergine increases cerebral blood flow, aids the breakdown

of lipofuscin, is an effective antioxidant, and stimulates neuronal metabolism. It also appears to have properties similar to those of nerve growth hormone. It appears to be most effective when combined with administration of piracetam.

In the United States, the traditional dosage of hydergine is 3 mg daily. Studies indicate, however, that it is generally more effective at 9 mg daily, which is the standard dosage in Europe. In the one case in which I have prescribed it, I have achieved a more positive reaction at the higher dosage.

This concludes not only the information on medications, but also the information on the entire multifaceted brain longevity program.

Now only one thing remains: putting it all together. In the final chapter I'll tell you how to combine all of the various components of a brain longevity program.

Doing so may be easier than you think.

A Case in Point

With Difficult Cases, You Must Be Aggressive

When S.B., seventy-three, entered my office for his initial consultation, he cut a splendid figure. He was tall, thin, distinguished looking, and stood broomstick-straight. He had a shiny mantle of silver hair, and his eyes sparkled like two blue stars. But he was just a hollow shell, a great-looking guy who was withering inside.

S.B., who had until recently managed three different businesses in two countries, had been diminished by cognitive decline. He still presented the image of a successful businessman, but his career was over—sooner than he preferred.

S.B., my intake testing revealed, was suffering either from early Alzheimer's or from severe age-associated memory impairment. He did very poorly on the recall test in which I name three objects, and then ask the patient to recall the objects a few minutes later. He could generally only recall one of the objects. Also, an MRI revealed that he had moderate cerebral atrophy, which may be consistent with Alzheimer's.

Because S.B. was a wealthy man, he had previously consulted with some of America's most noted physicians. His first doctor was a prominent neurologist in New York. But, according to the medical records S.B. provided, that doctor had offered him almost no hope. He had diagnosed S.B. with senile dementia, but had recommended no medical treatment. He had merely advised him to take an aspirin each day, to reduce risk of stroke. He had also told S.B. to stop smoking.

That advice fell drastically short of anything that might halt or reverse S.B.'s cognitive decline.

S.B. had been puzzled by the doctor's therapeutic passivity. As a self-made millionaire, and as an immigrant to America, S.B. disdained passivity. To him, it just seemed like laziness. He would have much preferred to try an experimental new drug, or any therapeutic modality that at least offered some chance for improvement. To S.B., doing virtually nothing was unthinkable.

S.B. had consulted with other doctors until he'd met one who had told him about my work. When S.B. heard about me, he flew straight to Tucson, and we went to work.

The first day we met, S.B. was ready to get down to action. I love patients like him. He took full responsibility for his own health and happiness, and didn't need a pep talk about making the necessary sacrifices.

S.B. had already given up smoking and drinking, and that had not been easy for him. He had been smoking a pack of cigarettes every day, and had been consuming four to five cocktails and a bottle of wine every evening. Because he had been a heavy drinker and smoker, quitting both of these habits cold-turkey had required real willpower.

Immediately after our first meeting, S.B. changed his diet considerably. That, too, was hard for him. He had enjoyed the rich foods that success had afforded him, and he hated giving them up.

He did not want to do a daily regimen of cardiovascular exercises and mind/body exercises—but he did it anyway.

He also began taking deprenyl, along with a full battery of natural medicinal tonics.

S.B. went on a full-scale, very aggressive program. At his stage of cognitive decline, that was the only approach that would work. The program was not easy. But S.B. was accustomed to working hard to achieve his goals, and now his ultimate goal in life was to revive his flagging cognitive function. He knew that his brain was the wellspring of all his success and happiness, and he was willing to do whatever it took to return his brain to health.

S.B. worked diligently at his brain longevity program, never wavering from it.

His progress was not spectacular. It was relatively slow, in fact, and sometimes characterized by temporary setbacks. It appeared as if he had suffered significant neuronal loss, and patients with that problem really have to work hard to get better.

But, gradually, S.B. improved. First his cognitive processing speed accelerated. This was followed by very noticeable improvements in his memory. His ability to focus increased, and his learning ability improved. He told me that his mind felt "younger" and "stronger." He also became more physically active, and is an avid swimmer. He even began driving his car safely again.

Thus far, S.B.'s cognitive decline has halted and perhaps even reversed. It's possible that in the future his decline might begin again. But I am hopeful that even if he does again start to decline, the progression of his decline will be much slower, and less pronounced.

S.B.'s brain longevity program has been a real challenge for him. But he prefers it that way. S.B. is a proud man, and now he has something new to be very proud of: his regenerative brain.

At his age, it's doubtful that S.B. will "conquer new territories" in the business world. But he doesn't care about that, these days. Now he's "conquering new territory" in his fight for brain longevity. And this fight, he says, is the most satisfying of his life.

20

Forty Days to a Better Brain

In this chapter we'll look at the practical application of everything you've learned about achieving brain longevity.

First we'll run through the average day of a person on a brain longevity program. As you'll see, nothing in this day is particularly difficult or unpleasant. In fact, the daily regimen may sound very inviting to you, because it's a pleasant lifestyle of reduced stress, good food, active recreation, and mental stimulation.

Then I'll give you a chart that shows you everything you'll need to do on your own program. This chart describes a regimen for four basic types of patients: (1) those who want to prevent brain degeneration; (2) those who want to achieve optimal cognitive function; (3) those who now suffer from age-associated memory impairment; and (4) those who now suffer from a form of senile dementia, including Alzheimer's.

The last half of the chapter will describe what you might expect to achieve during your first forty days on a brain longevity program. Your first forty days, you'll find, will be an exciting time of healing and brain regeneration. At the end of that time you will, in all likelihood, have a "better" brain—one that's regenerating, not degenerating.

A Day in the Life of a Brain Longevity Seeker

The average daily regimen of a person seeking brain longevity is not substantially different from that of any person who lives a healthy lifestyle.

All persons hoping to achieve brain longevity have two essential goals each day. The first goal is to avoid further degeneration of their brains through stress, poor nutrition, and lack of physical and mental exercise. The second goal is to stimulate regeneration, through the basic elements of a brain longevity program: dietary therapy; supplementation with concentrated nutrients; use of natural medicinal tonics; stress management; meditation; physical, mental, and mind/body exercises; and use of appropriate pharmaceutical medications.

Every brain regeneration program is unique, because each is tailored to the personal needs, goals, and biochemistries of each patient, but there are many similarities.

What follows is a general description of a *daily brain longevity program*. This general regimen, of course, would be customized for individuals.

When my patients first awaken in the morning, they generally try to engage in a few simple routines that help them greet the day with vigor and calmness. As a rule, if people start the day "on the right foot," the rest of their day goes more smoothly.

To start the day off right, many have found that it helps to not just immediately drag themselves out of bed, but to lie in bed quietly for a few minutes. As they lie there, they stretch gently, breathe deeply, and contemplate the day ahead in a positive way. They try to get "into the flow" of the day, and to face the day as their own "best self"—their courageous, optimistic, energetic self.

Some people like to say an affirmation before they get out of bed. Others do a little meditation.

I advise my patients to avoid the typical modern wake-up routine: fall out of bed, chain-drink coffee, immerse yourself in the world's latest catastrophes (through the newspaper and TV), and then sprint for work like a rat in a maze. This routine sets people up for stress, and causes their cortisol secretions to surge.

Often, my patients find that the morning is the best time for their mind/body exercises and meditation. Doing the mind/body exercises at the beginning of the day not only helps build a "protective wall" against stress, but also helps stimulate and balance the secretions governed by the pituitary, which is relatively more active early in the morning.

The most appropriate mind/body exercises to do in the morning are the basic spinal energy series, followed by the kirtan kriya. Both are described in chapter 18.

Many people begin the mind/body exercises by chanting one of the most powerful mantras of naad yoga: *Ong Namo Guru Dev Namo*. This means: "I bow before my highest consciousness." When they repeat this mantra several times, it reminds them that they have a higher purpose in life than just to suffer through another day and make a few more dollars.

Some also like to do cardiovascular exercise in the morning. A brisk workout, even if just for ten or fifteen minutes, pumps blood to the brain, and stimulates secretion of the catecholamine neurotransmitters, including norepinephrine.

When they take their morning shower, many of my patients enjoy adjusting the water temperature to cool during the middle of the shower. This can be very invigorating; it stimulates the nervous system.

For breakfast, most prefer a relatively light meal, which will not require much energy to digest. It's important, however, that this breakfast be rich in nutrients, and that it provide a stable source of food energy throughout the morning.

Many people enjoy a breakfast of fruit and yogurt, with cereal sprinkled on top. This breakfast is well balanced in food components, providing complex carbohydrates, simple carbohydrates, protein, and a modest amount of fat. The simple carbohydrates (or sugars) will immediately furnish the brain and body with glucose. The complex carbohydrates (or starch) will generally provide a somewhat slower-burning fuel. The protein will be oxidized even more slowly than the carbohydrates, and the fats will burn slower still. Because of the varying "glycemic indexes" of these various food components, this breakfast will provide a stable base of energy for the brain all morning long. This energy stability is critically important, of course, since glucose is the brain's only source of fuel.

A breakfast of fruit, nonfat yogurt, and grains is also rich in a diverse assortment of vitamins, minerals, enzymes, peptides, and amino acids.

You might try blending fruit and nonfat yogurt into a fruit "smoothie," to which you can also add lemon juice, a mild diuretic that helps the body to detoxify.

Any healthy breakfast, however, is acceptable. You should simply try to avoid a notably *unhealthy* breakfast, such as a high-fat breakfast of eggs, bacon, and heavily buttered toast.

Try to take the majority of your supplements with breakfast. I generally encourage my patients to "front load" their supplements, tonics, and medications, by taking most of them at the beginning of the day. This gives them the full use of these substances for the entire day. Also, some of the nutrients, tonics, and medications are stimulating, and can cause insomnia if they are taken too late in the day.

Many of my patients take a powerful multivitamin and mineral tablet. It can be difficult, however, to receive enough nutrients from just multiple vitamins. Often it makes more sense to take many of the vitamins in separate tablets or capsules. Different patients take different nutrients, in varying dosages, but most use the following nutrients: vitamin A, vitamin B complex, vitamin C, vitamin E, magnesium, selenium, and zinc. Often these supplements are taken *in addition to* a multivitamin, which provides lesser amounts of a broad range of nutrients and micronutrients. Some patients also take protein powder, or take the following amino acids: phenylalanine, glutamine, methionine, and arginine.

At the same time that they take their supplements, most also take one or more natural medicinal tonics, the most important of which are *Ginkgo biloba,* lecithin, ginseng, phosphatidyl serine, acetyl L-carnitine, and coenzyme Q-10.

If you are already oriented toward natural health and healing, this regimen of supplements may seem quite moderate to you. If, however, you are new to this medical approach, this may seem like a staggering number of pills to take. They will require only a couple of minutes a day to take, and their cost will not be excessive. But it would be *impossible* for you to receive this wide range of nutrients and tonics, at these dosages, solely from food-stuffs.

Morning is also the best time to take your "green juice" drink. This drink, loaded with amino acids and peptides, will almost certainly give you a powerful burst of physical and mental energy. If you mix your green drink with protein powder, nonfat yogurt, the juice of half a lemon, and a small amount of pure water, it can be a full breakfast; it will provide a high level of energy that will last most of the day.

If you really enjoy your daily "caffeine fix," drink a caffeinated beverage in the morning. Tea is far superior to coffee, because tea contains catechins—strong antioxidants that potentiate the strength of other antioxidants.

However, the longer my patients are on their brain longevity programs, the less they tend to rely on caffeine; they simply don't need it. They have more natural energy, and they also receive stimulation from various elements of their programs, such as their "green drinks" or DMAE.

Morning is also generally the appropriate time to take most brain longevity medications, since some of them tend to be mildly stimulating. The most common pharmaceutical medications are deprenyl, pregnenolone, and DHEA. Other pharmaceutical medications taken by brain longevity aficionados around the world include piracetam, Lucidril, Hydergine, and Vinpocetine.

If my patients take deprenyl, I advise them not to take it after

2:00 P.M., because it can cause insomnia if it's taken too late in the day.

During your regular daily routines, whether working or not, you should make a conscious effort to reduce your stress. Try to avoid stressors when possible, and to control your stress when you can't avoid stressors.

When you begin to feel stress, use the three best "stress-buster" strategies: *control, support,* and *release* (all of which are described in chapter 14).

You can also control stress with quick bouts of meditation during the day, or by occasionally practicing the Breath of Fire. These meditation sessions may last only a few minutes, and may even be done at a desk. They may consist of something as simple as a minute of deep breathing, or just repetition of an affirmation. Anything that replaces the stress response with the relaxation response helps tremendously.

When you keep your daily stress to a minimum, you not only promote the *long-term* health of your brain, but also achieve *immediate* enhancement of cognitive function. When stress is kept under control, the brain's glucose metabolism and neurotransmitter function are both immediately improved.

Try to make lunch the largest meal of the day. By eating a relatively large lunch, you can ingest a sufficient amount of food energy to carry you through an active day. Also take some of your supplements or tonics at lunch, particularly if you are taking a supplement or tonic that requires more than one administration per day.

Many of my patients eat a lunch that is relatively higher in proteins than in starches. As noted in chapter 13, this increases the output of stimulating catecholamine neurotransmitters.

Throughout the day, try to remain aware of your higher goals in life. Don't just slog through the day on "automatic pilot." Living life *fully* enables you to feel "like yourself." And the more you feel like yourself, the healthier you will become—in mind, body, and spirit. One piece of advice that I give to all of my patients is, "No matter what happens to you during the day, *you* should be *you.*"

Evening is a time to "recharge the batteries," a time for family, relaxation, personal fulfillment, and contemplation. I advise my patients not to indulge in the all-too-common practice of turning their evenings into a "second shift" of work. Of course, for many busy people, it's tempting to cram the evening with cleaning, shopping, cooking, and personal finances. However, if you allow these tasks to consume the small amount of leisure time you have, you'll end up with no leisure at all. You may end up being somewhat more productive, but what will you ultimately produce? A heart attack? A neglected family? A life of drudgery?

Most brain longevity seekers learn that they can actually get the *most* work done by working a little *less*, because that gives them more energy. Unfortunately, many of them learned this ironic lesson the hard way: by "burning out" so badly that their brains suffered degeneration.

Some like to do their meditation and mind/body exercises in the evening. Others do cardiovascular exercise. For many of them, this routine has replaced the cocktail that they used to need for relaxation.

You may want to make your evening meal somewhat smaller than lunch. Eating a smaller evening meal may help you to sleep well, and also helps to control your weight, if these are issues for you. The evening meal should be richer in carbohydrates than in protein, because this will stimulate production of the calming neurotransmitter serotonin, as described in chapter 13.

Many people take some of their supplements with their evening meal. Some supplements, such as vitamin C, are assimilated most effectively when they are taken several times a day, instead of all at once.

Also, most of them try to relax deeply before they go to bed. They take a hot bath, get in a hot tub, or get a massage from their spouse. A properly done foot massage seems to be especially helpful for promoting relaxation and a sound sleep. A small dosage of melatonin, when desired before bedtime, is effective for promoting sleep.

As a rule, brain longevity seekers sleep very peacefully. Because of their stress-management techniques, their nutritional programs, and the melatonin that most of them take, insomnia is relatively uncommon among them. Thus, they get a rejuvenating night's sleep, and wake up rested and refreshed, ready to enjoy another day.

As you can see, participation in a daily brain longevity program is simple, relatively easy, and pleasant. This is a program that virtually anyone can do, at any stage of his or her life.

A Chart for General Treatment

As you've noticed, brain longevity programs have four essential treatment goals: (1) they *prevent* brain degeneration; (2) they *optimize* cognitive function; (3) they *improve* cognitive function in people with age-associated memory impairment; and (4) they *may slow the progression* of dementias, including Alzheimer's.

Each of my patients falls into at least one of those four categories of treatment.

For some patients, two categories apply; for example, a patient might wish to prevent degeneration, and also to achieve optimal cognitive function.

The four categories of treatment require an ascending level of clinical aggressiveness. The treatment category requiring the least aggressive treatment is the *prevention* category. Next comes the *optimal function* category. More aggressive treatment is required to treat *age-associated memory impairment*. And the most aggressive treatment is required for patients with *full-blown dementias, including Alzheimer's.*

Below is a chart that outlines, in broad strokes, the treatment protocols that I generally apply to the four different treatment categories.

Of course, no two patients' programs are exactly alike. But there are often similarities in the program of patients who fall in the same treatment category. *Not all elements, however, are required by all patients.*

Again, you should always consult your health care provider before embarking on any brain longevity program. Also remember that as your brain cells regenerate and you begin to improve, you may need to adjust dosages of various nutrients or drugs.

BASIC TREATMENT CHART

Treatment Protocol	Applicable to patients seeking to prevent brain degeneration	Applicable to patients seeking to optimize cognitive function	Applicable to patients with age associated memory impairment	Applicable to patients seeking to slow progression of dementias, including Alzheimer's
Dietary modification	yes	yes	yes	yes
Control of stressors in lifestyle	yes	yes	yes	yes
Meditation, or elicitation of relaxation response	yes	yes	yes	yes (if possible. Or substitute music, family videos, relaxed walking, etc.)
Mind/body exercises	yes	yes	yes	yes (if possible; if not, same as above.)
Cardiovascular exercise	yes	yes	yes	yes
Mental exercise	yes	yes	yes	yes

Multiple vitamin/mineral tablet (with magnesium, selenium, and zinc)	1 tab, 1x daily	1 tab, 1–2x daily	1 tab, 1–2x daily	1 tab, 1–2x daily
Vitamin E	400 units, 1x daily	400 units, 1–2x daily	400 units, 1–2x daily	400 units, 2x daily
Coenzyme Q-10	100 mg, 1x daily in A.M.	100 mg, 1x daily in A.M.	100 mg, 1x daily in A.M.	100 mg in A.M. and 100 mg in P.M.
Vitamin C	1 gram, 3x daily	1 gram, 3x daily	2 grams, 3x daily	2 grams, 3x daily
Amino acids (including phenylalanine, glutamine, methionine, and arginine)	if recommended by doctor or nutritionist	if recommended by doctor or nutritionist	if recommended by doctor or nutritionist	if recommended by doctor or nutritionist
Vitamin B complex	50 mg, 1x daily	50 mg, 2x daily	50–100 mg, 2x daily	50–100 mg, 2x daily
Chlorophyll-based "green drink"	1x daily in A.M.	1x daily in A.M.	1x daily in A.M.	1x daily in A.M.
Phosphatidyl choline (derived from lecithin)	1,500–2,000 mg, 1x daily	1,000–1,500 mg, 2x daily	1,500–2,000 mg, 2–3x daily	2,000–2,500 mg, 3–4x daily
Phosphatidyl serine	100 mg, 2x daily	100 mg, 2x daily	100 mg, 2x daily	100 mg, 3x daily
Acetyl L-carnitine	250 mg, 3x weekly	250 mg, 1–2x daily	250–500 mg, 3x daily	500 mg, 3x daily
Ginseng	500 mg, 1x daily	750 mg, 1x daily	750 mg, 1–2x daily	750–1,000 mg, 2x daily

Treatment Protocol	Applicable to patients seeking to prevent brain degeneration	Applicable to patients seeking to optimize cognitive function	Applicable to patients with age associated memory impairment	Applicable to patients seeking to slow progression of dementias, including Alzheimer's
Ginkgo biloba	30 mg, 3x daily	40 mg, 3x daily	40–80 mg, 3x daily	40–80 mg, 3x daily
Deprenyl	1 mg, 2x weekly	1–2 mg, 1–2x daily	3–4 mg, 2x daily	3–5 mg, 2x daily
Melatonin	no, except for treatment of insomnia (1–3 mg for insomnia)	1/4–1/2 mg, 1x daily (more for insomnia) at bedtime	3 mg, 1x daily, at bedtime	3–6 mg, 1x daily, at bedtime
DHEA	if age 50 or older, or if DHEA levels are low: 25–50 mg, 1x daily, or every other day	50 mg, 1x daily (after levels are checked by physician)	50–200 mg, 1x daily (after levels are checked by physician)	50–200 mg, 1x daily (after levels are checked by physician)
Pregnenolone	no	no	(generally more effective for females) 50–100 mg, 1x daily (under medical supervision)	50–100 mg, 1x daily (under medical supervision)

Piracetam	no	400–600 mg, 3x weekly (under medical supervision)	600–1,200 mg, 1x daily, or every other day (under medical supervision)	1,200–2,400 mg, 1x daily (under medical supervision)
Lucidryl	no	100 mg, 3x weekly if recommended by physician	1,000 mg daily if recommended by physician	2,000–3,000 mg daily if recommended by physician
Vinpocetine	no	5 mg, 3x weekly if recommended by physician	5 mg daily if recommended by physician	5–10 mg daily if recommended by physician
Human growth hormone	no	no	dosage to be determined by physician	dosage to be determined by physician
Acupuncture, or electroacupuncture	if recommended by physician	if recommended by physician	if recommended by physician	if recommended by physician
Hydergine	no	no	3–9 mg daily if recommended by physician	9 mg daily if recommended by physician

The First Forty Days

As I've mentioned, most of my patients respond relatively quickly to their brain longevity programs. In fact, most achieve notable levels of improvement after a period ranging from about one month to forty days.

This initial improvement, however, is by no means the *end* of most patients' physical and mental regeneration. In fact, during the first thirty to forty days, they can reasonably hope to achieve only about one-fourth to one-third of their total, long-term improvement. Often it takes more than a year to achieve *all* of the improvement that can be gained from a brain longevity program. Some patients have continued to improve even after two to three years.

The first, forty-day stage of recovery, however, is often the most dramatic phase of improvement. The changes that patients experience can be quite exciting, because they generally occur in stark contrast to the long decline that has preceded them.

To begin a brain longevity program, you should find a doctor to monitor your progress, order necessary tests, and prescribe appropriate medications. Finding the right doctor may be somewhat difficult because, as I've mentioned, many doctors are not very familiar with some of the cutting-edge modalities I recommend. You may want to make a special effort to find a physician who practices complementary medicine. Of course, you can also consult your own family doctor, or a local neurologist.

In your initial meeting with the doctor, you may want to ask a few questions about his or her general approach. This will help you to determine if this doctor is appropriate for this endeavor.

Don't be afraid to "interview" this doctor in much the same way you would interview any other potential consultant, such as a stockbroker or an insurance agent. The doctor will know more about medicine than you do, but that's no reason to be intimidated. After all, it's your body, and it's your money.

Here are some questions you might want to ask:

- What test do you recommend to differentiate various types of memory loss?

- Would you send me to a neuropsychologist for a complete battery of cognitive testing, or do you rely on your own examinations and evaluations?

- Would you advise me to have an MRI or CAT scan?

- What types of therapy do you advise for patients with memory loss? Do you commonly recommend tacrine or aricept?

- Do you refer patients to university centers for investigational new drugs studies?

- Are you familiar with the adjunctive therapies of complementary medicine?

- Are you knowledgeable about recent developments in hormone replacement therapy?

- Have you attended any national or international conferences on memory loss?

- (For a general practitioner.) Would you recommend I also consult with a neurologist?

After you actually begin your brain longevity program, it is likely that your first noticeable improvement will be a marked increase in physical energy. Quite often, patients come to me with a serious deficit of physical vigor. Frequently they are not even aware that their low level of energy is abnormal. They believe that profound loss of physical energy is a natural and unavoidable aspect of aging. When I tell them this is not true, they are often initially skeptical.

Soon, though, their skepticism turns into enthusiasm, as they experience the initial surges of energy that are common among beginning brain longevity patients. Often this increase in energy will take place during the first week to ten days on a program.

The initial resurgence of energy is not due to rebuilding of the brain, because regeneration of neurological structures does not occur this early in a brain longevity program. Rather, the increase in energy is generally a sign of *improved efficiency* of neurons, neurotransmitter systems, and endocrine glands.

This improved efficiency is usually a result of the ingestion of specific concentrated nutrients, natural medicinal tonics, mind/body exercises, and pharmaceutical medications. These elements can almost immediately revive the function of neuro-transmitter systems, and can enhance neuronal metabolism. They can also quickly stimulate proper function of the endocrine glands.

For example, "green juice" products often immediately boost physical energy, because the peptides they provide stimulate the activity of the energizing catecholamine neurotransmitters. In-gestion of ginseng, too, can immediately boost physical energy, by improving the function of the adrenals.

Also, certain nutrients, such as B-complex vitamins, can quickly increase physical energy, particularly if a patient has been suffering from a chronic nutritional deficiency.

Some of the pharmaceutical medications I prescribe also elicit a sharp, sudden increase in energy. Medications like de-prenyl and piracetam have such a positive impact on neuronal metabolism that patients often feel immediately energized.

Similarly, many patients feel a notable upgrade in their en-ergy levels when hormonal deficiencies are corrected. Often, ad-ministration of DHEA or pregnenolone will quickly restore physical energy.

The second phase of improvement—which often begins after about two weeks on a brain longevity program—is generally char-acterized by improvement in the patient's sense of emotional well-being. As improvements in physical energy become consoli-dated, improvements in mood and emotional status usually be-come subjectively and objectively apparent.

Many of the same factors that enhance physical energy also contribute to improvements in mood, emotional stability, and general sense of well-being. Patients usually become aware of in-creased physical energy, however, before they become aware of improvements in well-being, partly because well-being is a some-what subtler index of health.

If, however, the patient has been suffering from a serious mood disorder, such as clinical depression, this improvement in well-being may be very easily recognized. Some clinically depressed patients have told me that the cessation of their depressive symptoms felt like a weight being lifted off them.

For most people, brain longevity programs do not create altogether *new* feelings of well-being, but instead restore *old* feelings of well-being—much like the feelings that patients experienced during their youths. A very common expression of this restoration of well-being is the comment that "I feel like a kid again." Many patients have said that to me. By this they usually mean that, once again, they hop out of bed in the morning feeling optimistic and unhurried, and keep this positive feeling throughout their day, even when confronted by significant stressors. Often these stressors no longer feel like calamities, but like challenges.

Some of this sense of enhanced well-being stems merely from patients' heightened energy, and from increases in their cognitive abilities. Patients simply have more energy and brain power with which to solve their problems. Their lives become a little easier. *Most* of the sense of enhanced mood, however, stems from *physical improvements* in the function of the brain, nervous system, and endocrine system.

The primary factors that contribute to improvements in mood include elevated function of the adrenals, increased energy production within neurons, improvements in neurotransmitter function, and improved balance of hormones. As I've shown, all of these physical factors can have a profound impact upon mood.

Sometimes my patients begin to undergo a positive shift in mood, but are not fully aware of it. For example, after one of my patients had been on a brain longevity program for about three weeks, I asked her if she had experienced any improvements. The patient, a seventy-two-year-old woman with mid-stage Alzheimer's, told me, "I still forget, so I guess I'm not any better."

Her husband, who was with her, disagreed strongly. "You *are* better," he said. "You have more energy; these days you don't just sleep all the time. You're more active. You pay attention to things. You make jokes. You *smile* more."

She nodded. It was all true; she just hadn't noticed it. Changes are sometimes more apparent to family members than to patients.

The third and final phase of improvement, for most people, is an increase in *cognitive function*. The first aspects of cognitive function to improve may be concentration and alertness. This often precedes improvements in memory.

Improvements in cognitive function are sometimes very sudden and dramatic, and sometimes gradual and subtle. Individual reactions depend upon the existing degree of cognitive decline, and upon the specific causes.

For example, if a person has a gross deficit of the memory neurotransmitter acetylcholine, he or she might achieve quick and dramatic increases in cognitive function from ingestion of substances that increase acetylcholine—such as phosphatidyl choline, phosphatidyl serine, or DMAE. Within just a few days the person might experience marked improvement in concentration, alertness, and memory.

If, on the other hand, his or her problems were caused mostly by extensive death of neurons, improvements would almost certainly occur much more slowly, and would be more subtle.

Most people, however, do experience significant improvements in cognitive function during their first thirty to forty days on their programs. The most common changes are increased ability to focus; increased length of concentration; decreased mental lassitude; improvements in working memory; moderate improvements in short-term memory; enhanced ability to recall long-term memories; improvements in learning ability; improved access to existing vocabulary; and a heightened sense of creativity.

Of course, these cognitive improvements vary from one person to another, and may take months, or even years, to develop fully.

Often, as cognitive abilities improve, people also experience unexpected ancillary improvements. For example, many experience a significant improvement in sex drive, in ratio of body fat to muscle, and in ability to sleep well. These kinds of changes, while not of primary importance to some people, can add significantly to quality of life.

As you can see, actually applying a brain longevity program is not very difficult. It's mostly a matter of *being good to yourself.*

At the beginning of this book, I promised to take you on a fascinating journey—a journey deep into the inner workings of your own brain.

Now that journey is at an end.

But now an even greater and richer journey is beginning: your journey through the rest of your life.

Now that you have learned the science and the art of brain longevity, I believe you are better equipped than ever before to make that journey.

A Case in Point

There's No Such Thing as False Hope

In 1993, L.G., sixty-one, went to her family doctor, fearing that she had Alzheimer's. Her doctor referred her to a neurologist, who performed a complete medical workup.

The neurologist discovered, through an MRI scan, that she suffered from lack of blood flow (or ischemia) to the area around her brain's paraventricular and subcortical white matter. This generally indicates Alzheimer's, because it means that the brain's open spaces, or ventricles, are becoming larger, while the brain is becoming smaller. Atrophy of the brain is a primary indicator of Alzheimer's.

L.G. had been diagnosed with dementia of the Alzheimer's type. She'd been told by her neurologist that no existing drug could significantly improve her condition, and it was suggested that perhaps she should enroll in a clinical study for one of the new experimental drugs being tested for Alzheimer's.

L.G. discussed this option with her family doctor, who, she said, advised her not to do it. She told me her doctor felt that it was not very likely that one of the new drugs would yield satisfactory results, and that participating in the study might give L.G. false hope.

Discouraged, she decided not to pursue this option. She received no treatment and steadily declined over the next two years.

Then L.G. went to a specialist in internal medicine, for treatment of a health problem that was not related to her cognitive decline. However, when the internist discovered that she had been diagnosed with Alzheimer's, he recommended that she consult with me.

The internist was well aware of my approach to senile dementias, and was very supportive of it. He had heard me speak at a medical conference, and had been intrigued by my work. He'd been particularly interested in my use of natural medicinal tonics and concentrated nutrients. Because he was treating a number of patients with serious heart disorders, I had recommended to him that he prescribe the nutrient coenzyme Q-10 to them, because it often is very helpful for circulatory ailments.

He had put three patients, all of whom were waiting for heart transplants, on coenzyme Q-10. As an apparent result of administration of coenzyme Q-10, all three had improved markedly. They had previously all been on oxygen, but after taking coenzyme Q-10, all had been able to discontinue use of supplemental oxygen. They had improved in status from "class 5" to "class 2," which indicated that they might no longer need transplants.

After this happened, the internist had enthusiastically referred a number of patients to me.

During my initial consultation with L.G., it was obvious that she was suffering from severe cognitive decline. A former middle-school principal, she seemed to be only moderately aware of her surroundings, and of what I was saying to her. She was accompanied to the consultation by her best friend, who did most of the talking. L.G. was simply not able to respond coherently to most of my questions.

She did very poorly on various mental-status exams. Her short-term memory was extremely weak, and her cognitive processing skills were badly compromised. She was a stage 5 on the Global Deterioration Scale.

Her friend told me that L.G. now needed help in her daily activities, and that she constantly misplaced things. They had stopped playing golf together, because L.G. no longer knew which club to use; for example, she might tee off with her putter.

According to L.G.'s friend, she had been functioning well until about five years before, when she suffered severe pneumonia. Her fever had spiked to dangerous levels, and there had been doubt that she would survive. L.G. had recovered from the illness, but never regained full control of her mental faculties. It was possible that she had suffered from oxygen deprivation during this illness, or that the high fever had caused extensive neuronal loss.

After the illness, L.G. returned to work, but her job became extremely stressful for her, because of her cognitive difficulties. She endured the stress for about a year, and then retired. After her retirement, her cognitive impairment seemed to wax and wane, but the essential progression was downhill.

I put her on an aggressive brain longevity program, in which I prescribed deprenyl, and placed her on high dosages of phosphatidyl serine, *Ginkgo biloba*, and acetyl L-carnitine. I urged her to reduce significantly her consumption of dietary fat, in order to optimize the blood circulation to her brain.

L.G. did not enthusiastically engage in the mind/body exercises at first, but she did get a significant amount of cardiovascular exercise. She had three dogs, and every day she walked them, one at a time.

Six weeks after L.G. began her program, her friend drove her to my office for a follow-up consultation.

I began asking the friend about L.G.'s progress. But when I'd ask a question, L.G. would interrupt her friend, and would answer the question herself. This was quite different from our first meeting, when she had barely responded.

"It sounds like *you're* the one I should be talking to," I told her.

"Of course," she said, "I'm the patient." She started telling me how much better she felt. She said that she felt much "stronger" mentally, and not nearly so "fuzzy-headed." She said her memory was much better, and that she was much more actively involved with her daily routine.

She was far more animated than she had been at the first consultation. She made eye contact, laughed and smiled, and followed everything that was going on.

Her friend told me that L.G. seemed "very much improved."

Even so, L.G. said she still often became "mentally tired." So I increased her dosage of deprenyl, and also her dosage of acetyl L-carnitine. I also urged her to get more mental exercise. I recommended that she and her friend read the newspaper together, and talk about it.

She continued to improve.

The progression of her disease seemed to be slowed, and possibly even reversed.

By L.G., who'd had the courage and the common sense to keep trying to get better—when there appeared to be no hope—I was reminded of an important lesson: There's no such thing as false hope. Hope is gone only when you give up.

As my uncle Leo, who was a great clinical cardiologist, used to say, "Where there's life, there's hope."

Epilogue:
The Best Is
Yet to Come

Now that you have read this book, you have probably already started doing some of the elements of the brain longevity program. Perhaps you've started using certain nutritional supplements, or taking some natural medicinal tonics. Maybe you've begun doing the mind/body exercises, or possibly you've asked your doctor to place you on one of the cognitive-enhancing medications.

If so, now you know that this approach is very effective.

It's exciting, isn't it?

But the best is yet to come.

It will come when you begin a *full-spectrum* brain longevity program. When you fully integrate the entire multi-modality program into your life, you will reach your own peak performance levels of cognitive function. You'll feel smarter. You'll feel younger. You'll feel like "your old self" again.

When this happens, you will have achieved a "twenty-first-century mind": a mind that is regenerating instead of degenerating. You will have discovered that degeneration of the brain from aging *is not inevitable*.

Recently I was talking to one of my longtime patients, a woman who has made tremendous progress on her brain longevity program. I love talking to this patient, because she's a fireball of energy and wit.

When she first consulted with me, however, several years earlier, she was a different type of person.

Back then her doctor, she said, had told her that she was suffering from age-associated memory impairment and from a spinal condition that would soon rob her of the ability to walk. He had said that virtually nothing could be done for either condition. The first time she'd come into my office, she considered herself nothing more than just another victim of the aging process: a helpless, tired old woman with incurable problems. She'd thought her life was over.

But when I offered her a glimmer of hope, she grabbed onto it. For the next several years, she worked extremely hard on her brain longevity program. And her program reignited the spark in her brain. She regained most of her cognitive powers.

The last time we talked, though, she told me that her doctor had discontinued a course of exercise therapy for her spinal condition because he felt that further decline was "inevitable."

I began to commiserate with her.

"Hold on!" she interrupted. "I started exercising on my own, and even joined a class, and I'm stronger than ever. That's one thing I learned from you: *Nothing is inevitable.*"

She was absolutely right.

Nothing is inevitable.

There was an article in the newspaper recently about a report issued jointly by the U.S. Census Bureau and the National Institute on Aging. The tone of the article was gloomy.

It said that the number of Americans older than sixty-five will almost double in the next twenty-five years, as the baby-boom generation passes midlife. The article said that this will be a catastrophe for our society. Already the government spends 50 percent of all tax dollars on the elderly. In about ten years this will increase to 75 percent.

People in the sixty-five-plus age group, the article said, generally require about 300 percent more medical care than people who are younger than sixty-five. Therefore, when the first of the baby boomers hit sixty-five—less than fourteen years from now—Medicare and Social Security will be bombarded. For the programs to survive, the current Social Security tax of 15 percent will have to be raised to 40 percent.

Regardless of what the government does, the article said, the life savings of millions of families will be decimated.

The article also said that the number of Americans older than eighty-five will increase at an even *faster* rate than the segment of sixty-five-year-olds. This unprecedented increase in the "oldest of the old" will be particularly devastating to our country. Currently, the article said, almost 50 percent of all people older than eighty-five have Alzheimer's, and 24 percent of them live in nursing homes.

In the near future, the article said, *many millions* of the oldest Americans will not be just poor and sick, but will become virtual outcasts, destitute, homeless, and demented.

This will be our parents. Then it will be us.

That was the bad news.

There was no good news.

But I do not share the sense of foreboding that pervaded this article—for one simple reason: *Nothing is inevitable.*

This report was based on the assumption that current disease trends among the elderly will continue. But I do not believe they will. I believe that millions of us, working together, and working on our own, will reverse these trends. We will take control of our own destinies. As we age, we will remain healthy. We will remain productive. This can happen. It *must* happen.

We already have the knowledge that we'll need to achieve this reversal. And I believe we also have the *will* that we'll need to achieve it.

When we do achieve this reversal, our world will change. And we will change with it.

One of my patients, mentioned earlier in a Case in Point, a wealthy, hard-driving executive, recently told me that his brain longevity program had helped him achieve his "first real success in life."

I thought he meant career success, but he quickly corrected me.

"I mean success in *life*," he said, "success in my marriage, with my children, with my friends. But mostly, success with myself. Finally, I've got the kind of success that *really* feels good. You know what they say: Nobody on his deathbed ever said he wished he'd spent more time at the office."

"Do you mean that you're no longer as interested in your career?" I asked.

"I love my work as much as ever," he said. "But now there's just more of me to go around. I don't come home at night feeling dead. These days I can't wait to get home and see my family and listen to all their stories. I've always loved my family, but I used to come home feeling like my nerves were shot, and I didn't really enjoy seeing them. And they didn't enjoy me much either."

"I remember when I first met you," I said. "Your main interest was in getting your brain sharp again, so that you could get your new business off the ground."

He smiled. "People change," he said.

People *do* change. That's the beauty of the human race. We adapt. We learn. We grow. We become more spiritual.

As I have helped patients to achieve brain longevity, I have *seen* them change. Many of them changed in ways that they did not expect. Most of them begin their brain longevity programs hoping to become smarter, stronger, and faster. And they did achieve those things. But most of them achieved much more.

They also became more intuitive. They became more creative. They became more sensitive. They became less afraid.

They became themselves—their *true* selves. They became the selves that they had always hoped to be, but had never had the energy or the cognitive power to be.

If your brain is now beset by neurotoxins, hormonal imbalances, and metabolic dysfunction, it will be almost impossible for "*you* to be *you*."

But when you begin your brain longevity program, and your

brain becomes infused with health and vitality, it will be relatively easy for you to be your true self. In fact, it will be hard for you to be anything else.

When your brain starts to feel strong, *you* will feel strong—strong enough to be whatever you want to be.

When you do become your true self, you will rediscover the world. You will return to the world that you knew as a child: a world where time stops when you lose yourself in an activity. A world of energy and joy. A world of clarity.

And when you rediscover this world, you will also rediscover the *truth* that you knew as a child. By truth, I simply mean *reality*. You will see the world as it really is. Your view will no longer be distorted by exhaustion, confusion, anger, and anxiety.

And when you return to this truth—as a mature adult—you will find what all aging people dream of finding: wisdom.

Wisdom comes naturally to older people. It is the natural product of experience. Your neurons are biologically *built* for wisdom. As the years of your life have unfolded, each of your neurons has sprouted new dendrites, and has made new dendritic connections with other neurons. If you have already reached midlife, you have developed an abundance of multibranched dendrites, with billions of connections to other neurons.

Living long is the *only* way to achieve this abundance of multibranched dendrites, with billions of connections.

If you are in midlife or beyond, you have something that no young person can possess: a rich, wide, variegated view of the world, created by a dense network of interconnected neurons. Compared with the brain of a young person, yours has an almost limitless horizon. That is your gift from nature. It is your reward for staying alive.

But not everyone who ages achieves wisdom. Some people use their ever-branching dendrites merely to soak up one worthless fact after another.

If a new piece of knowledge does not help you to become your *true self*, and to achieve your highest goals as a human being, it is ultimately meaningless. It is trivia. It may be knowledge, but knowledge is not wisdom.

Wisdom is knowing who you truly are.

It's possible that, for many years, your brain was simply too battered and beaten to enable you to discover who you truly were.

But it could well be that that has now changed. It is very likely that your brain longevity program has given you the *physical tools* you need to discover your true self, and to find the wisdom that your experience holds.

Even something as simple as reading this book has probably enriched your experience of life, and made you wiser.

Consider all the fascinating things you've learned recently.

You've learned that aging isn't always a process of degeneration, but can be an opportunity for regeneration.

You've learned that your brain has plasticity, and can renew itself.

You've learned ways to put mind over matter, and matter over mind.

You've learned how to keep your mind young, and how to keep your body brimming with vitality.

You've learned that the brain is flesh and blood. That's why the brain is vulnerable—but it's also why the brain is *renewable.*

You've learned that if you nurture your brain, you can be intelligent and happy during *every* stage of your life.

You've learned that controlling your stress can make you smarter—now, and forevermore.

You've learned that no matter how depleted your brain power is, you can always improve it.

You've learned that the brain has an almost limitless capacity for learning. And for joy.

You've learned that there's no such thing as false hope.

Yesterday, when I was talking to one of my patients—an elderly man who has experienced a profound recovery from age-associated memory impairment—he told me that he felt very grateful to me.

But I told him that it was I who should be grateful. I told him that it's easy for a doctor to recommend that patients make major adjustments in their lives. But it's very *difficult* for patients to enact those changes.

Occasionally, when I am introduced at medical conferences, I am referred to as a "medical pioneer." But it's not I who am the pioneer. My patients are the pioneers.

Every day, each of my brain longevity patients stands alone at the frontier of medical science, forging new paths for others to follow.

For many of these patients—elderly, ill, and frail—forging these paths is terribly difficult. I often wonder where they get the strength to continue.

But they do continue.

I celebrate these brave pilgrims of medicine. They are the source of *my* strength.

If you begin your own brain longevity program, you will be among those pioneers.

I pray for your success.

I honor your pilgrim's spirit.

Together, all of us—patients and doctors, families and friends—will find the way to long lives of health and happiness. I believe this with all my heart.

Don't give up.

The best is yet to come.

Your life, as always, lies ahead.

Resources and Referrals

All who wish to explore the Alzheimer's Prevention Foundation services or support its mission in the prevention and reversal of memory loss are welcome to write or call:

The Alzheimer's Prevention Foundation
11901 E. Coronado Road, Tucson, AZ, 85749
Phone: (520) 749-8374; Fax: (520) 749-2669
E-Mail: Drdharma@aol.com; www.brain-longevity.com

Excellent source of information about Dr. Khalsa's complementary medical program for the prevention and reversal of memory loss. Also product information, and information about ongoing speaking engagements.

OTHER INFORMATIONAL AGENCIES

Alzheimer's Association
919 N. Michigan Avenue, #1000
Chicago, IL 60611-1676
(800) 272-3900

Good source of general information on support groups and ongoing investigational drug studies. You can also contact your local chapter.

American Academy of Anti-Aging Medicine
1341 West Fullerton Street, Suite 111
Chicago, IL 60614
Phone: (773) 528-4333; Fax: (773) 528-5390
E-Mail: rklatz@worldhealth.net;
http://www.rklatz@worldhealth.net

Good source of information on anti-aging medicine, and annual conference.

Cognitive Enhancement Research Institute (CERI)
Box 4029-2016, Menlo Park, CA 94026-4029
Phone: (415) 321-2374; Fax: (415) 323-3864
E-Mail: noos@ceri.win.net; www.ceri.com

Excellent source of information on cognitive enhancement, especially through their newsletter.

IKYTA (International Kundalini Yoga Teachers Assoc.)
Rt. 2, Box 4, Shady Lane, Espanola, NM 87532
Phone: (505) 753-0423; Fax: (505) 753-5982
Internet: yogibhajan.com

For information about Kundalini yoga and meditation, or to locate a teacher in your area.

Life Extension Foundation
Box 229120, Hollywood, FL 33022-9120
(800) 841-5433

Good source of new health and medical findings from around the world. Also *Life Extension* magazine, buyers' club, and database phone line for members.

Santa Fe Institute for Medicine and Prayer
906 Canyon Rd., Santa Fe, NM 87501
Phone: (505) 982-5414; Fax: (505) 982-5310
Tony Rippo, M.D., Medical Director

U.S. Office of Alternative Medicine
National Institutes of Health
9000 Rockville Pike, Bldg. 31, Room 5B-38
Bethesda, MD 20892
(301) 402-2466

Clearinghouse for alternative medical therapies. Information available about funding of research.

BUYERS' CLUBS

International Anti-Aging Systems, Ltd.
#8 Rue Imberty
Monaco 98000 (France)
phone and fax 377-93-251-251
e-mail: iasltd (W) @attmail.com
(Pharmaceutical products.)

Life Extension Foundation
Box 1097-B, Hollywood, FL 33022
(800) 333-2562
E-Mail: Brain.@lef.org
Web Site: http://brain.lef.org
(Non-pharmaceutical products only.)

Life Services Supplements
3535 Highway 66, Building 2, Dept. R.S.
Neptune, NJ 07753
(800) 542-3230
(Non-pharmaceutical products only.)

RETAIL PRODUCTS

The following are known for high-quality formulations. Call for product lists, including "brain nutrients." These products can be found in health food stores.

Naturally Vitamins   (800) 899-4499

Quantum, Inc.   (800) 448-1448
                                   E-Mail: Annequant.com
                                   Web Site:
                                   http://www.quantumhealth.com

Retail Anti-Aging Compounds

Baxamed Medical Center
Hauptstrasse 4
4102 Binnigen, Switzerland
Phone: 011-41-61-422-1292; Fax: 61-422-1286

Great source for growth hormone and cell therapy products.

Books

Herbert Benson, M.D., *The Relaxation Response*, William Morrow and Co., New York, 1975.

Herbert Benson, M.D., *Timeless Healing*, Scribners, New York, 1996.

Yogi Bhajan and Guru Charan Singh Khalsa, *Shabad Guru, Quantum Technology for Awareness*, Shabad Guru Team, Espanada, NM, 1995.

Jean Carper, *Stop Aging Now*, HarperCollins Publishers, Inc., New York, 1995.

Larry Dossey, M.D., *Prayer Is Good Medicine*, HarperCollins Publishers, Inc., New York, 1996.

Daniel Goleman, Ph.D., *Emotional Intelligence*, Bantam Books, New York, 1995.

Ronald Klatz, D.O., and Robert Goldman, D.O., *Stopping the Clock*, Keats Publishing, Inc., New Canaan, Connecticut, 1996.

Vernon Mark, M.D., with Jeffrey Mark, *Reversing Memory Loss*, Houghton Mifflin Company, Boston, 1992.

Robert Sapolsky, Ph.D., *Why Zebras Don't Get Ulcers*, W.H. Freeman and Company, New York, 1994.

Roy L. Walford, M.D., and Lisa Walford, *The Anti-Aging Plan*, Four Walls Eight Windows, New York, 1994.

Andrew Weil, M.D., *Spontaneous Healing*, Alfred A. Knopf, New York, 1995.

Journals

Herbalgram   (512) 331-8868

Life Services News   (908) 922-5329

Index

thought chemistry in, 124, 128

treatable problems that mimic, 180–93

amino acids, 251–52, 263

amygdala, 92–93, 111, 115, 136–37, 149, 153, 174, 176, 305

antioxidants, 50, 158–59, 225, 410

supplements and, 246–47, 250–51, 265

brain, 85–132

as flesh and blood, 85–87

hemispheres of, 108–9

joy and pleasure capacity of, 90–93

as just another body organ, 360–62

limitless powers of, 87–90

lobes of, 105–7

major divisions of, 102–10

mystery of, 95–97, 130–32

plasticity and renewability of, 93–95, 97–100

weight of, 107–8

why it deteriorates with age, 151–57

brain longevity programs:

basic elements of, 46–63

day in life of persons on, 419–25

essential treatment goals of, 425

in first forty days, 430–35

principles of, 83–100

results of three patients treated with, 67–79

brain waves, 311–15

caffeine, 265–66, 422

calcium, 39–40, 51, 141, 153, 204, 249

calories, 201–2, 229–31, 341

cerebellum, 102–4, 134, 163, 175–76

cerebrum, 102–5, 108

chunking, 139–40, 354–55

coenzyme Q-10 (CoQ), 266–68, 324, 436

cognitive function, 7, 13–14, 41–43, 45, 48, 64–65, 68, 73, 79–80, 83, 85–86, 107, 115–17, 124, 129, 131–32, 180, 182, 192, 243, 268, 361, 423, 425, 434, 436–37, 439–40, 442

age-forty-five-plus brains and, 146–47, 150–52, 154, 159, 161

Alzheimer's disease and, 18, 167–70, 173, 175, 177–78

exercises and, 72, 323–24, 327–28, 331, 333, 337–42, 351, 355–60, 364, 368–69, 372

in lifestyle errors, 186–90

memory and, 135, 142–44

in multiple minor strokes, 184–85

nutritional therapy and, 49, 198, 208–9, 212, 215, 219–21, 223–24, 239–40

pharmacology and, 59–60, 343–45, 393, 395–96, 398, 402–4, 407–8, 410–17

stress and, 34, 36–39, 70, 120–21, 272–75, 279, 282, 295, 298–300, 303, 312, 314, 320

supplements and, 245, 250, 253–55, 257–59, 261–62, 264, 267

testing for decline in, 16–17

in younger adults, 98–99

complementary medicine, 8, 10, 13, 35, 45, 431

corpus callosum, 103, 109, 408–9

cortisol, 8–10, 13–14, 19, 44–45, 47, 87–88, 91, 186, 343, 420

age-forty-five-plus brains and, 153–57

in Alzheimer's disease, 8–9, 14, 28, 166

exercises and, 57, 330, 333

hippocampus vulnerable to, 111

memory and, 32–33, 39–40, 137, 142

nutritional therapy and, 49, 199, 204

pharmacology and, 61, 74, 401–2, 406, 412

stress management and, 8, 10, 19, 52–54, 70, 121, 272, 276, 278–80, 286, 305, 309–10

supplements and, 260

thought chemistry and, 128

dehydroepiandrosterone (DHEA), 20, 62–63, 65, 73–75, 80, 117, 167, 217, 233, 361–62, 400–403, 432

stress and, 299, 310, 401

dendrites, 51, 94–95, 322, 443

in Alzheimer's disease, 163

exercises and, 325, 328, 350, 352, 360

nutritional therapy and, 229–30

stress management and, 277

in thought chemistry, 124

deprenyl, 60–61, 73–76, 80, 99, 127, 144, 160, 178, 192, 233, 299, 393–400, 422–23, 432, 437

depression, 15–16, 48, 152, 180–84, 190, 279, 361, 432–33

Alzheimer's disease and, 16, 167, 177–78, 182–83

(continued)